Notes on Surgical
Nursing

Notes on Surgical Nursing

William C. Fream, M.B., B.S.
S.R.N., B.T.A.Cert.(Hons), S.T.D., F.C.N.A.

General Practitioner and Medical Officer of Health
Warrnambool, Victoria, Australia
Formerly Senior Nurse Tutor
Ballarat Base Hospital, Victoria, Australia

SECOND EDITION

CHURCHILL LIVINGSTONE
EDINBURGH LONDON AND NEW YORK 1978

CHURCHILL LIVINGSTONE
Medical Division of Longman Group Limited

Distributed in the United States of America by
Churchill Livingstone Inc., 19 West 44th Street, New
York, N.Y. 10036 and by associated companies,
branches and representatives throughout the world.

First Edition 1971
Second Edition 1978
  Reprinted 1980

ISBN 0 443 01682 8

British Library Cataloguing in Publication Data

Fream, William Charles
  Notes on Surgical Nursing — Second Edition
  1. Surgical Nursing
  I. Title
  610.73´677   RD99   77-30135

Printed in Singapore by
Singapore Offset Printing (Pte) Ltd.

Preface

Present day students are under tremendous pressures. The explosion of knowledge in every field has led to a situation wherein no one person can possibly take in more than a small fraction of the available information. The best that can be hoped for is that they can gain a working level of competence in broad basic skills and can lay a firm foundation on which further advances and special skills can be built.

My book on Surgical Nursing has been deliberately designed to offer to the student a quick and easy reference to basic knowledge so that it will be fresh in the mind when the all important examinations come round. Because it deals with fundamentals I have found little reason to make major alterations for this second edition.

I hope it continues to meet the special needs of the senior student and I am pleased if others continue to find it useful.

Australia, 1978   W. C. Fream

Contents

Chapter 1

PRE- AND POST-OPERATIVE CARE

PRINCIPLES OF PRE-OPERATIVE PREPARATIONS

AIMS

To eliminate or minimize complications during and after surgery by ensuring (1) that the patient is in best possible mental and physical condition (2) that nurse can anticipate and prevent complications.

TYPES OF SURGERY

Elective. Planned operation allowing time for preparation.

Emergency. Immediate operation without which death or serious disability would result. Time for minimal preparation only.

PLANNED PREPARATION

1. REMOTE

May commence many weeks prior to operation and extend to within 12 hours of operation.

(a) Psychological factors. *Fear of unfamiliar surroundings and people.* Admit 2–3 days prior to operation (longer in special cases, e.g. Thyroidectomy). If possible arrange bed position with patients of own age group and similar condition.

Establish satisfactory nurse-patient relationships by (i) attitude to patient and relatives: warm, friendly, kind, considerate, unhurried, efficient, (ii) introduction of self and other patients, (iii) explanations of hospital routines and procedures.

Fear of operation, anaesthetic, disfigurement and death. Reinforce doctor's explanations, avoiding flippancy or over-dramatization. Arrange visit with successful case.

(b) Socio-economic factors. Encourage patient to talk about these. If wanted arrange visits with medico-social worker

1

and spiritual adviser; encourage visits from relatives and friends.

(c) Investigations. *General.* For most operations: chest X-ray to exclude lung conditions, e.g. pneumonia, tuberculosis, abnormalities of heart size.

Determination of haemoglobin level, white cell count (increased in infections). Blood grouping and crossmatching if blood loss anticipated.

Specific. Ordered according to condition of patient.

(d) Nutrition. *Diet.* High calorie if patient underweight, low calorie if overweight. Easily digested, low residue. Glucose to prevent liver damage.

Fluids. Copious, to prevent shock and dehydration. In major surgery, added protein and vitamin C may be indicated to promote healing.

(e) Treatment of existing abnormality. e.g. dental caries, skin lesions, constipation, respiratory and cardiac conditions, etc.

(f) Hygiene. Ensure cleanliness of skin, nails, umbilicus (especially in abdominal surgery), mouth.

(g) Physiotherapy. Increases ventilation where there is respiratory impairment. Advise against smoking at least for 2—3 days pre-operatively. Short frequent walks (especially for elderly patients) aid lung expansion and prevent respiratory and vascular complications. Breathing and leg exercises have the same three objectives.

(h) Rest. Physical: exhaustion deteriorates general health. Mental: exhaustion aggravatcs shock. Sedation may be necessary.

(i) Specific preparation. Depends on type of surgery, e.g. bowel preparation, passage of Ryle's tube, catheters, etc.

2. IMMEDIATE

Includes all care 12 hours before surgery. Applies to elective and emergency surgery.

(a) Anaesthetic consent form. Signed by patient if able to comprehend its import, or by parent or guardian if patient a minor, or by next of kin if patient unconscious or irrational. In some countries a witnessed telephone call or telegram is legally acceptable in emergencies.

(b) Time of operation. Notify relatives; in emergency may also be necessary to notify minister of religion.

(c) **Observations.** *Vital signs.* Temperature, pulse, respirations, blood pressure – as base-line for future observations and comparison. To detect abnormalities which may entail postponement of operation, e.g. pyrexia, pulse rate over 120 or below 60, abnormality of blood pressure for that particular patient.

Urine test. To detect abnormalities which may have arisen since admission test.

Weight. As base-line for future comparison. To calculate drug and anaesthetic doses.

(d) **Alimentary tract preparation.** Six hours' fasting prior to operation (danger of inhalation of vomitus under anaesthesia). In emergency, aspiration of stomach contents may be necessary.

Bowels. Empty rectum eliminates (i) incontinence during anaesthesia, (ii) discomfort of post-operative abdominal distension. Excess purgation is contra-indicated – results in dehydration and disturbed rest. Aperients may be ordered 2 nights before. Suppositories or small enema on morning of operation. (Special preparation needed in surgery of the bowel.)

(e) **Skin preparation.** *General.* Bath, shower or full sponge with special attention to nails, umbilicus and perineum. Cosmetics removed as these disguise colour changes, e.g. pallor or cyanosis of lips, cheeks, nails. (In some hospitals anaesthetist may condone use of cosmetics in special cases.) Hairpins removed to prevent injury during anaesthesia.

Local shave. Removes hairs (which may harbour micro-organisms, superficial epithelium and dirt) from extensive area from well above incision line to well below, with good margin on each side. Avoid cutting or scratching during shave as this causes pain and may facilitate infection.

Antiseptic. Applied in theatre in most hospitals.

3. FINAL PREPARATION

(a) **Clothing.** Gown: covers trunk and arms; easily removable without turning patient; usually cotton material to provide warmth without overheating. Cap: completely covers hair and prevents soiling with blood and vomitus.

(b) **Jewellery.** May cause burns if it contacts metal part of table during diathermy, therefore remove and keep in safe place. If removal impossible cover with adhesive tape.

3

(c) **Dentures**. Removal prevents dislodgement during anaesthesia. Store in suitable receptacle in patient's locker.

(d) **Other prostheses**. Remove artificial limbs, glass eyes, etc.; keep safe.

(e) **Identification**. Suitable label attached to patient; name, age, ward, operation – type, time and site if necessary. (Type and time of pre-operative medication may be added.)

(f) **Pre-operative medication**. Usually consists of combinations.

Sedatives and analgesics. Opiates, e.g. morphia 10–15 mg, pethidine 50–100 mg, omnopon 10–20 mg. Barbiturates, e.g. nembutal 100–200 mg, sodium phenobarbitone 30–120 mg; 'Tranquillizers', e.g. chlorpromazine 25–100 mg, promethazine 25–100 mg.

These drugs minimize shock by reducing apprehension, thus ensuring sleep. Also reduce amount of anaesthetic required, post-operative pain and vomiting.

Anticholinergics. Atropine 0.25–1 mg, scopolamine 0.3–0.6 mg.

These drugs dry up secretions or prevent overproduction when inhalational anaesthetics used, especially ether; improve heart's action and suppress vagal influence on heart.

Time. Must be given ½–¾ hour pre-operatively to ensure above effects. Time of giving to be recorded accurately. If omitted or delayed – inform anaesthetist. Do *not* give under the maxim 'better late than never'.

(g) **Micturition**. Bladder emptied before patient transferred to theatre, by catheter if necessary, to avoid (i) injury to bladder in lower abdominal and pelvic operations, (ii) incontinence during operation, (iii) restlessness in the early post-operative stages.

(h) **Journey to theatre**. Minimal noise as hearing acute after premedication. All movements in transport to be gentle, steady, unhurried. Nurse takes clinical notes, charts, X-rays and accompanies patient until anaesthetized.

PRINCIPLES OF POST-OPERATIVE CARE

AIMS

1. By skilful observation and application of knowledge to prevent, recognize and treat complications during unconsciousness and up to the time of discharge from hospital.

4

2. To ensure patient's comfort.

3. To restore patient to individual maximal health and independence.

PREPARATION

Bed. Type — routine post-operative with clean linen. Warm without overheating to prevent shock.

Specific beds depend on type of case, e.g. divided for amputation, frames and extensions for traction.

Position. Easily accessible to staff. Quiet. Well ventilated but free from draughts. Good lighting.

Equipment. Routine post-anaesthetic instruments; oxygen; suction apparatus; bedblocks. Special equipment as needed, e.g. intravenous infusion stand, bedcradle, drainage tubes and bottles, gastric aspiration tray, thyroid tray.

CARE OF THE ANAESTHETIZED PATIENT

Must never be left alone during this stage because of danger of asphyxiation, shock and haemorrhage.

Maintenance of airway. Can be obstructed by tongue, mucus, vomitus, blood, teeth, packs, swabs.

Position. Varies with operation. Basic principles:

1. Head turned to one side. Prevents bulky tongue falling by gravity over pharynx and blocking airway.

2. Head lower than shoulders. Prevents flow of fluid into trachea. Allows secretions to pool in cheek thus making removal easier, preventing obstruction and pneumonia.

Usual position — modified Sims' — upper knee and hip flexed, upper shoulder blade resting against a pillow. No pillow under head.

Control of tongue. Position as above.

1. Use of airway — flanged rubber and metal tube held between teeth or gums with flange resting externally against lips. Tube follows curve of tongue to pharynx thus keeping tongue forward. Should be retained until return of swallowing reflex when patient rejects airway.

2. Support of jaw. Tongue and muscles of floor of mouth are attached to mandible. Lifting mandible forward by means of

5

thumbs behind angle of jaw or by fingers under chin, prevents tongue falling back.

3. Tongue forceps or clips used only when tongue cannot be retrieved by above methods. They are placed 2.5 cm (1 in) from tip of upper surface of tongue thus avoiding blood vessels on under surface.

Suction. Visible mucus, vomitus and blood swabbed from mouth. Excess secretions removed by gentle suction intermittently applied to pharynx using rubber or polythene catheter or metal nozzle. Powerful or continuous suction can damage mucous membranes and predispose to pneumonia.

Observations. *General condition.* Restlessness may be due to haemorrhage, asphyxia, full bladder, change in conscious state.

Inertia may be due to shock, asphyxia, cardiac arrest, deep anaesthesia.

Colour. Pallor may be due to shock, haemorrhage, asphyxia, cardiac arrest.

Cyanosis may be due to respiratory obstruction, shock, cardiac arrest.

Flushing may be due to blood transfusion, circulatory overloading, over-clothing, carbon dioxide retention.

Vital signs. Pulse and blood pressure recorded ¼−½ hourly, to assess degree of shock and early signs of deepening shock, haemorrhage and cardiac arrest. Report pulse over 120 or under 50 beats per minute, blood pressure below 90 or if it is unusually high for that particular patient.

Respirations should be inaudible and regular in depth and rhythm. Noisy (stertorous) respiration indicates partial obstruction. Sighing respirations indicate haemorrhage. Chest and diaphragmatic movements observed for exaggeration, or absence.

Temperature taken 2−4 hourly as guide to degree of shock.

Dressings. If excessive seepage, reinforce dressing. If fresh blood appears, report immediately.

Drainage tubes. Connect to appropriate receptacle and establish drainage. Record amount, type and colour.

Intravenous infusion. Observe − rate of flow, type of fluid, whether apparatus is airtight and patent; site of insertion, dislodgement, whether leaking or infected.

Moving the patient. All movements minimal, gentle,

unhurried. During anaesthesia blood pressure compensatory mechanism inhibited, any sudden alteration of position may lower blood pressure.

CARE OF CONSCIOUS PATIENT
Immediate

Analgesia. Pain usually prominent feature with return to consciousness. Pethidine 50–100 mg; omnopon 10–20 mg; morphia 10–15 mg. Followed by period of sleep.

Sponge. After sleep and if condition satisfactory, hands and face sponged, jacket changed, hair combed, mouth wash or sips of fluid if allowed.

Physiotherapy. Deep breathing, coughing, leg movements encouraged hourly to prevent chest and vascular complications.

Position. Depending on blood pressure, pulse and colour, gradually elevate to semi-upright or upright position, to allow maximum expansion of lungs (abdominal organs fall by gravity), facilitates abdominal drainage, following peritonitis encourages pus to drain into pelvis where it can be treated more effectively.

Continuing Care

Specific care, e.g. Ryle's tube, catheters, intravenous fluid, underwater drainage, etc.

Fluids. Sips of water given on demand and gradually increased as tolerated until copious (2½–3 litres daily). If unable to tolerate oral fluids replace losses by rectal or intravenous fluids. Discontinue when oral fluids tolerated.

Diet. Commenced when oral fluids tolerated. Light, easily digested, well balanced, gradually increasing on demand to normal diet. Add roughage to encourage bowel action. (In some cases protein and vitamin C may be increased to facilitate healing.)

Drugs. Analgesics as in Immediate Care (above). As need for these decreases milder analgesics given. Panadol 0.5–1 g; codeine; Mist morph. et aspirin. Sedatives for first few nights, Nembutal 100–200 mg; sodium amytal 100–200 mg, etc.

Antibiotics. To combat existing infection or to provide prophylaxis if infection anticipated or a particular danger. Varies

7

according to infecting organism. Penicillin usual as prophylactic measure.

Drainage tubes. Placed in cavity, canal, organ or wound to (1) provide escape of blood or serum following surgery to prevent infection, e.g. nephrectomy; (2) reveal possible concealed haemorrhage; (3) allow escape of pus when infection present; (4) allow escape of body fluid by an alternative route—bile via 'T' tube.

Removal: when drainage diminished or absent, average 2–5 days. Most tubes shortened 1–3 cm daily before final removal to prevent fistula or sinus formation.

Dressings. Checked frequently for excessive drainage and fresh blood. Undisturbed until (1) sutures removed: average 7–10 days (face and neck 4–5 days; areas subjected to strain 12–14 days); (2) excessive drainage: constantly wet dressings become infected easily; (3) evidence of wound infection: pyrexia or pain over wound or purulent discharge.

Hygiene. Skin care: daily sponge, later bath or shower. Pressure area care, 2–4 hourly position change; use of aids as indicated (air cushion, pillows, ripple mattress, sheep skins); massage.

Mouth: mouth wash; mouth toilet; care of teeth; ice to suck; later – copious fluids.

Eyes: toilet or irrigation with elderly or debilitated patients.

Nose: nasal toilets if intragastric tube or intranasal oxygen in use.

Bladder. Regular emptying encouraged. Should pass urine within 12 hours of operation otherwise nursing measures employed: position of patient (male: sit on side of bed or stand well supported beside bed; female: swing legs over side of bed or sit on commode); privacy often all that is needed; persuasive psychology – sound of running or splashing water; copious fluids. If these fail either catheterization under strict aseptic precautions or injection of antispasmodic drug – carbachol, esmodil.

Bowels. Once diet started bowel action can be expected. If not in 3–4 days aperient may be given. If patient complains of abdominal discomfort or if aperient unsuccessful, suppositories or small enema may be required. High fibre diet usually eliminates need for enema.

Physiotherapy. While in bed, deep breathing, coughing and leg exercises encouraged. Ambulate after 1–3 days, advantages: reduces pulmonary and vascular complications by ensuring deep breathing and improved circulation; improves muscle tone and reduces nausea and vomiting; facilitates easier bladder and bowel control. Reduces possibility of pressure sores; improves patient's morale. Encourage movement rather than just sitting when out of bed. (Sitting with legs hanging down increases risk of femoral vein thrombosis.)

Contra-indications to early ambulation: shock; exhaustion; if thrombosis has already occurred; infection, e.g. peritonitis; obesity — strain on heart and wound; associated heart conditions.

Charts and records. Vital signs gradually increasing time interval from ¼ to ½ hourly to hourly, then 2-hourly, 4-hourly, 12-hourly according to patient's satisfactory progress.

Fluid balance, time, type and amount of intake and output.

Any abnormalities recorded and reported.

Treatments, recorded as performed and effects of same.

Socio-economic needs. Establish satisfactory nurse-patient relationships. Visits encouraged from relatives and friends. As required: visits from medico-social worker and spiritual adviser.

Convalescence. Gradual improvement in ambulation and independence. Diversional and occupational therapy as indicated. Rehabilitation: improvement of affected area and re-education of other areas of body as necessary.

Discharge. To suitable environment when patient is at maximal level of health and independence. Instructions as required *re* diet, dressings or other treatments, date to return to doctor or follow-up clinic, drugs, when to return to work, any prostheses (e.g. legs, breast, eye).

POST-OPERATIVE DISCOMFORTS

1. Flatulent Abdominal Distension

Cause. Decreased peristalsis resulting in stasis of bowel contents with increased gas production. More common when there has been much handling of gut during operation.

Prevention. Encourage movement while in bed. Early ambulation.

Treatment. Change of position in bed. Passage of rectal

(flatus) tube — overcomes anal spasm and initiates reflex response. Occasionally, small enema may be given. Occasionally Prostigmine 0.5 mg of 0.05% solution intramuscularly acts as a parasympathetic stimulator and encourages peristalsis.

2. Hiccough

Irritations of diaphragm causing contractions associated with spasm of larynx on inspiration.

Cause. 'Indigestion'; hot or cold fluids; gas in stomach or bowel. More serious: dilatation of stomach; paralytic ileus; incipient uraemia; peritonitis; subphrenic abscess.

Prevention. Avoid abdominal distension as above; avoid drinking water other than in sips too soon post-operatively; avoid faulty eating habits.

Treatment. Relief of abdominal distension. Relax diaphragm — deep breathing; hold breath; increase carbon dioxide intake — inhale own CO_2 from paper bag; intranasal 10—15% CO_2.

Sedation: sodium phenobarbitone 60—100 mg; chlorpromazine 10—25 mg.

3. Nausea and Vomiting

Post-anaesthetic, first 24 hours.

Cause. (a) Inadequate pre-operative fasting, (b) fear and apprehension (pylorospasm), (c) anaesthetic, (d) sensitivity to drugs, e.g. morphia.

Vomiting after 24—48 hours may be due to more serious causes, e.g. paralytic ileus, dilatation of stomach.

Prevention. Ensure complete fasting 6 hours pre-operatively. Minimize fear and apprehension pre-operatively. Careful choice of anaesthetics and analgesics. Encourage deep breathing. Do not hurry re-introduction of foods.

Treatment. Hold head. Support wound. Hold vomit bowl. Bed rest — avoid 'jerking' movements. Withhold copious fluids but encourage frequent sips.

Anti-emetic drugs: chlorpromazine 10—25 mg; dramamine 50—100 mg; torecan 6.5 mg; metochlopramide 10 mg I.M.

If vomiting persists: pass intragastric tube, aspirate contents of stomach every 15 minutes and rest alimentary tract. Give intravenous fluids if necessary.

4. Thirst
Cause. Inadequate hydration pre-operatively. Little or no oral intake. Atropine pre-operatively. Sweating.

Prevention. Ensure adequate hydration pre- and post-operatively. Theatres not overheated.

Treatment. Ice to suck. Frequent mouth rinses. Sips of water. Mouth toilets. Fluid replacement by alternative routes. Encourage salivation — chewing gum, peppermints.

5. Parotitis
Inflammation of parotid gland due to infection ascending from the mouth via Stensen's duct. (Rare with modern care.)

Cause. Dry mouth due to thirst as above. Dental caries and infected gums. Oral antibiotics upsetting natural ecology of mouth flora.

Prevention. Prevent and treat thirst as above. Mouth cleanliness.

Signs and symptoms. 3–10 days post-operatively: pyrexia, stiffness and tenderness of jaw, swelling at angle of jaw.

Treatment. Heat: local application of Plastine. Chemotherapy: e.g. penicillin, 1 mega-unit 6-hourly.

If abscess forms: incision and drainage. Frequent cleansing of mouth. Dental extraction of septic teeth.

6. Constipation
Cause. Reduced peristalsis. Restricted food and fluid intake. Atropine pre-operatively.

Prevention. Physiotherapy while still in bed. Early ambulation. Stop analgesics as early as possible. Copious fluids as soon as possible. Increase roughage in diet. Encourage regular habits. Use of commode or lavatory rather than bedpan.

Treatment. Aperient, preferably patient's own choice. Suppositories. Enema. Manual removal — impacted faeces.

7. Urinary Retention
Inability to pass urine from bladder.

Causes. Painful abdomen. Shock (poor muscle tone). Abnormal position in bed (men often cannot pass urine lying down). Bruising and swelling of urethra following vaginal or perineal surgery.

11

Prevention. Psychological preparation of patient pre-operatively. Catheterization pre-operatively where operations on pelvic floor are likely to lead to retention.

Treatment. See page 8.

8. Urinary Infection

Cause. Urinary stasis; dehydration. Incomplete emptying of bladder. Catheterization (probably carries infection from urethra). Urinary drainage tubes and bags.

Prevention. Copious fluids. Early ambulation. Aseptic technique for catheterization following inunction of urethra with antiseptic cream. Cleansing urethral meatus regularly with antiseptic once catheter is in situ.

Drainage into closed pre-sterilized container with a filtering air inlet.

Drainage bottle to contain formalin 40% to maintain sterility.

Measure residual urine after operations on pelvic floor.

Treatment. Rest in bed. Copious fluids. Culture urine and give appropriate antibiotic. Bladder washouts.

9. Pain

Main sources. (a) Wound. (b) Back. (c) Head.

Prevention. In abdominal surgery avoid abdominal distension and urinary retention. Hold wound when vomiting or coughing. Analgesics before physiotherapy. Avoid tight binders, bandages and strapping. Avoid wound infection.

Backache: support curves of spine adequately with pillows. Change position 2- to 4-hourly. Place footboard, firm pillow or sandbag at feet to prevent sliding down. Air cushion.

Headache: provide adequate ventilation. Keep hair arranged tidily. Delay sitting up after operation for 12 hours especially after spinal anaesthesia.

Treatment. Loosen and readjust binders, bandages and strapping. Investigate for sepsis if accompanied by pyrexia. Some pain inevitable immediately after surgery and analgesics should not be denied.

Backache: change position. Avoid slumping. Massage back. Rearrange pillows.

Headache: shade light. Suppress noise. Apply cold compress to forehead.

12

POST-OPERATIVE COMPLICATIONS

SHOCK

Reaction of body to stress. State of depression of all body functions. Results from reduction of volume of circulating blood.

PHYSIOLOGY

Because of relatively limited amount of blood in the body, economy of distribution is essential. The autonomic nervous system controls muscle layer of arterioles; contraction narrows lumen and lessens blood supply, relaxation widens lumen and increases blood supply to tissues according to demands (heart, brain and kidneys excepted).

Normally arterioles dilate in active organs, at the same time arterioles constrict in inactive organs; e.g. vasodilation in digestive organs after meals, vasoconstriction in skeletal muscle vessels. (Hence 'cramp' occurs if exercise taken immediately after meal.)

Blood pressure maintained by (1) contraction of left ventricle, (2) elastic recoil of great arteries, (3) net peripheral (arteriolar) resistance, (4) total volume of blood, (5) viscosity of blood.

Compensatory mechanisms. Impairment of any of the factors maintaining blood pressure decreases circulation. This affects vasomotor control centre in medulla oblongata and causes (a) sympathetic impulses to travel to skin vessels which constrict and increase peripheral resistance, (b) increased heart rate to ensure better distribution of lesser volume of circulating blood. Thus patient appears pale, cold and clammy, pulse rate increased but blood pressure maintained.

PATHOLOGY

If cause of shock unrelieved, compensatory mechanisms fail. General vasodilation occurs, peripheral resistance reduced. Same quantity of blood has now to fill a greater volume so each individual vessel contains less blood. This is peripheral circulatory failure. Accelerated and made worse if blood volume further decreased as in haemorrhage, or if toxic products such as histamine are released due to tissue hypoxia, or cell damage as in burns. Blood pressure continues to fall. Capillary permeability increased, further reducing circulating fluid leading to haemocon-

13

centration with increased viscosity. If not corrected vital functions fail: kidneys — oliguria, anuria, uraemia; brain — unconsciousness, coma, respiratory failure; heart — tachycardia, weak systole, irregular beat, failure.

CLASSIFICATION AND CAUSES

Primary (neurogenic). Sudden outflow of autonomic impulses to arterioles resulting in a shunt of blood. Usually self-limiting, e.g. fainting.

Causes. Pain, fear, emotional upset, anaesthesia.

Secondary. 1 TOXIC. Due to release of histamine; results in increased capillary permeability and leads to (2) below.

Causes. Burns, crush injuries, wounds — surgical or accidental, antigen-antibody reaction (anaphylactic shock).

2. OLIGAEMIC OR HAEMATOGENIC. Loss of fluid either from body or from circulation.

Causes. Haemorrhage, loss of plasma or serum, vomiting, diarrhoea, paralytic ileus.

SIGNS AND SYMPTOMS

Increasing pallor. Cold, clammy skin. Subnormal temperature. Pulse — increasing rate, weak volume. Blood pressure — falling. Respirations — shallow and rapid; later becoming deep and sighing (air hunger). Muscles — hypotonic. Mental state — apathetic at first, later apprehensive, finally unconscious.

Shock aggravated by age, exposure to cold, rough handling, starvation.

PREVENTION

Psychological preparation. Allay fear and anxiety by encouraging patient to talk freely, providing relevant, sensible explanations, nurses' calm efficient attitude.

Physical prevention. Pre-operatively, correct dehydration, electrolyte imbalance, anaemia, infections.

Avoid unnecessary movement, rough handling, exposure to cold, overheating. (Heat causes vasodilation thus combating compensatory mechanism. Also encourages sweating and therefore loss of fluid.) Minimal operation trauma and exposure for surgery. Pain relief by nursing measures and intelligent administration of analgesics. Careful choice of anaesthesia. Blood and plasma readily available.

TREATMENT

Aim. Maintain or restore circulation to ensure adequate oxygen to brain.

Maintenance of circulation. 1. Rest (a) Physical: recumbent position; avoid unnecessary movement, (b) Mental: allay fear and anxiety as in prevention above.

2. Elevate foot of bed on blocks. Bandage lower limbs to aid venous return to heart and brain.

3. Warmth (because patient feels cold) without overheating. (See prevention above.)

Restoration of blood volume. 1. Oral, warm, sweetened drink in mild shock.

2. Rectal infusion of tap water.

3. Intravenous infusion when oral route contra-indicated: glucose, electrolytes, plasma, serum, whole blood according to cause.

Oxygen. By polythene face mask, 6–7 litres per minute to ensure increased concentration. (If patient frightened of mask – discontinue as fear increases shock and oxygen administration is not essential.)

Treatment of cause. Relieve pain; arrest haemorrhage, etc.

Stimulant drugs. Increase blood pressure by vasoconstriction, e.g. metaraminol, angiotensin, 1–noradrenaline.

HAEMORRHAGE

Loss of blood from circulatory system as result of injury or disease.

Types. Arterial: bright red (oxygenated) spurts out in time with heart beat. Venous: dark red (deoxygenated) wells rapidly. Capillary: bluish-red; oozes.

Most haemorrhages a mixture of all three with one type predominating.

Time. *Primary.* Occurs at time of injury or operation, i.e. direct result of injury.

Reactionary. After operation or injury, usually within 12–24 hours. Caused by return of blood pressure to normal with dislodgement of clot and/or ligatures.

Secondary. During second week after operation or injury. Infection weakens clots or erodes blood vessel walls.

Signs and Symptoms

Acute. Can lose 500 ml without noticeable effect (e.g. blood donors). Loss of greater volume results in shock, restlessness, anxiety, increasing pallor spreading to mucous membranes; subnormal temperature; skin cold and clammy; falling blood pressure; pulse rapid and weak; thirst; respirations shallow and rapid, later becoming deep and sighing (air hunger). Later signs in extreme blood loss — tinnitus; blurred vision; coma; dilated pupils.

Chronic. Continued small losses over long period. Body compensates by replacing volume from tissue fluid and fluid intake. Haemoglobin not replaced as quickly as lost therefore anaemia develops. Patient languid, easily tired; pallor gradually develops; breathlessness and faintness on exertion. Thirst.

Sites and Special Types

EXTERNAL. From a wound or abrasion. Obvious visible blood.

INTERNAL. From an organ or cavity; may be revealed or concealed.

Revealed. Blood escapes through an orifice, e.g. epistaxis (nose bleeding); haemoptysis (bright frothy blood from lungs); haematemesis — vomited blood which may be swallowed blood from mouth, nose or oesophagus, or fresh from gastric wall. In appearance resembles brown flakes due to alteration by gastric juice (coffee-ground vomit). Melaena — dark tarry stool due to presence of digested blood from small intestine (e.g. duodenal ulcer). Mixtures containing iron, bismuth or manganese may change colour of stool — not to be confused with melaena. Bright blood in stools — colonic or rectal bleeding, e.g. neoplasm, haemorrhoids, ulcerative colitis; occult blood — blood present but not visible to naked eye, detected by chemical test. Haematuria — blood in urine, small amounts — urine appears smoky; larger amounts — macroscopic blood — urine appears red; menorrhagia — excessive menstrual bleeding; metrorrhagia — abnormal uterine bleeding especially between periods.

Concealed. Intraperitoneal: liver, spleen, ruptured ectopic gestation. Retroperitoneal: kidney. Pleural cavity: haemothorax. Joints: haemarthrosis. Interstitial: haematoma, ecchymosis, extravasation.

Natural control. (Haemostasis.)

1. Contraction of tunica media (muscle layer) of cut vessel and of tunica intima (squamous lining) causing 'incurling' of cut edge.

2. Slowing down of blood in vessels as result of above, and, if bleeding persists, general lowering of blood pressure.

3. Clotting. Following trauma enzyme, thromboplastin (thrombokinase), released from platelets. In presence of calcium salts this acts on prothrombin to form thrombin. This in turn acts on fibrinogen to form strands of fibrin. These form network in which red and white cells and platelets become enmeshed forming the clot. Prothrombin made by liver cells in presence of vitamin K. Fibrinogen also manufactured in liver.

Aids to natural arrest of haemorrhage. (1) Blood vessel contraction: application of cold or pressure. (2) Blood pressure reduction: physical and mental rest. (3) Clotting: application of heat (hastens enzyme action); contact with rough surface, e.g. gauze; drugs − vitamin K; calcium salts; thrombin.

Artificial control. 1. ELEVATION OF PART. Venous bleeding, e.g. ruptured varicose veins.

2. PRESSURE. (a) *Direct* (pressure on bleeding ends of vessels). Pad and bandage over wound; swabs or gauze held in place during surgery; artery forceps applied to cut ends of vessels press edges together.

(b) *Indirect* (pressure on vessel supplying area). Digital on nearest pressure point: face − facial artery two fingers' breadth from angle of jaw; neck − common carotid artery pressed against transverse processes of cervical vertebrae at level of cricoid cartilage; upper limb − subclavian artery pressed against first rib behind midpoint of clavicle; or brachial artery against humerus at inner aspect of upper arm; lower limb − femoral artery midway between pubes and crest of ilium or popliteal behind knee.

(c) *Tourniquet.* Strong band of material, cloth or rubber, applied round limb with sufficient force to compress main artery. Should be used only when other methods have failed to arrest

17

haemorrhage. Temporary measure only. Dangers: (i) If applied with insufficient force to compress artery it merely compresses veins, venous congestion occurs, bleeding made worse. (ii) Damage to skin if applied without towel or cloth intervening between tourniquet and skin. (iii) Damage to peripheral nerves — paralysis. (iv) Ischaemia and possible gangrene if blood supply restricted for too long. (Tourniquet should be released every half-hour.) (v) Arterial thrombosis resulting from damage to arterial wall especially if already affected by arteriosclerosis.

3. HEAT. Hot packs. Hot vaginal douche (44–48°C). Hot bladder washout. Irrigation of wound. Diathermy — seals smaller vessels by heat.

4. LIGATION. Various materials — silk, thread, catgut, nylon, etc., tied round end of bleeding vessel.

5. SUTURE. May be inserted into damaged vessel.

6. DRUGS APPLIED TO WOUND. Adrenaline-soaked gauze causes vasoconstriction. Styptics (astringent action), e.g. Tincture benzoin compound, tannic acid.

Treatment. (1) Arrest haemorrhage (as above). (2) Treat shock (p. 15). (3) Replace fluid (p. 15, Fluid balance). (4) Save specimen for inspection by doctor (e.g. haematemesis, melaena, etc.).

ASPHYXIA

Interference with process of gas exchange resulting in oxygen deficiency (hypoxia) and increase in carbon dioxide (hypercapnia).

CAUSES

1. Obstruction in air passages : (a) tongue, teeth, packs, swabs; (b) inhalation of vomitus, mucus, blood; (c) laryngeal or glottal spasm or oedema; (d) swelling, e.g. post thyroidectomy or other neck surgery haemorrhage.

2. Paralysis of respiratory centre — muscle relaxant drugs, e.g. curare (tubarine), gallamine (Flaxedil), suxamethonium (Scoline).

SIGNS AND SYMPTOMS

Restlessness. Respirations may be noisy (partial obstruction), shallow (partial paralysis) or absent (complete obstruction or paralysis). Chest movements: exaggerated and accessory muscles used (partial obstruction), or absent (complete obstruction or paralysis). Colour: cyanosis (hypoxia), red and moist (hypercapnia). Pulse rate: increased as heart tries to compensate.

PREVENTION
See p. 5. Ensure adequate pre-operative fasting.

TREATMENT
Position. On side with head lower than shoulders.

Control of tongue. Support jaw; pull tongue forward with gauze on fingers; use tongue forceps only if failure of above.

Suction. See p. 6.

Artificial respiration. Only after airway cleared.

MOUTH TO MOUTH OR MOUTH TO NOSE RESUSCITATION. (Advantages — easy to learn; no complicated apparatus needed though Safar and Brook airways are available — aesthetically desirable but not essential; effective).

Method. Patient lies on back if possible. Mucus removed from mouth. Chin lifted, neck extended to lift tongue from pharynx. Mouth covers patient's mouth ensuring adequate sealing to prevent air leakage. (In adults nose may be pinched. In children mouth may cover child's nose and mouth.) Breathe into patient until chest seen to rise, then remove mouth to allow patient to breathe out passively. Repeat inflation of chest 10–20 times per minute. If chest fails to rise, reposition head as airway may be obstructed. If stomach fills with air, usually due to too forceful inflation; empty by gentle pressure on epigastrium. Mouth to nose breathing less apt to distend stomach. Continue until patient breathes spontaneously or help arrives.

MECHANICAL DEVICES. *Negative pressure.* 'Iron lung' (Drinker respirator), complete cabinet imitates lung action — chest expansion leads to lung expansion through negative pressure in pleural space. Of value in complete respiratory paralysis. Involves complex nursing care.

Positive pressure. Method of choice for prolonged asphyxia, e.g. 'Ambu' bag — manual operation, alternate pressure and relaxation on rubber bag. Bird's respirator — advantages: regulation of pressure and volume; low resistance to expiration; makes use of any limited respiratory power of patient; can be used with face mask, endotracheal tube or tracheostomy tube; can be used manually or automatically.

Tracheostomy. See p. 191.

CARDIAC ARREST

May rapidly result from asphyxia or from heart conditions, e.g. coronary artery disease, ventricular fibrillation.

Warning signs. Cyanosis; falling blood pressure; slow feeble irregular pulse.

Clinical death. Absence of pulse (carotid, femoral); absence of respirations (apnoea); absence of blood pressure (no bleeding from wounds); dilated pupils; unconsciousness.

Biological death. Occurs after 4–6 minutes when, as a result of oxygen deficiency, irreversible damage has been done to brain and heart.

Resuscitation. Must be prompt.

AIM. Ensure oxygen supply to brain within 4–6 minutes of clinical death.

THREE STEPS. (1) Restore airway (p. 5). (2) Ventilate lungs: mouth to mouth or mouth to nose resuscitation. (3) Restore heart beat: external cardiac massage. Pressure over lower half of sternum compresses heart and forces blood into circulation (artificial systole). Release of pressure allows expansion of heart thus creating negative pressure, blood drawn from circulation into atria (artificial diastole).

Method for external cardiac massage. 1. Have patient lying on flat firm surface with head lower than feet if possible (not essential), e.g. fracture boards under mattress, patient lying on floor.

2. Place heel of hand over lower half of sternum and place other hand on top.

3. Depress sternum 5–10 cm by a rapid thrust, then release instantly. Should be sufficient force to produce a pulse beat at carotid or radial artery. (To gauge strength of thrust practise on 'Ambu' mannikin. Should raise pressure 60–100 mm Hg.)

4. Repeat depression of sternum and immediate release once per second.

5. Stop every 30 seconds to allow for ventilation (mouth to mouth). If alone: 3–6 breaths to every 20–30 compressions.

(For children pressure of two fingers or thumb on sternum is sufficient force.)

If this fails to initiate heart beat, some surgeons prefer open cardiac massage especially if cardiac arrest occurs in theatre. Incision made in chest wall or below left costal margin, heart compressed between fingers or against anterior thoracic wall.

VASCULAR COMPLICATIONS
TERMINOLOGY

Venous thrombosis: presence of blood clot in vein. (Thrombus — clot; plural — thrombi.) Cause: venous stasis; damage to vein wall; inflammation.

Embolus. A moving blood clot or other material (e.g. air, fat) inside blood vessels.

Embolism. Embolus carried in circulation until it reaches a vessel too small to allow further onward passage. Vessel thereupon blocked by embolus thus preventing continuance of circulation through that vessel. If embolus in veins — will be carried to pulmonary circulation. If embolus in pulmonary veins, left side of heart or arteries — will be carried to brain, coronary vessels, kidneys or skin.

Infarction. Embolus or thrombus cuts off blood supply to a volume of tissue which undergoes degenerative changes. Such volume termed an infarct. Vessels commonly affected: (1) femoral vein, (2) long saphenous vein, (3) pulmonary artery.

PHYSIOLOGY

Factors which aid venous return from lower limb: (1) cardiac diastole, (2) pumping action of muscles surrounding veins, (3) negative pressure in thorax during inspiration (deep breathing therefore aids venous return), (4) valves in veins prevent backflow of blood.

FEMORAL (DEEP) VEIN THROMBOSIS

Predisposing factors. 1. Venous stasis: (a) Immobility from pain, fear, type of surgery, fractured pelvis; (b) Impaired circulation, e.g. congestive cardiac failure, old age, reduced volume (shock, haemorrhage), anaemia; local pressure: on calf of leg, pillow, theatre table, old-fashioned 'donkey' used in original

Fowler's position; tight abdominal binder; abdominal distension; pressure pneumothorax; pregnancy.

2. Injury or infection to veins: may result from intravenous infusion.

3. Blood disease: increased coagulability of blood (rare, e.g. polycythaemia).

Signs and symptoms. May occur at any time but most commonly between 5th and 10th days. Tightness and tenderness of calf of leg, especially when foot pulled up (dorsiflexion). (Due to inefficient clearance by circulation of waste products in muscles.) Slight rise in temperature and pulse after same have been normal. Oedema, slight at first, along tibia and ankle (may need to measure to confirm in early stages). Leg appears pale (later: 'white leg').

(Four 'P's: pain, pyrexia, puffiness, pallor.)

Treatment. AIM. To prevent embolism and further clot formation.

1. Movement of affected leg forbidden to prevent dislodgement of clot. Absolute rest in bed.

2. Foot of bed elevated, aids venous return by gravity, prevents further clot formation.

3. Crepe bandage from toes to groin to support superficial veins.

4. Bedcradle to take weight of bedclothes from leg.

5. Copious fluids to prevent venous stasis.

6. Anticoagulant drugs to prevent further clot formation: Heparin (inhibits action of thromboplastin; effective immediately). Intravenous injection 10,000—15,000 units, 4—6 hourly, 2 days. Phenindione (Dindevan) (prevents liver manufacturing prothrombin. Ineffective while body's stocks last — about 24 hours). Oral administration 1st day 100 mg, 12-hourly; 2nd day 50 mg, 12-hourly, then dosage according to prothrombin estimations. Warfarin (Coumadin, Marevan) 2—10 mg. daily according to P.T. Danger of these drugs is uncontrolled haemorrhage from wounds, intestines, urinary tract, uterus.

SUPERFICIAL VEIN THROMBOSIS

May occur in arm or leg veins; most commonly long saphenous of leg and antecubital of arm. Usually results from infection or injection of irritating substances (e.g. thiopentone, glucose) or injury or spontaneous thrombosis in varicose veins.

Signs and symptoms. Pain and inflammation along course of vein. Slight pyrexia and pulse rise. Ankle oedema if saphenous vein involved. Veins feel taut and cord-like.

Treatment. Encourage movement and ambulation to prevent formation in deep vein. Local application of heat to aid absorption of clot (plastine, infra-red lamp). Crepe bandage to localize clot. Copious fluids.

PULMONARY EMBOLISM

May be first sign of presence of deep vein thrombosis. Most common time 9—14 days. May be heralded by early warnings, often unnoticed, brief feelings of faintness, tightness in chest, breathlessness, lasting for a few minutes only.

MASSIVE EMBOLUS. Bifurcation of pulmonary artery.

Signs and symptoms. Urge to defaecate; severe substernal pain; dyspnoea; sudden collapse and death.

SMALLER EMBOLI. Substernal pain. Shock — pallor. Dyspnoea. Cyanosis. Followed by increase in temperature, cough and sputum, often haemoptysis. Small emboli. May simulate pneumonia.

Treatment. 1. Position: recumbent if shock predominant feature; upright if dyspnoea predominant feature.

2. Oxygen: intranasal or face mask; tent may be necessary.

3. Reassurance: by presence, calm efficient attitude, relevant explanations.

4. Respiratory stimulants may be necessary, e.g. Nikethamide.

5. Anticoagulant therapy.

Prevention. Encourage circulation: massage and passive leg movements. Deep breathing exercises pre- and post-operatively. Early ambulation. Treat existing cardiac conditions. Prevent shock, haemorrhage and dehydration. Support circulation with crepe bandage (narrows lumen of superficial vessels thus increasing pressure and avoiding venous stasis). Avoid tight abdominal binders and abdominal distension. Avoid pressure on calf: during surgery minimal time in Trendelenburg and lithotomy positions, ensure correct position of legs on table, ankles not crossed. Knee pillow forbidden. When sitting out of bed elevate legs and avoid long sessions of sitting still.

PULMONARY COMPLICATIONS

LUNG COLLAPSE (ATELECTASIS)

Cause. Inhalation of plug of mucus or vomitus, occasionally foreign body, e.g. tooth. More common in right bronchus which is shorter and more oblique than left. If plug completely blocks main bronchus whole lung may collapse (massive collapse). If in lobular bronchus whole lobe may collapse. If in smaller bronchiole several small areas of collapse (patchy atelectasis).

Signs and symptoms. Majority occur 24–48 hours after surgery.

Massive collapse: sudden onset of pyrexia, dyspnoea, cyanosis, cough, sputum, increased pulse rate. May be absence of chest movements on affected side. X-ray shows consolidation, displacement of mediastinum towards affected side, elevation of diaphragm.

Lobar or patchy atelectasis: similar to pneumonia (below).

Treatment. AIMS. To dislodge obstruction and re-inflate lung.

1. Encourage coughing. Morphine 15 mg, ½ hour prior to coughing helpful in thoracic surgery as it makes coughing less painful and more effective.

2. Postural drainage and percussion. Patient lies with affected side uppermost and during coughing chest slapped vigorously over affected part.

3. Bronchoscopy and direct removal of plug by suction if above measures fail.

4. Smaller areas: steam inhalations or inhalation of atomised water, bronchodilation (ephedrine, aminophylline), mucolytic drugs by inhalation (detergents, sodium ethasulphate). Attempt to liquefy and dislodge plugs.

5. Antibiotics. To prevent or limit infection.

PNEUMONIA

Cause. (1) Result of inhalation of mucus, blood, vomitus or septic material during anàesthesia (inhalational pneumonia). (2) Stasis and stagnation of fluid in lungs due to inadequate use of lung tissue in breathing (hypostatic pneumonia).

Signs and symptoms. Tightness in chest; cough and sputum; dyspnoea and cyanosis; pyrexia.

Treatment. Oxygen administration, by tent in severe cases.

Upright position to aid breathing. Physiotherapy to help re-expand or make maximum use of lung tissue. Copious fluids. Antibiotics. Steam tent may be used if cyanosis not marked to ensure that inspired air moist, warm and soothing.

PREVENTION OF PULMONARY COMPLICATIONS

Pre-operatively. Recognition and treatment of oral sepsis, upper respiratory tract infections, bronchitis, asthma, emphysema, congestive cardiac failure. Encourage patient to give up smoking (inhibits ciliary movement). Encourage deep breathing to ensure maximum expansion of lungs and in preparation for post-operative period. Encourage ambulation. Ensure fasting for 6 hours or if necessary aspirate stomach contents.

During surgery. Anaesthetist will avoid prolonged deep anaesthesia. Avoid pressure on chest by collection of used instruments or by tired assistant. Adequate suction of respiratory passages.

Post-operatively. Avoid exposure to cold and draughts. Adequate suction. Change position 2-hourly, elevate to upright or semi-upright position as soon as condition allows, passive physiotherapy while patient anaesthetized; deep breathing exercises as soon as patient conscious; adequate analgesia to ensure deep breathing exercises not inhibited by pain; avoid use of respiratory depressant analgesics; encourage early ambulation.

WOUND COMPLICATIONS

INFECTION

Successful invasion by pathogenic organisms due mainly to faulty asepsis or lowered resistance of patient.

Causes. 1. Environment: dust, droplets, occasionally vector, e.g. flies.

2. Skin: inadequate preparation before incision, poor nutritional state.

3. Dressings: inadequate sealing of wounds, too early interference by doctor, nurse or patient.

4. Dressing technique: use of contaminated equipment, inadequate washing of dresser's hands, faulty dressing technique, e.g. swabbing from contaminated areas towards wound; inadequate immediate disposal of soiled dressings.

5. Stitch abscesses.

6. Existing underlying infections, e.g. urinary infection prior to suprapubic prostatectomy.

Signs and symptoms. Local tenderness; pyrexia and increased pulse rate after same have been normal; on examination of wound there may be redness, swelling and discharge; general malaise.

Treatment. Rest in bed and local rest of part, e.g. arm — splint. Remove sutures to encourage drainage if obvious stitch abscess. Appropriate antibiotic. Local application of heat — plastine, surgical fomenation, hot water bottle. Copious fluids. Reinforce preventive measures.

Prevention. Eliminate causes.

1. Environment. Dust: bedmaking completed at least ½ hour before dressing exposed. Wet vacuuming and damp dusting best methods of ward cleaning, but all dusting, sweeping and mopping to be completed at least ½ hour before dressings commenced. Traffic through ward to be at a minimum. Smoking prohibited. Separate room best. Droplets: correct use of masks. Laughing and shouting prohibited. Talking kept at a minimum. Vectors — prohibited.

2. Skin: thorough washing, shaving, application of alcoholic disinfectant, e.g. alcoholic chlorhexidine 0.5%. Diet: increased proteins, vitamins, copious fluids.

3. Dressings: larger than wound, completely cover area. Plastic skin such as Nobecutane may be used as alternative to dressing. Wound *not* inspected until sutures due to come out, unless there is excessive drainage or suspicion of infection. Patient warned against investigating wound.

4. Dressing technique: sterile equipment, completely aseptic technique, adequate washing, disinfecting and drying of hands, dressings received into disposable receptacle and incinerated as soon as possible. All underlying infections treated before surgery.

BURSTING (DISRUPTION, DEHISCENCE)

Complete or partial separation of wound edges with or without evisceration.

Causes. 1. Premature removal of sutures.

2. Delayed healing. *Local factors:* infection; drain tube; foreign body; sequestrum; tissue loss or damage; haematoma or

excessive serum collection; sutures too tight or too loose or ineffectively tied. *General factors:* obesity; old age; poor nutritional state; decreased blood supply, e.g. anaemia, arteriosclerosis, oedema.

3. Increased intra-abdominal pressure: excessive coughing; vomiting; distension; straining at stool; vigorous movement.

Signs and symptoms. *Complete disruption.* Sudden brown serous discharge on dressing; patient may complain of tearing sensation; gaping wound with or without evisceration.

Minor disruption. Gaping in the wound seen when dressing removed. May be some serous discharge.

Treatment. *Complete disruption.* Act quickly and calmly without alarming patient. Cover area with sterile towel, seek medical aid. Prepare patient for theatre for resuturing.

Minor disruption. Bedrest. Eliminate cause wherever possible. Either secondary sutures inserted or strapping 'corset' or 'gate' or 'butterfly' sutures to draw edges together. Binder.

Prevention. Sutures not removed until wound healed (unless they are serving no useful purpose).

Encourage wound healing. *Local factors:* avoid infection as above; placement of drain tubes through separate stab wounds, not through main suture line; ensure wound edges in apposition by eliminating foreign bodies, blood clots, damaged tissue, sequestra and by ensuring correct tension of sutures; apply suction to areas where fluid accumulation is expected. *General factors:* correction of factors as listed in causes. Advise patient to support suture line when coughing or vomiting. Avoid straining at stool or vigorous movements.

HERNIA

Incisional or ventral. Protrusion of portion of abdominal contents through abdominal wall, either through small part of wound or along its entire length.

Causes. More common in lower than in upper abdominal wounds. Inadequate closure of deeper layers of wound; wound infection; burst abdomen; obesity.

Signs and symptoms. Visible bulging or protrusion under skin; discomfort in area.

Treatment. Abdominal belt sometimes satisfactory. Surgical repair.

Prevention. As for prevention of wound disruption.

GASTRO-INTESTINAL COMPLICATIONS

PARALYTIC ILEUS

A form of paralytic intestinal obstruction where a segment of small intestine, usually ileum, fails to transmit peristalsis.

Cause. Actual cause unknown. Thought to be interference with neuromuscular junctions in sympathetic nerve plexuses of Auerbach.

Contributory causes. Peritonitis; shock; prolonged anaesthesia; excessive handling of gut during surgery (e.g. freeing of adhesions); extraperitoneal haematoma or abdominal wall injury; electrolyte imbalance (potassium essential for effective neuromuscular mechanism).

Pathology. Gastric, duodenal, pancreatic juices and bile will continue to flow into alimentary tract above area of paralysis. This fluid plus swallowed air causes distension of bowel wall thus rendering it less likely to recover from paralysis. Large quantities of fluid lost from circulation in this way. Dehydration, electrolyte imbalance results. Fluid accumulating in paralysed area stagnates and decomposes with bacterial action. Toxins produced are absorbed causing severe toxaemia.

Signs and symptoms. Abdominal distension and discomfort. Absolute constipation of faeces and flatus. (No bowel sounds heard through stethoscope.) Vomiting without nausea or retching; may be associated with hiccoughs. Vomit: clear fluid at first, then bile stained, then thin brown foul-smelling faecal fluid; copious. Increased pulse rate which continues to rise. Respirations: thoracic. Patient very quickly shows signs of dehydration and toxaemia if condition not treated early. Diagnosis confirmed by plain abdominal X-ray showing gas and fluid levels.

Treatment. AIMS: deflate and rest alimentary tract to allow muscles to regain tone. Meet patient's nutritional requirements by alternative route. Limit absorption of toxins.

Alimentary tract. (1) Nothing by mouth until bowel sounds present, (2) removal of fluid in stomach via intra-gastric (Ryle's or Levin's) tube or intestine by Miller-Abbott tube with continuous or intermittent aspiration.

Fluid replacement. (1) Amount determined by past loss, normal daily requirements and amount of fluid aspirated (i.e. present loss), (2) intravenous infusion – method of choice because fluid, electrolytes, calories and blood can be given by this route.

Antibiotics.

Specific points in nursing care. Upright position – aids in respiration. Passage of rectal (flatus) tube.

Prevention. When paralytic ileus anticipated (see causes), alimentary tract rested, alternative routes of fluid replacement chosen.

ACUTE DILATATION OF STOMACH

Paralysis of stomach.

Cause. Same as paralytic ileus.

Signs and symptoms. Rising pulse rate. Vomiting after 48 hours. Thin, dark green or brownish-black fluid. Tense tender abdomen. Gross distension of stomach – outline may be seen on abdominal wall. Dyspnoea may occur if gastric distension embarrasses action of diaphragm. Dehydration and toxaemia develop very quickly.

Treatment. Early recognition and treatment essential as condition deteriorates rapidly. Death rate high. Nil orally. Aspirate stomach contents. Fluid replacement by alternative route. Nurse patient face down. Metochlopramide (Maxolon) 10 mg I.M.

Prevention. As for paralytic ileus.

RESIDUAL ABSCESSES

Following abdominal surgery if infection present pus may localize in three main areas:

1. Pelvic abscess: pouch of Douglas, fold of peritoneum between rectum and vagina in females, bladder in males.

2. Subphrenic abscess: fold of peritoneum between liver and diaphragm.

3. Iliac abscess: para-colic gutters, folds of peritoneum on lateral sides of ascending and descending colon. Pus collects either in right or left iliac fossa.

Signs and symptoms. Return of pyrexia 3–6 days post-operatively; swinging temperature which may be masked by antibiotics. Increasing pulse rate. Pallor, decreased haemoglobin. Malaise. Increased white cell count (leucocytosis).

Local symptoms. 1. Pelvic abscess. Mucus in stools; diarrhoea may be present. Fullness in rectum. Tenderness on vaginal or rectal examination, bulging mass felt on anterior rectal and posterior vaginal walls. Hypogastric pain.

2. Subphrenic abscess. Pain in right hypochondrium, referred to shoulder. Tenderness and rigidity of abdomen over area may be present. X-ray of chest shows elevation and immobility of diaphragm.

3. Iliac abscess. Pain and rigidity of left or right iliac fossa.

Treatment. *General.* Rest in bed. Copious fluids. Antibiotics.

Local. 1. Pelvic abscess (easiest to treat). Encourage localization by hot rectal or vaginal douches, may discharge spontaneously through rectum, observe stools for pus. Incision and drainage via posterior vaginal wall (colpotomy) or anterior rectal wall. Suprapubic approach rare — only when large abscess which can be palpated abdominally. Sometimes instead of incision through rectum or vagina, sinus forceps may be inserted to puncture area.

2. Subphrenic abscess. Aspiration via needle (only possible when infection has sealed pleura otherwise pneumothorax may result). Laparotomy — incision and drainage.

3. Iliac abscess. Laparotomy: incision and drainage.

Prevention. In cases of peritonitis or anticipated infection give adequate antibiotic cover after surgery; insert drainage tube at time of surgery; encourage pus to drain into pelvis by maintaining upright position as soon as condition permits.

ADHESIONS

Bands of fibrous tissue, forming as result of infection or injury may cause bowel obstruction (p. 114).

Cause. Peritonitis or trauma.

Prevention. As above.

Treatment. Rest bowel as in paralytic ileus (p. 28). Surgery: laparotomy and freeing of adhesions.

INTRAVENOUS INFUSION

Introduction of water and certain chemicals (especially salts) into body via vein.

Indications. Dehydration. Dilution of toxins. To keep vein patent if further blood loss anticipated.

Type of fluid. (Those in common use.)

Glucose (Dextrose). 5%, isotonic, 200 calories per litre. 10–20%, hypertonic, 400–800 calories per litre (has diuretic effect; may cause thrombophlebitis).

Electrolyte fluids. Normal saline. 0.9%, isotonic, 155 mEq sodium chloride per litre. Hypertonic saline, 3–5%, 510–850 mEq per litre. Sodium lactate, 1/6 normal saline, 166 mEq sodium ion and 166 mEq lactate per litre (lactate converted to bicarbonate in the body). Hartmann's and Darrow's solution, 5 mEq per litre of potassium ion as well as sodium and chloride. Intestinal and gastric replacement fluids: various concentrations of electrolytes. Ringer's solution: similar to electrolyte composition of plasma. Dextrose 4% with 1/5 normal saline – isotonic fluid.

Parenteral feeding. Increase calorie supply, e.g. alcohol, 56 calories per 10 ml, can be added to litre dextrose 5%; Parenamine 6% – amino acids, 240 calories per litre; Levugen 10% – fructose in water, 400 calories per litre; Amigen 5% – casein hydrolysate, protein, 170 calories per litre.

Blood plasma substitutes. e.g. Dextran, to raise blood pressure.

Aims. Correct past deficiencies. Supply normal daily requirements. Replace current loss.

Normal daily requirements. Water – 2.5 litres; calories – 1,700 (maintain basal metabolism while at rest in bed). Sodium chloride 5 g. Potassium chloride 3–6 g.

METHODS
1. TROLLEY
Set observing scrupulous asepsis. Accessory equipment gathered: drip stand, fluids, etc.

2. PREPARATION OF PATIENT
Adequate explanations – patient may associate intravenous infusion with reports of desperate illness or death. Ensure physical comfort – warmth and privacy. Offer bedpan. Remove arm from sleeve of night attire. Shave if necessary. Place on mackintosh-covered pillow. In case oedema occurs place wedding ring on right hand if left arm used for infusion.

3. CHOICE OF SITE

Left arm as thrombophlebitis less likely because greater amount of movement prevents venous stasis; commonly used veins — basilic (upper arm), cephalic (forearm), long saphenous (near ankle) commonly used in children, dorsal venous arch.

4. TECHNIQUE

Arm or leg placed on splint temporarily. Chosen vein distended by application of sphygmomanometer cuff inflated to slightly above diastolic pressure (tourniquet may be used, lightly applied to prevent compression of arteries). Fluid to be administered checked. Tubing connected to flask and air expelled. Skin antiseptic applied. Local anaesthetic may be injected round site. Needle inserted into vein (skin, if tough, may be nicked with scalpel). Sphygmomanometer released. Fine polythene tubing may be passed through needle (Intracath) and attached to tubing from flask. Fluid infused into vein. Check site for oedema: indicates perforation of vein or needle in subcutaneous tissues. Flow regulated to 30—60 drops per minute. Needle and tubing attached to arm or leg with adhesive strapping or elastoplast. Splint may be removed, or may be bandaged on if necessary. Equipment removed. Patient left clean, dry and comfortable. 'Cut-down' technique. Uses: collapsed, small or deep veins or veins that have been used previously. After local anaesthetic has taken effect, small incision made over site. Vein dissected out with use of mosquito forceps and aneurysm needle. After incision of vein with fine scissors, needle, tubing and cannula introduced; may be held in position with catgut sutures.

5. MAINTENANCE OF INFUSION

Regulation of rate flow. Time per flask ordered by doctor. Calculations. 15 minims (drops) = 1 ml, therefore 15,000 drops per litre.

(a) Rate (drops per minute) $= \dfrac{\text{Volume in minims}}{\text{Time in minutes}}$

e.g. 1 litre to be given in 10 hours:

32

$$\text{Rate} = \frac{15000}{10 \times 60} = 25 \text{ drops per minute}$$

(b) To determine how long an infusion will continue.

$$\text{Time (in hours)} = \frac{\text{Volume in minims}}{\text{Rate (drops/minute)}}$$

e.g. How long will it take to administer 1 litre at 50 drops per minute?

$$\text{Time} = \frac{15000}{50 \times 60} = 5 \text{ hours}$$

(c) To determine amount that can be given at a certain rate in a certain time:

$$\text{Volume} = \text{Rate (drops per minute)} \times \text{Time (in minutes)},$$

e.g. How much fluid can be given in 5 hours at 25 drops per minute?

$$\text{Volume} = 25 \times 5 \times 60 = 7500 \text{ minims} = \frac{7500}{15000} \text{ litres} = \frac{1}{2} \text{ litre.}$$

Observations. (a) Apparatus. Flask: quantity, quality, patency of air inlet. Filter chamber: airtight, not blocked. Tubing: kinks, patency, airlocks. Needle or cannula: position, attachment to tubing. (b) Site. Redness, oedema, pain, leakage, strapping or bandage not impeding flow, discomfort. (c) Fluid balance chart — accurate recording of intake and output. (d) General condition. Pulse, blood pressure, respirations, temperature, colour, cough.

Comfort of patient. (a) Position. Depends on condition: semi-recumbent or semiupright. Arm adequately supported, leg on splint with bedcradle to take weight of clothes and small blanket to keep leg warm. (b) Oral care: mouth rinse, ice to suck or mouth toilets. (c) May require assistance with meals, sponging and use of bedpan. (d) Encourage patient to report pain or discomfort.

Stoppage of flow. *Causes.* Empty flask, blocked air inlet disconnection or clogging of filter chamber, obstruction by sphygmomanometer, flexed arm, tight bandage or strapping, needle or cannula blocked with debris or clots, vasospasm, perforation of vein, imbedding of needle in vein wall, air embolus.

Treatment. Check flask, air inlet, filter chamber, tubing, etc. Ensure firm joints. Alter position of arm. Remove and reapply bandages or strappings. Inspect site for oedema or haematoma. Overcome venous spasm by gently stroking vein, application of warmth, gentle positive pressure by opening tubing clamp. Doctor may inject normal saline or local anaesthetic round site. Doctor or sister may alter position of needle slightly. Doctor may aspirate air from tubing.

Changing flasks. Fluid must never drain completely from flask. Check flask with doctor's orders and patient's name. Ensure flask has a hanger. Wash hands. Do not contaminate needle, stopper or air inlet. Keep bottles above level of needle. Change filter if necessary. Keep clamp very slightly open. If no orders for new fluid put up 5% dextrose until orders obtained. Never follow blood or serum immediately with glucose (causes agglutination).

6. REMOVAL OF INFUSION

Indications. Completion of therapy; blockage of needle; irritation of vein; circulatory overloading.

Method. Small dressing prepared. Bandage, splints and strapping removed. Needle or cannula gently and smoothly withdrawn. Dressing applied under pressure for few minutes. Pressure bandage if bleeding persists.

7. COMPLICATIONS

(a) THROMBOPHLEBITIS. Due to chemical irritation, e.g. from glucose.

Signs and symptoms. Inflammation extending along course of vein.

Treatment. Slow down infusion, inform doctor. Remove infusion, transfer to new site. Apply warmth, e.g. plastine, infrared rays.

(b) HAEMATOMA (local oedema.) May sometimes necessitate aspiration.

(c) EXCESSIVE OR TOO RAPID ADMINISTRATION.

Signs and symptoms. Dyspnoea, bubbly cough, frothy sputum, engorged neck veins, increased pulse volume (full and bounding), rising blood pressure, mental confusion, convulsions (if extreme).

Treatment. Slow down infusion, inform doctor who may discontinue infusion. Measures taken to clear lungs, e.g. postural drainage. Occasionally — venesection, forced diuresis.

(d) SALT RETENTION. May occur with associated renal insufficiency or renal failure. (i) Sodium: collection of fluid in injured sites, e.g. suture lines, sites of anastomosis. (ii) Potassium: variable signs and symptoms, e.g. anxiety, muscle twitching, falling blood pressure, slowing pulse rate, cardiac irregularities. Cardiac arrest may occur.

TRANSFUSION

Transfer of blood, plasma, or packed red cells from circulation of one person (donor) to another (recipient).

Indications. To restore blood volume, e.g. after haemorrhage, shock, burns, crush injuries. To replace blood parts, e.g. in anaemia, leucopenia, clotting disorders. To exchange blood, e.g. Rh incompatibility, carbon monoxide poisoning.

METHODS

Direct. Unchanged blood transferred directly from donor to recipient. Small pump required to prevent clotting of blood in transit.

Indirect. Blood taken from donor into flask, bottle or plastic bag. Anticoagulant added, e.g. citrate. May be stored for up to 3 weeks at low temperature (not freezing) before use.

COMPATIBILITY

Certain factors in blood can cause red cells to become 'sticky'. Agglutination occurs, may block lumen of small blood vessels. Haemolysis occurs with release of haemoglobin into urine. During concentration of urine, haemoglobin may be thrown out of solution causing blockage of nephrons.

To avoid incompatibility serum of recipient carefully cross-matched with red cells of donor.

Main groups

1. ABO grouping. Four groups A, B, AB and O. AB recipients have no agglutinins and can receive from any other group (universal recipient). Group O contains two agglutinins (anti-A

35

and anti-B), in such small quantity that it can be given to any other group (universal donor). In a group O recipient there are enough agglutinins to cause agglutination with all except group O blood. Groups A and B contain one agglutinin (anti-B, anti-A respectively) and can receive only from their own group (or from group O).

2. Rh grouping. 85% of population possess red cells which will cause production of an agglutinin if they come in contact with blood of other 15%. Those people with this type of red cell are called Rh positives. The other 15% are called Rh negatives. Once a Rh negative is sensitized he cannot receive Rh positive blood.

3. Several other agglutinins are known but their occurrence is rare. They can cause agglutination, hence the need for careful crossmatching even between blood of the same main groups. Other groupings — MNS, Lutheran, Kell, Lewis, Duffy, Kidd.

Types of fluid. Whole blood. Packed cells (whole blood with much of plasma removed). Plasma. Pooled human serum. Human serum albumen (concentrated, 25%, 5% in Hartmann's solution). Stabilized plasma proteins solution. Dried fibrinogen. Platelets.

Procedure. Blood taken from recipient for grouping and crossmatching. Blood stored between 1° and 6°C. Must *not* be: stored in freezer, kept out of refrigerator for long before use, warmed before use, more than 15 days old.

Two people should check before administration: doctor's written order; name of patient, name on container; blood groups; Rh group; serial number on flask with compatibility report; date of expiry or date of collection of blood; whether blood is frozen; appearance — serum should be clear, straw coloured. Do not give if there is bluish or pink tinge (haemolysed), or if cloudy (infected).

Management. As for infusion.

Complications (in addition to those of infusion).

INCOMPATIBILITY. *Signs and symptoms.* Restlessness, anxiety; increased pulse rate; falling blood pressure; rising temperature often accompanied by rigor; headache; skin rash (allergic response). Pain in loins, haematuria, oliguria, anuria. Substernal pain (clogging of coronary vessels). Excessive bleeding (impaired clotting power). Jaundice (late sign of haemolysis).

Treatment. If any of above occur, stop transfusion, inform doctor. Save all specimens of recipient's and donor's blood. Do not wash bottles or tubing. Treat for shock. Treatment of renal failure may be necessary.

RIGORS may also be due to (1) blood: old, cold or given too fast, or (2) pyogenic infection: blood acts as culture medium, organisms multiply rapidly. Precautions taken when collecting or giving blood to prevent contamination. Septicaemia may develop rapidly.

Chapter 2

INFLAMMATION AND INFECTION

INFLAMMATION

Response of body tissues to injury or an irritant.

Causes. *Trauma.* Intentional, e.g. surgery. Accidental, e.g. blow, bruise, wound, crushing injury. Foreign objects, e.g. splinter, bullet, drain tube. *Infection.* Micro-organism invasion, destructive agents, e.g. heat, electricity, friction, cold, X-rays, ultraviolet rays. *Irritants,* e.g. chemicals, allergens. Tumour cells.

Pathology. Intensity varies with cause, state of tissues and general resistance of body.

Vascular changes. Dilatation of vessels to and from area causing increased volume of blood (hyperaemia). Ensures increased nutrients, oxygen, electrolytes, white cells, antitoxins and antibodies. Slower flow of blood through part (stasis) ensures more time for action of body defences. Increased permeability of capillaries allows accelerated exchange between blood and tissue fluid. Leucocytes migrate through capillary walls, ingest foreign bodies and cellular debris (phagocytosis).

Tissue changes. Occur later than vascular changes. Destruction or devitalization. May be due to severe irritants, bacterial toxins, occlusion of blood supply by increased amount of fluid exudate in area, e.g. central core of necrosed tissue in boil or carbuncle. Later, granulation and fibrosis walling off inflamed area.

Signs and symptoms. *Local.* Five cardinal signs and symptoms. Red, hot, swollen, painful and useless area. Redness and heat mainly due to hyperaemia. Some mild heat produced by chemical reactions. Later, purple discolouration from venous stasis and congestion. Swelling due to increased amount of blood and exudation into tissues. Pain, throbbing in nature, due to momentary increase in pressure during systole and pressure of exudate on sensory nerve endings; irritation by toxins or exposure of damaged tissues. Loss of function due to pain and swelling.

General. (1) Pyrexia. Raised temperature alters ideal state for multiplication of bacteria thus making it easier for them to be overwhelmed. (2) Increased pulse rate circulates more blood to infected area in an endeavour to rid body of toxins (in severe infections temperature may fall, body may attempt to raise it by intense muscular activity — rigor). (3) Toxins from bacteria and damaged tissue circulate in blood (toxaemia) and depress many body activities, hence — malaise, anorexia, lethargy, headache, mental depression, constipation, oliguria.

POSSIBLE RESULTS OF INFLAMMATION

Resolution. Body overcomes invader without residual damage. Occurs when (1) infecting agent of low virulence; (2) resistance of patient high; (3) degree of local injury slight. Inflammatory processes reverse, redness and heat subside, function returns as pain and swelling subside. Treatment of all inflammation is aimed at this result.

Repair. Damage to or loss of tissue is repaired by formation of fibrous scar.

Suppuration. Pus formation. Indicates some death of tissue. Pus consists of collection of fluid heavily laden with micro-organisms, dead white cells and dead tissue cells. Usually body 'walls off' and hence localizes pus — i.e. forms an abscess (p. 40). Occasionally body defences may not be adequate and pus may be liberated into blood stream (pyaemia, p. 45).

Spread. Into (1) tissues immediately surrounding original site of infection, e.g. cellulitis; (2) neighbouring organs; (3) lymphatic channels; (4) blood stream.

Chronic inflammation. Body unable to overcome low virulence organisms. Changes less marked in blood vessels than in tissues, i.e. little hyperaemia and capillary fragility but marked proliferation of tissues.

Causes. Inadequate rest of area; inadequate drainage; presence of foreign object; excessive fibrosis thus limiting blood supply to part; type of organism, e.g. syphilis, gonorrhoea, tuberculosis.

Treatment. *Local.* 1. Remove cause if possible, e.g. foreign object.

2. Rest: essential to allow body to overcome invader. Assisted by splints, slings, sandbags, etc. Internal organs rested by general rest of patient or reduction of function, e.g. low protein diet in acute nephritis. Prolonged immobilization avoided, movement or activity encouraged as soon as acute phase over.

3. Heat: aimed at imitating natural process. Heat should cause vasodilation to increase blood supply to part thus hastening resolution or localization. Effects disputed, but patient gains much comfort. Methods — hot fomentations; kaolin (plastine) poultice (contains methyl salicylate which has 'counter-irritant' effect, retains heat longer than fomentations); short waves, e.g. infrared or ultraviolet diathermy, delivers heat below skin surfaces; hot douche, e.g. rectally or vaginally, to help to localize pus in pelvic abscess.

4. Drainage of pus.

General. 1. Rest, under sedation if necessary.

2. Reduction of pyrexia — if severe, by tepid sponging to assist cooling by evaporation; if mild, by antipyretic drugs, e.g. aspirin may suffice.

3. Copious fluids: dilute toxins, help to reduce temperature.

4. Diet: sufficient calories to ensure energy; protein and vitamin C to aid healing. Light, tempting meals needed because of anorexia.

5. Aperients to overcome constipation and aid further excretion of toxins.

6. Specific antibiotic therapy.

7. Analgesics for pain and headache.

INFECTIONS

LOCAL INFECTIONS

ABSCESS
Localized collection of pus.

Cause. Successful invasion by pyogenic micro-organisms, usually *Staphylococcus aureus.*

Signs and symptoms. Local inflammation. Hard brawny swelling until pus forms. Swelling softens in centre and becomes fluctuant. General signs and symptoms of inflammation as above.

40

'Hectic' or swinging temperature indicates pus formation. Leucocytosis — bone marrow produces more white cells when body needs them.

Possible results. (1) Absorption of pus by body defences. (2) Pus travels along line of least resistance until it reaches a surface and then ruptures spontaneously. Cavity unable to marshal sufficiently powerful forces to overcome organism and organisms not sufficiently powerful to extend further.

Treatment. General treatment as above.

Drainage. (1) If abscess ruptures spontaneously, edges kept open with drain tube or gauze wick until adequate healing occurs at base of cavity. (2) Incision, drainage for several days. Forestalls spontaneous rupture, incised wound less ragged, cavity smaller. (3) Aspiration with syringe and wide-bore needle. Healing of cavity.

PARONYCHIA

Infection under fold of skin at base of nail usually causing localized suppuration.

Causes. Spread from cuticle; most commonly follows removal of 'hang-nail'. Infection of haematoma under nail.

Signs and symptoms. Redness, heat, swelling, pain, loss of function around base of nail. Suppuration may occur under nail.

Treatment. *Conservative.* Rest. Splint may be necessary. Antibiotics. Copious fluids. Local heat. Keep finger dry.

Surgical. Drainage. (1) Incision of nail bed. Single or double incision with nail folds elevated over gauze for 48 hours to ensure adequate drainage. (2) Removal of proximal half of nail (distal portion protects finger, patient able to use hand more quickly). (3) Removal of entire nail if infection extensive.

BOIL (FURUNCLE)

Abscess in sweat gland or hair follicle. Furunculosis — multiple boils.

Cause. Most commonly *Staphylococcus aureus.*

Predisposing causes. Low resistance to infection. Diabetes. Hormonal imbalance, e.g. at puberty. Poor personal hygiene. Friction.

Signs and symptoms. Pain and tenderness, becoming intense until bead of pus erupts, relieves tension; 1–2 days later central core of necrotic material (slough) extruded.

Treatment. Avoid squeezing. Incision left until area fluctuant, otherwise infection may spread instead of remaining localized. No dressing unless pus discharging as skin may become moist and soggy thus encouraging growth of staphylococci. Hot packs, analgesics if pain severe. Prevent spread by cleansing round area with antiseptic, e.g. pHisoHex. Antibiotics not usually necessary.

In furunculosis predisposing causes must be eliminated. Antibiotics may be used. Patient washes twice daily with hexachlorophene soap. In some cases autogenous vaccine may help.

Specific complication. Boils of face above level of mouth may cause spread to cavernous sinus of brain. Special care taken to avoid pressure (e.g. squeezing) which may precipitate spread. Antibiotics given.

CARBUNCLE

Infection of several hair follicles usually extending to subcutaneous tissues.

Cause. Staphylococci, streptococci. (Sometimes both.)

Predisposing causes. More common in patients with diabetes mellitus.

Sites. Anywhere, but most commonly back of neck.

Pathology. Swelling of hair follicles impedes blood supply to tissues between them. Area of gangrene results. Central cores of several sloughs are extruded leaving craters, often large.

Treatment. As for boils. Antibiotic therapy aids subsidence of process, reduces extent of surgery. Investigate for diabetes, treat if present. Incision and drainage, cruciate (cross-shaped) incision and the four quadrants of skin elevated so that these can be excised if necessary. Subsequent skin grafting may be required.

SINUS

Abnormal tract leading from deeper tissue (blind end) to open on to skin or mucous surface.

Cause. (1) Complication of abscess which fails to heal completely; (2) foreign object: sequestrum, hair, infected ligature, drain tube, keeps sinus open until removed.

Signs and symptoms. Opening discharging pus or serum on to surface. Probe may be passed along tract to locate blind end.

42

Treatment. Removal of foreign object. Widen sinus by incision and drainage. Excise tract completely.

PILONIDAL SINUS

Sinus due to penetration of hair into subcutaneous tissues.

Site. Most commonly on back in midline over sacrococcygeal junction. Occasionally on hands (especially barbers), or umbilicus.

Cause. Trauma forces hair into subcutaneous tissues, causes infection. In sacrococcygeal area this occurs where a congenital fault in coalescence of skin exists.

Signs and symptoms. More common in young (late teens or early twenties). Dark hirsute males. Acute abscess. Chronic draining sinus. Several sinuses may result on either side of mid-line.

Treatment. *Conservative.* Antibiotics and general measures (p. 40). Rarely successful alone.

Surgical. Acute abscess — incision and drainage; excision usually required. Dye (e.g. methylene blue) injected. Elliptical incision made, widened according to extent of blue stained tissues. Wound closed if no infection present — primary closure with deep tension sutures. Danger of recurrence if only minute area of infection remains. Open method — wound packed, not sutured. Pack removed in 5 days and sitz baths twice daily. Heals by granulation in 3 weeks.

FISTULA

Abnormal communication between 2 epithelial surfaces, e.g. between 2 organs or between an organ and skin or mucous surface. *Examples:* vesico-vaginal, vesico-rectal, gastro-colic, faecal fistula, anal fistula.

Cause. (1) Infection, especially abscess bursting in two directions; spread from one organ to another. (2) Foreign object — as for sinus. (3) Tissue damage. Trauma, e.g. following instrumentation; necrosis, e.g. following radium implant. (4) Congenital.

Signs and symptoms. Vary with site. (See separate sections.)

Treatment. Also varies with site. Principles — remove cause; widen and drain, i.e. remove roof of tract; excise completely.

SPREADING INFECTIONS

Cellulitis. Spreading inflammation (usually non-suppurative) among tissues, classically subcutaneous tissues.

CAUSE. Most often — haemolytic streptococcus, highly virulent organism in patient with low resistance.

PATHOLOGY. Original wound may be so slight as to be non-evident. Body defences inadequate to contain invader which may be discharging enzymes which break down confining barriers, e.g. collagen.

SIGNS AND SYMPTOMS. Area bright red, shiny, distinct demarcation from normal tissue. Tenderness, pain, heat swelling. General signs and symptoms of toxaemia.

TREATMENT. Open and drain if wound evident, otherwise conservative measures. Rest, local heat, copious fluids, antibiotics especially penicillin.

Erysipelas. Acute form of cellulitis involving mainly skin.

CAUSE. Infection with haemolytic streptococci. May spread to other parts with wounds. Elderly and debilitated patients more susceptible.

SITES. Face and legs more commonly.

SIGNS AND SYMPTOMS. Inflamed area, scarlet, hot, painful, swollen, raised above surrounding skin with clearly defined edge. Blisters may form on top of inflamed area. Signs and symptoms of toxaemia.

TREATMENT. As for cellulitis. Penicillin specific. General condition must be improved with high protein diet and vitamin C. Patient may be isolated.

Lymphangitis. Inflammation of lymph vessels or channels.

CAUSE. Inadequate body defences. Highly virulent organisms.

SIGNS AND SYMPTOMS. Painful red streaks, e.g. on arm from infected finger.

TREATMENT. Treat primary focus.

Lymphadenitis. Inflammation of lymph nodes.

CAUSE. Spread of infection from focus along lymph channels.

PATHOLOGY. Lymphoid cells attempt to overcome invader. Node may become swollen and tender. If cells fail, node itself becomes infected and suppurates.

TREATMENT. Treat primary focus. Incise and drain node if it suppurates.

Toxaemia. Liberation of toxins into blood stream.

44

CAUSE. Successful invasion by micro-organisms in any part of body. Organisms usually remain localized.

SIGNS AND SYMPTOMS (p. 39).

TREATMENT. Treat infection. Palliative measures (p. 40).

Bacteraemia. Bacteria in blood stream, usually transient.

Septicaemia. Micro-organisms multiplying in blood stream, i.e. infection of blood itself.

SIGNS AND SYMPTOMS. Toxaemia with rigors, high swinging temperature at first, later remains high. Pulse, at first full and bounding, later weak and thready. Patient flushed and anxious at first, later becomes delirious and unconscious. When kidneys involved urine contains albumin and blood.

DIAGNOSIS. Confirmed by blood culture.

TREATMENT. In addition to treatment for toxaemia (p. 40). Vigorous antibiotic therapy. Combined antibiotics started immediately, changed if necessary on result of blood culture. Organisms causing septicaemia often resistant to commonly used antibiotics. Special nursing measures required as patient weak, debilitated and will be confined to bed for a long time.

Pyaemia. Circulation in blood stream of pus-forming bacteria.

CAUSE. Sepsis, e.g. pus in mastoid antrum followed by septic lateral sinus, brain or kidney abscess from distant septic focus.

PATHOLOGY. Wherever emboli (colonies of bacteria) lodge, abscesses will form.

SIGNS AND SYMPTOMS. Rigors. Swinging temperature. General symptoms of pus formation, toxaemia. Local symptoms depending on sites of lodgement.

TREATMENT. May be prolonged. Incision and drainage of abscesses. Vigorous measures as for septicaemia.

SPECIFIC INFECTIONS

Tetanus. Infection of central nervous system by exotoxin of *Clostridium tetani.*

CAUSAL ORGANISM. *Clostridium tetani.* Anaerobic, spore-forming bacterium, normally inhabits intestine of herbivorous animals, hence likely to be present in soil containing manure.

TYPES OF WOUNDS. Deep puncture wounds (anaerobic). Dead or devitalized tissue especially jagged wounds, compound fractures, extensive burns.

PATHOLOGY. Organism uninvasive, remains at point of entry. Toxins given off, carried via blood stream to central nervous system. Toxin acts at synapses by suppressing normal inhibition. Causes mild spasms around wound, more severe spasms of voluntary muscles (beginning with jaw muscles) until whole body thrown into repeated spasms. Death may result from exhaustion, or asphyxiation from prolonged spasm of diaphragm.

INCUBATION PERIOD. Usually 7—14 days although symptoms may occur within 24 hours of injury or as long as 8 months after injury.

SIGNS AND SYMPTOMS. Early tingling in wound. General irritability, restlessness, insomnia. Usual sequence of skeletal muscle involvement (1) jaw (trismus) — so-called 'lock-jaw', (2) difficulty with mastication followed by dysphagia. (3) Angles of mouth retract causing hideous grinning grimace — risus sardonicus. (4) Back of neck causes head retraction. (5) Abdominal, limb and back muscle produce severe arching of back. In severest form, head and heels only may be touching bed (opisthotonos). (6) Respiratory muscles.

Muscular stiffness succeeded by spasm. Slight and transient at first with long respites between. Later becomes more frequent, more prolonged and eventually patient may pass from one attack to another without respite. Consciousness not lost, in fact awareness heightened. Spasms initiated by mild stimulation, e.g. light, noise, movement, draught.

TREATMENT. Intensive treatment started as soon as early manifestations noted.

Immunization. 1. Active (prophylactic): best during childhood. Tetanus toxoid 0.5 ml. Three injections, second after 6 weeks, third after 9 months. First injection results in significant amounts of antitoxin within 7—21 days but manufacture falls without second and third injections. Booster doses every 4—5 years and at time of injury.

2. Passive. If danger of infection present in patient not previously immunized, ready-made antitoxin (tetanus antitoxin, antitetanus serum) can be injected. (Antitoxin manufactured in body of animal usually horse, by course of injections of toxin into animal. Serum extracted contains proteins of horse's blood.) Danger of allergic reactions: (*a*) anaphylactic shock with broncho-

spasm, laryngeal oedema, hypotension. Can cause death in minutes or hours; (*b*) delayed serum sickness starting 7—21 days after initial injection. Various manifestations: giant urticaria, asthma from bronchospasm, eczema, swelling of lymph nodes, oedema, joint pains, pyrexia, headaches, nausea, vomiting, diarrhoea. Adrenaline, antihistamines, cortisone derivatives used in treatment. Patient may need to be desensitized.

Because of this danger modern trend is to avoid passive immunization, concentrate on thorough cleansing and debridement of wound and start active immunization. If passive immunization is used ask patient if previously immunized with horse serum, e.g. diphtheria antitoxin, or if he has any allergy; have adrenaline, antihistamine and cortisone ready; give test dose (500 units), observe for any reaction in next 30 minutes; if none occurs, give remaining dose. Antitoxin does not affect toxin already in nerve cells, hence need for early injection while toxin still in blood stream. Antitoxin may be injected around wound prior to surgery.

Penicillin. Bacteriostatic. Massive doses to prevent liberation of toxin from organisms.

Wound care. Bathe wound with hydrogen peroxide. Lay wound open, excise all dead and devitalized skin, subcutaneous tissue, muscle, fat. Delay closure if contamination heavy. Irrigate with hydrogen peroxide or pack with zinc peroxide paste.

Control of muscle spasm. Patient isolated in quiet, warm, darkened room. Spared all unnecessary movements. Sedation with barbiturates or chlorpromazine may control mild spasms. Anaesthetic or muscle relaxants, e.g. curare in severe cases.

General measures. Constant and expert nursing care to prevent complications, e.g. pneumonia, asphyxia, injury, urinary infection, constipation, dirty mouth, damaged eyes. Fluid balance and nutritional maintenance by intragastric or intravenous feeding. Respiration: tracheostomy may be required for laryngeal oedema. Mechanical artificial respiration may be needed for days or weeks. Antibiotics do not arrest tetanic spasms but may prevent pneumonia.

Gas gangrene. Infection and destruction of tissue by *Clostridium welchii* or its relations.

CAUSAL ORGANISM. *Cl. welchii, perfringens, sporogenes.*

Anaerobic, spore-forming organisms that give off gas as a waste product of metabolism. Live in guts of herbivorous animals. May be found in human intestines and vagina.

PATHOLOGY. Organisms thrive in devitalized, bloodless, deoxygenated tissues especially muscle. Organisms produce enzymes which digest muscle tissue. Bubbles of gas form, muscle tissue becomes discoloured, necrotic and finally becomes a soft, gas-filled pulp. Subcutaneous tissue also affected. Overlying skin becomes pale, cold at first, later, dusky, purple mottled. Blisters may appear on surface. Exotoxins cause a severe toxaemia which may be fatal.

TYPES OF WOUND. (1) Lacerated, especially if muscle involved. (2) Contaminated wounds, especially gunshot wounds in which pieces of clothing carried deep into tissues. Also compound fractures. (3) Bloodless field surgery. (4) Abdominal wounds contaminated with faeces. (5) Following septic abortion.

SIGNS AND SYMPTOMS. Incubation period 1–4 days but may appear within 6 hours of injury. Pain in wound. Pulse rate increased out of proportion to temperature. Sero-sanguineous discharge — watery and brown, 'mouse-like' odour, not unlike acetylene gas in low concentrations. Discolouration of skin around wound. General severe toxaemia. Anaemia due to extensive haemolysis. Crepitus felt in swollen limb due to gas bubbles, may be demonstrated by X-ray before it is palpable.

TREATMENT. *Prophylactic.* (1) Debridement of wound especially damaged muscle fat. Heavily contaminated wound left open. (2) Antibiotic therapy especially penicillin and tetracycline. (Antitoxin of no value in prophylaxis.)

Curative. (1) Massive does of antibiotics. (2) Anti-gas gangrene serum (gas-gangrene antitoxin) 40,000–80,000 units, given after skin test for hypersensitivity. (3) Extensive debridement. Wound left open. If disease is spreading rapidly amputation may be needed. (4) Blood transfusion. (5) Measures to overcome shock, toxaemia.

Chapter 3

WOUNDS, ULCERS, BURNS, SKIN GRAFTING

HEALING

STAGES OF HEALING

Granulation. Raw surface covered with blood clot and tissue fluid. Clot organizes, i.e. small capillary buds grow into it bringing white blood cells for liquefaction and absorption of unwanted clot and tissue. The capillaries give a granular appearance, hence the name — granulation tissue. Easily damaged. Bleeds freely if injured.

Fibrosis. Fibroblasts lay down long fine fibres which help to draw edges of wound together. Rich blood supply ensures that fibres increase in number and thickness. Eventually fibres nip off blood supply and remain as dense mass which slowly contracts and makes wound smaller. Over-contraction in large wounds, e.g. burns, can cause deformity.

Epithelialization. Epithelium grows in from wound edges to cover granulation tissue. Discharge usually given off by granulation tissue until epithelium covers it. A scab of dried blood and tissue fluid may form. Plays no part in healing but provides temporary protective cover. Epithelium will not grow over granulations if they project above surrounding skin level (proud flesh). Excess granulations cauterized with silver nitrate or copper sulphate.

METHODS OF HEALING

First or primary intention. Edges of wound in close apposition either because of nature of wound or because of assistance by sutures or clips. Scar tissue minimal and process described above is not so evident.

49

Second intention or granulation. Open wounds where tissue lost by injury, infection or disease, skin edges cannot be approximated. Much larger area of scar tissue results, above process evident.

FACTORS NECESSARY FOR HEALING

Local. (1) Adequate haemostasis (for clot formation). (2) Rest of area (assures formation of clot). (3) Apposition of skin edges if possible. (4) Adequate blood supply to area to ensure nourishment and oxygen. (5) Freedom from infection.

General. Healthy tissue. Depends on (1) Age. Younger people have more active cells. (2) Nutrition. Protein, vitamins A and C essential for healing; vitamin K for blood clot (indirectly). (3) Adequate circulation. Depends on heart action, state of blood vessels, composition of blood, e.g. adequate haemoglobin, white cells, fluid, oxygen, food substances.

CAUSES OF DELAYED HEALING

Local. (1) Haemorrhage. (2) Inadequate immobilization, e.g. vigorous exercises, straining of abdomen from chronic cough or constipation. (3) Presence of (*a*) foreign object, e.g. sequestrum, drain tube; (*b*) fistula or sinus; (*c*) neoplasm; (*d*) excessive haematoma. (4) Excessive tissue damage or skin loss. (5) Edges of wound inverted. (6) Sutures too loose allowing too much movement between edges. (7) Sutures too tight cutting down blood supply. (8) Wound infection. (9) Inadequate venous drainage of area.

General. (1) Old age. (2) Malnutrition especially when associated with malignant disease. (3) Obesity. (4) Jaundice. (5) Existing disease such as congestive cardiac failure, atherosclerosis, anaemia, dehydration, oedema, uraemia, pulmonary pathology, diabetes. (6) Cortisone therapy.

WOUNDS

Breaks in surface epithelium.

TYPES

Incision. Edges of wound evenly separated; made with sharp instrument, e.g. knife, piece of glass. Tends to gape; usually bleeds freely; heals by first intention.

50

Laceration. Tissues torn, edges of wound jagged and may become necrotic, e.g. wound made with barbed wire.

Puncture. Deep, narrow wound, e.g. from knife point, needle, bullet, insect bite.

Contusion. Surrounding area bruised. Delays healing, e.g. blow from blunt instrument.

COMPLICATIONS

Haemorrhage. Shock. Infection. Damage to deeper structures. Evisceration, especially through abdominal wound. Incisional hernia.

TREATMENT

Clean, fresh wound. Arrest haemorrhage. Close by sutures or clips. Apply sterile dressing or plastic skin.

Lacerated wound. *1. Fresh.* Arrest haemorrhage. Excise dead or devitalized tissues. Close wound by direct suturing. Relieving incision may be necessary, i.e. skin incised parallel to wound so that skin can be drawn across wound. Incision allowed to heal by granulation (occasionally used to close skin over compound fracture where this assists immobilization). Skin grafting may be needed. Sterile dressing. Immobilization with splint or plaster if necessary.

2. Over 12 hours' duration (infection possible). Arrest haemorrhage. Clean thoroughly with detergent substance, e.g. cetrimide. Remove foreign objects. Excise all dead and devitalized tissue. Suture with enough tension to approximate edges and allow discharge to escape. If closure impossible (due to oedema) wound left open, closed later (delayed primary suture). May be allowed to heal by granulation. If 'dead space' left in depth of wound, drain tube inserted and brought through surface via separate 'stab' wound. May be packed. Sterile dressing applied. Area immobilized. Prophylactic systemic antibiotics.

Infected wound. Tissues not excised because of danger of spreading infection. Area immobilized. Infection treated (p. 39—40). Observe for complications — abscess, cellulitis, lymphangitis, gas gangrene, secondary haemorrhage. Wound irrigated with antiseptic solution. Slough removed. When wound clean, closed by secondary suture or skin graft.

Stab wounds. If infected laid wide open, treated as above.

51

SUTURES

Stitch introduced into body tissues on a surgical needle to maintain appositicn of wound edges until healing occurs. Ligature: material tied round vessel or piece of tissue. Introduced by slipping it under area with aneurysm needle or tying it round a cut vessel held by artery forceps.

Materials

Depends on (1) individual surgeon's choice, (2) tissue being sutured (e.g. delicate: eye, peritoneum, bowel; strong: muscle, skin; viscera: absorption necessary), (3) desired cosmetic result, (4) strain to be imposed on area.

Classification

Absorbable. Must be non-irritant to tissues; easily, quickly and cheaply sterilized; fine, strong, pliable, easily handled, reliable.

CATGUT. Obtained from submucous layer of sheep's intestine. Processed, sterilized and supplied either in double wrapped foil or in glass tubes containing chemical, e.g. xylol, to retain in perfect condition, free from water.

Size range. 6/0 — extremely fine, to 4 — very thick. Fine used for delicate tissues, e.g. peritoneum. Medium for aponeurosis, liver, kidney, uterus. Thick for repair of levator ani muscle, etc.

Types. (1) Plain (unhardened). Absorbed during 2nd week (may lose tensile strength in 4—5 days). (2) Chromic (hardened with chromic acid). Absorbed during 3rd week. Retains tensile strength until 2nd week.

Precautions. Should not be exposed for long periods. Becomes friable with drying. Rinsed in sterile water or drawn through wet swab before insertion to reduce irritant effect on tissues. Glass containers broken with special breaker to prevent scattering of glass fragments.

DEXON. Synthetic. Various sizes, with and without needle. Various absorbtion rates.

Non-absorbable. SILK. Sterilized by autoclave or boiling.

Wound on large diameter spools to prevent shrinkage and loss of tensile strength.

Sizes. 6/0 to 4. May be dyed different colours to distinguish different strengths.

Types. (1) Floss. Thick but soft. Usually for ligatures, e.g. haemorrhoids, patent ductus arteriosus. Chinese — for repair where strength is needed, e.g. intestinal anastomosis. Waxed — for skin. Non-irritating to tissues but knot tends to slip. Disadvantages: irritant to tissues (except waxed). Must not be used in already infected wounds. (2) Silkworm gut. Produced from body of silkworm. Mainly for skin sutures. Knot tends to undo readily.

NYLON. Synthetic resin. Completely non-irritating to tissues. Sterilized by autoclaving or boiling. (Repeated autoclaving tends to make it hard and brittle.)

Sizes. 5/0 to 2.

Disadvantages. Knot tends to slip unless nylon specially braided. Dissolved by carbolic in any form.

Uses. Skin sutures or ligatures, e.g. root of lung.

LINEN. Made from flax. Tends to absorb moisture therefore less effective in tissues but strong, reliable, cheap, easily sterilized.

Sizes. 3/0 to 3.

Uses. Ligation especially of bleeding points. Not usually used on skin.

HORSEHAIR. Rarely used. Easily sterilized by autoclaving or boiling. (Claimed that tetanus and other spores could be present and they not killed by usual methods of sterilization.) Cheap and durable.

COTTON. Prepared from fibres in seed pods. Sterilized as for silk.

Sizes. 24 and 40 most commonly used.

Uses. Skin sutures. Does not unravel easily and knot remains firm. Less likely to be invaded by granulation tissue.

WIRE. Silver, stainless steel, tantalum. Sterilized by boiling or autoclave.

Sizes. 25–40.

Uses. Abdominal wall layers. Repair of hernia. Repair of tendons. Immobilization of bone.

Advantages. Great tensile strength. Does not irritate tissues.

Disadvantages. Difficult to handle especially if kinked. Ends of knot must be cut very short to prevent damage to surrounding tissues.

CLIPS. e.g. Michel's. Spiked clips. For skin wounds only. Applied with special forceps which arch clip while spikes approximate wound edges.

FASCIA. Taken from thigh (fascia lata) or aponeurosis of external oblique muscle. Taken from patient (autogenous) or from another person (homologous).

Uses. Hernia repair; reconstructions, e.g. pelvic floor.

Needles

Made of stainless steel. Does not break easily when bending force applied. Small needles threaded while holding in needle holder. Holder grips needle about ⅓ of length from eye (strongest point). Each has three parts – eye, body, point.

Varieties. *Eye.* (1) Atraumatic. Needle tubular at end and suture gripped into tube. No eye, therefore needle does not expand at end. Used for fine work. (2) Eye may be round, square, oval, pear-shaped. May pass from front to back or from side to side. (3) Self-threading spring eye.

Body. Cross section – round, triangular or flat. Shaft straight or curved. Curve may by ¼, ⅜ or ½ circle.

Point. May have cutting edge – triangular, trocar, taper. May be blunt and rounded.

Types of suturing. (1) Approximation: bringing wound edges together. (2) Tension: larger and bolder stitches through deeper layers; takes tension off skin sutures.

Forms. (1) Continuous. Simple oversewing, blanket, mattress. (2) Interrupted. Each stitch tied separately, e.g. simple loop. Mattress and vertical mattress. Buttons or rubber tubing may be threaded on to that part of tension suture that lies outside, to prevent cutting of skin.

Removal of sutures

Reasons. (1) Wound healed, sutures no longer necessary. (2) Stitch abscess. (3) Sutures too tight or too loose. (4) Accumulation of fluid under skin, e.g. following mastectomy or thyroidectomy.

54

Aims. To prevent infection from skin or from that part of suture which has remained outside tissues. To cause as little discomfort as possible.

Time. Average 7–10 days. Face (good blood supply), 3 days. Tension sutures, about 14 days.

Method. 1. Disinfect skin with antiseptic lotion, e.g. alcoholic chlorhexidine 0.5%, to minimize risk of infection.

2. Grasp knot with forceps, gently lift up small area that has been buried in tissues (ensure that no part of suture which has been outside skin is pulled through wound).

3. Press rounded end of scissors gently down into skin and cut through part previously buried.

4. Apply gentle traction on knot until buried part of suture comes through tissues. Force not necessary.

5. When all sutures removed apply antiseptic paint, e.g. mercurochrome 1%, to prevent infection and aid drying. Or spray with plastic skin, e.g. nobecutane. Some wounds may require supportive dressing, e.g. gauze and pad supported by elastoplast or binder.

Michel clips. Usually removed earlier than sutures 3–5 days.

1. Disinfect.

2. Insert specially made blade of remover under central arch of clip, press blades together. Clip straightens out and spikes disengage skin.

3. Cover wound as for sutures.

DRAINAGE TUBES

Purposes. Placed in cavity, canal, organ or wound. (1) Escape route for blood or serum following surgery, to prevent infection and aid in healing. (2) Reveals possible concealed haemorrhage. (3) Escape route for pus if infection present. (4) Escape route for body fluids, e.g. bile.

Materials. Usually rubber or polythene. Must be soft, not rigid. Various sizes. Tubular, corrugated, occasionally flat, e.g. 'glove' drain (strip of material from rubber glove). Paul's tubing (Penrose drain) (originally intended for use with Paul's tube for colostomy drainage). Collapsible tubing. Long length extends from site. Knot tied at distal end. Drainage collects in tubing. Knot cut off, drainage expelled, knot retied. Provides a closed circuit, prevents entry of organisms. Not recommended when drainage excessive.

Gauze may be used as drain (in form of wick). Fluids pass out by capillary action; can therefore drain against gravity. Danger when gauze thoroughly impregnated that no further drainage will occur and gauze becomes plug instead of drain.

Drainage tubes may be anchored with skin stitch to prevent displacement. Safety pin usually inserted crossways to prevent tube slipping completely into wound.

Collection of drainage. *Into dressing.* Small amount of discharge. Dressing changed when necessary; wet dressings harbour infection.

Into plastic bag. May be attached to bedside on special hanger or to patient's body, e.g. leg bag for urinary drainage, or to binder, e.g. T tube from bile duct.

Under-water drainage bottle. 4–5 litre capacity bottle containing ½–1 litre disinfectant, e.g. formalin 40%, chloroxylenol (Dettol) 5%. Tube from patient connected to tube passing through stopper, distal end of which is under surface of disinfectant, hence no risk of infection passing up tubing. May drain by gravity or by gentle suction (electric motor or Wangensteen's apparatus).

Care of drain tube and tubing. Avoid kinks especially from patient reclining against tube. Avoid tension especially during movement of patient. Attach tubing to skin by strapping so that tension taken on strapping. Avoid blockage especially with thick drainage (care with selection of size of tube and connections). If tube blocks and gentle milking action fails to clear it, tube may be washed out. Fine catheter inserted into tube and sterile normal saline instilled. Small amount injected at a time and aspirated before more is instilled (pain may result if too much inserted).

Amount of drainage observed and recorded on fluid balance chart together with note of colour, consistency, constituents, odour.

Removal. Indicated when amount of drainage minimal. Any tube left in for more than 5 days treated by tissues as a foreign object; fibrous tract develops around it. Tissue necrosis may occur if tube remains too long. Average time 48–72 hours, sometimes 24 hours, sometimes 5–7 days. (T tube remains up to 3 weeks.)

Method. 1. Remove retaining skin suture. Leave safety pin in situ.

2. Gently rotate tube through 180°. Withdraw 1–1½ inches or according to instructions. (Rotation applied in case granulations grow into side holes. Tube shortened so that granulations may grow from depth before skin closure to prevent sinus formation.)

3. Sterile safety pin inserted through tube close to skin.

4. Tube cut between safety pins.

5. Narrow adhesive tape may be passed through pin and anchored to skin to prevent tube slipping into wound.

PACKING OF WOUNDS

Purpose. Assist granulation from base. Clear up infection or remove slough by applying antiseptics, e.g. Milton 2½%, Eusol 50%, hydrogen peroxide 25%, or antibiotics, e.g. sofratulle.

Materials. Ribbon gauze, gauze squares. Dry or impregnated with petroleum jelly, paraffin or antibiotics.

Insertion. Dry gauze may be soaked in prescribed lotion and packed into wound lightly from below upwards. Must be changed frequently. If individual pieces of gauze used they should be counted at insertion and removal. If ribbon gauze used avoid contamination by dragging over skin surface or dressing towels. Avoid loose threads.

Removal. Avoid damage to granulation tissue. If dry, moisten each progressive layer with hydrogen peroxide or normal saline.

DRESSING OF WOUND

Purpose. Protection from infection. Support to keep wound edges in apposition. To apply pressure over wound.

Materials. Gauze, dry or impregnated with petroleum jelly, paraffin, antibiotic. Cotton wool kept in place with bandage, binder, elastoplast, zinc oxide strapping. Plastic skin – nobecutane.

Method. Wound should be kept dry (micro-organisms thrive in warmth and moisture). Dressing should be disturbed as little as possible. Sterile equipment prepared; in separate room if possible, free from infection. Two people for dressing; assistant wears mask, and prepares patient – explanation, privacy, exposes dressing without unduly exposing patient, loosens bandages, strapping, etc. Dresser dons mask, surgically cleanses hands. Assistant removes equipment from packets with sterile lifting forceps. Dresser removes old dressing with sterile forceps and discards dressing and forceps. Area cleansed using swabs dipped in antiseptic, e.g. aqueous chlorhexidine 0.05%. Swabs held in forceps, used for one stroke only. Area dried. Applications applied if ordered. New dressing applied. Nothing touched with fingers. Clean bandages, etc. applied to keep dressing in place. Assistant ensures patient's comfort. Dressings and soiled swabs discarded into paper bag, incinerated.

Observations. Any signs of inflammation: discharge — amount, colour, consistency, odour. Rate of healing: any haematoma or unusual swelling. Loose or tight sutures: stitch abscess.

ULCERS

Break in continuity of surface epithelium with impaired healing.

Causes. Decreased circulation.

General. Obliterative arterial disease: impaired venous return; congestive cardiac failure; malnutrition; anaemia; degenerative changes.

Local. Pressure, e.g. bedclothes, splints, plasters, patient's weight. Neoplasm (outgrows blood supply); injury — heat, cold, electricity, chemicals, mechanical; infection with non-specific organisms, e.g. *Staphylococcus aureus,* or specific organisms, e.g. tuberculosis, typhoid, actinomycosis.

Observations. Site; size; shape; edges; floor; discharge.

Stages. *Extension* (spreading). Surroundings: red, hot, swollen, painful. Edge: clearly defined. Floor covered with dark yellow material: slough of tissue fluid and dead cells. Discharge: copious, thin, offensive.

Intermediate (transition between sloughing and granulation). Surroundings: oedematous, may be pigmented. Edges thickened and elevated. Floor: dark greenish colour (slough) smooth and shiny. Discharge: scanty, serous or purulent.

Healing (obvious granulations). Edges: blue, epithelium growing inwards. Floor: covered with red granulations (p. 49). Discharge: very scanty, serous.

Treatment

Conservative. Treat underlying cause, e.g. tuberculosis. Improve blood supply to area by elevating part (aids venous return and clears way for arterial supply), exercises, external support, e.g. elastic stocking, Viscopaste, crepe bandage. Improve general health, e.g. diet, iron. Rest of some areas, e.g. restricted diet for gastric ulcer. Treat inflammation and prevent further infection.

Remove slough with local applications, e.g. Eusol 1 in 2, Milton 5%, enzyme preparations, e.g. Trypure Nova. Curettage of floor may be necessary.

Encourage granulation — irradiation, ultraviolet or infra-red (never used together because of danger of burns); packing with petroleum jelly gauze (dry dressing never used because removal causes disturbance of new granulations). Occasionally gauze soaked in white of egg effective. Stimulating lotions may be applied — lotio rubra, tincture of benzoin, scarlet red ointment.

Surgical. (1) Excision of ulcer. (2) Excision of ulcer bearing area, e.g. partial gastrectomy. (3) Excision and skin graft. (4) Skin graft to clean ulcer.

SPECIFIC ULCERS

Peptic ulcer. See p. 102.

Varicose ulcer. See p. 232.

Decubitus ulcer (pressure or bedsore). Ulcer caused by prolonged pressure, aggravated by moisture, irritation, friction.

SITES. Bony prominences, e.g. ischium, sacrum, trochanter, heel, malleolus, elbow, spinous process, occiput, scapula.

CAUSES. *Local and mechanical.* (1) Patient's own weight in one position too long; splints, bandages, plasters, bedpans, foreign objects and wrinkles in bedding. (2) Moisture and irritation — incontinence, inadequate drying after sponging, sweating. (3) Friction: extreme restlessness, loose plasters, splints, bandages, careless lifting of patient and insertion of bedpan.

Generally predisposing. (1) Emaciation: carcinoma, tuberculosis, malnutrition. (2) Impaired general blood supply: anaemia, congestive cardiac failure, old age, obesity. (3) Dryness of skin: prolonged fever, dehydration. (4) Immobility: unconsciousness, paralysis, traction.

Those more prone. Aged, debilitated, emaciated, obese, immobilized.

PREVENTION. *Local.* 2-hourly changes of position. Use of bed aids — ripple mattress, pillows, sheepskins, air rings. Gentle massage to stimulate circulation. Careful attention to bed making — elimination of wrinkles, foreign objects. Changing wet beds immediately. Water-proofing skin with silicone cream. Absolute cleanliness. Thorough drying. Careful lifting of patient and insertion of bedpan. Careful application of bandages, splints, plasters.

General. Correction of predisposing factors, e.g. anaemia, malnutrition, obesity. Encourage early ambulation. Active and passive exercises while in bed. Diet: increase proteins, vitamin C, fluid intake.

Warning signs and symptoms. Redness. Complaint of numbness, heat, tenderness, smarting. Crops of pimple-like eruptions. Discolouration. If any of these occur preventive measures intensified.

SIGNS AND SYMPTOMS. Abrasion. Ulcer — stages as above. If neglected, extensive damage to skin and soft tissues. Bones may be exposed and become infected. Patient may die from toxaemia.

TREATMENT. (1) Preventive measures intensified to avoid extension of ulcer. (2) Pressure on area removed entirely. (3) Ulcer treated as infected wound — kept clean, dry and debrided. Slough removed, and granulation encouraged. (4) Surgical measures for large resistant areas — debridement, removal of bony prominence, closure of wound with skin graft.

BURNS

Destruction of tissues by extremes of temperature, chemicals, electricity, radiation. (Burn — dry heat; scald — moist heat.)

CAUSE

Dry heat: flame, hot objects especially metals, electricity, radiation. Moist heat: liquid, steam, molten metals, fat. Chemicals: strong acids, alkalies. Intense cold.

Burns may affect skin, deeper tissues, e.g. subcutaneous muscle, bone. Inhaled or swallowed agents affect mucous membranes. Majority of burns occur in very young and very old. Result of ignorance, infirmity or carelessness.

PREVENTION

Education of public: (1) Fixed fireguards round open fires. (2) Special care of children — inflammable clothing, pots and pans on stoves, pulling of tablecloths, use of matches and fireworks. (3) Smoking in bed. (4) Use of electrical equipment. (5) Industrial hazards.

CLASSIFICATION

Depth. Various classifications from 2 to 6 degrees; commonly 3 degrees.

1. *First degree burns.* Erythema only. Superficial partial skin thickness. Destruction of epidermis. Not involved: hair follicles, sebaceous and sweat glands.

2. *Second degree burns.* Erythema, blister formation. Deep partial skin thickness. Hair follicles, sebaceous glands destroyed. Deep sweat glands survive.

3. *Third degree burns.* Destruction of full thickness skin and often deeper structures: subcutaneous tissues, muscle, bone. Depth of burn determines rate and type of healing, method of treatment, liability to infection.

Extent. Area of burn. Expressed in percentage of total skin surface. Quick guide — palm of hand 1%.

Wallace's 'rule of nine'. Head 9%, arm 9%, front of trunk 18%, back of trunk 18%, leg 18%, genital area 1%. In a child: head 18%, arm 9%, front of trunk 18%, back of trunk 18%, leg 14%, genital area 1%. Extent determines degree of shock, amount and type of fluid to be replaced.

PATHOLOGY.

Healing. (1) Partial thickness burns (superficial, deep), epithelium grows again. First degree burns: dead cells flake off, healing rapid, new skin indistinguishable. Second degree: healing slower, new skin may have poor texture and elasticity. (2) Third degree: damaged surface separates as slough in 7—10 days. Healing takes place by granulation and inward growth of epithelium from surrounding edges. Final healing may be slow, epithelialization proceeds at approximately 1 mm per day. Scar tissue formation may be extensive. Deformities may result from contractures; may be prevented by early skin grafting.

EFFECTS OF BURNING

1. Death of cells by coagulation. Rarely sufficient involved to cause death of patient unless area vital, e.g. ingestion of chemical may destroy sufficient oesophagus to cause death, inhalation of potent gas or flame may destroy lung tissue.

2. Vasodilation and increased capillary permeability as result of heat (may cause death from shock). Rapid loss of fluid from vascular to extracellular areas in form of (a) blisters, (b) exudate from raw surfaces, (c) oedema in subcutaneous tissues. Capillaries recover tone and normal permeability in 36–48 hours.

3. Pain. Severe in first and second degree burns due to exposure of nerve endings or pressure of fluid on nerve endings. Third degree burns may be painless due to destruction of nerve endings.

4. Loss of red blood cells due to (a) destruction by heat, (b) increased fragility, premature haemolysis, (c) loss into tissue fluid when capillaries grossly incompetent.

5. Liberation of toxins into circulation, e.g. histamine, adenosine compounds, abnormal proteins released from burnt surface. Exact action not known. May cause renal failure, liver necrosis, duodenal ulcer (Curling's).

PROGNOSIS

Depends on age, previous health of patient, total area burnt, depth, effectiveness of treatment in overcoming shock and preventing complications.

COMPLICATIONS

Shock. *Causes.* Loss of fluid from circulation. Pain. Psychological factors associated with appearance and smell of burn. Severity depends not on depth but on total area of burn, e.g. over 15% (10% in children) may cause irreversible changes if fluid loss not replaced in first 48 hours. Over 35% in older patients and 50% in younger, usually fatal. Burns of face, hands and feet produce deeper shock than trunk.

Effects. Most marked on (1) kidney – oliguria resulting from (a) haemoconcentration following plasma loss from circulation, (b) fall in blood pressure. Anuria may be end result if fluids not replaced. (2) Intestine – severe hypoxia results in paralytic ileus.

Infection. Raw area with serum exudate acts as culture medium in which organisms find ideal conditions – warmth, moisture and dead tissue for food. Tetanus and gas gangrene can occur in deep burns.

Effects (a) Local – delayed healing, suppuration, prolonged hospitalization, unsightly scars. (b) General – toxaemia, septicaemia, toxic shock which may cause death.

Scars and contracture. Degree of scarring depends on age of patient, depth and site of burn. Hypertrophic activity of scar reaches maximum in 3 months after healing, gradually becomes paler, flatter and softer over 1–2 years. During stage of hypertrophy often unsightly and itchy. Keloid scars (very rare) differentiated from above when they fail to resolve in few months and continue to grow and invade healthy areas. Contractures may follow deep burns. Due to shrinkage of scar tissue. Maximal at 3 months, becoming more lax thereafter. Limitation of joint movement. Causes (1) skin contractures near joint, (2) prolonged immobilization resulting in secondary changes in joint.

Anaemia. Causes: destruction and haemolysis of red cells; protein loss and diversion of protein to tissue repair.

Dangers resulting from prolonged recumbency (p. 313).

TREATMENT

FIRST AID
Deep burns
1. Remove cause. (a) Smother flames. Lay patient down and envelop in rug, coat or mat. (b) Switch off electric current or remove victim from wire or wire from victim. Use wooden stick (beware of dampness or metal appliance. Wear rubber footwear or stand on dry rubber mat). (c) Flood area with water if chemical is the cause.

2. Care of wound. (a) Do not remove clothing which is burnt (clothing impregnated with chemicals should be removed immediately). (b) Cover wound from air (air increases pain) with

dry sterile dressing if available, otherwise use freshly laundered sheet or pillow case. (Avoid application of creams, lotions, paints, etc., which confuse later estimation of depth and degree of burn, may introduce infection or further damage tissue.) (c) Immobilization of area sometimes necessary, especially limbs.

3. Shock. (a) Reassure patient by constant attendance, efficiency, sympathetic attitude and manner, giving relevant explanations. (b) Give analgesics if available. Morphia if pain severe. (c) Withhold oral fluids in severe burning because of danger of paralytic ileus. (d) Transfer to hospital as matter of urgency.

Minor, first and second degree burns

Pain may be eased by placing area under cold running water.

DEFINITIVE TREATMENT

Patient received into specially prepared room. Facilities available for immediate resuscitation and prevention of infection. Burnt area covered with sterile towel, left untouched until shock treated.

Shock

Aims. Eliminate or minimize factors responsible for increased capillary permeability and vasodilation. Replace fluid lost and current loss for next 48 hours.

Relieve pain. Morphia 15—30 mg, intravenously if shock severe and circulatory failure obvious.

Provide warmth. Minimize heat loss. Overheating dangerous as it increases vasodilation of peripheral vessels and increases oxygen requirements.

Administration of oxygen. (Controversy as to its effectiveness.) May aid in tissue hypoxia but as the basic cause is a deficient oxygen-carrying capacity, it is best treated by blood transfusion.

Fluid replacement. Amount, type and rate determined by total area burnt.

Amount. (1) Normal insensible loss replacement of 2,000 ml. Given orally if possible otherwise intravenously — dextrose in water, lactated Ringer's solution. (2) Rough guide to replace-

64

ment: 1 ml colloid, 0.5 ml balanced electrolytes for each 1% body surface burnt per kg body weight in 24 hours; e.g. patient weighing 70 kg with 30% burns would need 2,100 ml plasma or blood, 1,051 ml electrolytes, 2,000 ml normal replacement — total 5,150 ml in 24 hours.

Type. (1) Colloid, for all burns over 15% (10% in children). If haematocrit (ratio of cells to plasma in blood — normal 45%) over 60%, plasma only given. If under 60% up to half replacement must be whole blood. Whole blood usually needed in deep and extensive burns because of haemolysis. (2) Electrolytes. If kidney function impaired normal saline may be dangerous due to sodium retention. Potassium loss high during acute phase and 3–4 g should be replaced daily.

Rate. Varies with individuals. Guide: half total volume in first 8 hours; half over next 16 hours. Patient's condition assessed at end of every 4 hours. Second day ¼–½ amount given previous day.

Route. Colloid replacement intravenously. Other fluids orally if no nausea or vomiting. [Intragastric tube and aspiration if patient has paralytic ileus. Amount aspirated (equivalent) replaced intravenously.]

Guide to fluid replacement. (1) Blood tests. Haematocrit. Haemoglobin. Serum electrolytes. (2) Urinary output. Catheterization may be necessary for accurate measurement if oliguria present. Output maintained at 30—50 ml per hour. Less, indicates need for more fluid; more, indicates overhydration. (3) Thirst. May be severe in dehydration.

Observations and records

Restlessness (pain and shock). Colour (state of shock). Vital signs: temperature, pulse, respirations, blood pressure (shock, onset of infection). Fluid balance, intake and output recorded. Test urine for specific gravity, chlorides, sugar, albumin, blood, ketones. Nausea and vomiting (paralytic ileus). Weight if possible.

Care of burnt area

Aims. Prevent infection. Restore skin to normal as quickly as possible with minimal disfigurement. Control oedema.

Prevention of infection. Patient isolated where air flow can be filtered. Attendants wear caps, masks, gowns. Patient may be nursed between sterile sheets. Swab taken from area as base line for assessment of infection; covered with sterile towels until shock treated.

Cleansing. May be done under general anaesthetic. Clothing cut away. Burnt area and surrounding skin gently washed with antiseptic detergent, e.g. cetrimide, chlorhexidine or hexachlorophene soap.

Debridement. All loose and dead tissue carefully snipped off.

Blisters opened. May be removed or left as protective covering.

Covering of area. Varies according to site and depth.

EXPOSURE METHOD. *Pathology.* Scab forms from dried exudate and layers of 'shed' skin within 24—48 hours of exposure to air. Protects underlying skin from infection while healing. Principles behind method — bacteria cannot survive combination of coolness, dryness and exposure to light. Less absorption of toxins from dry area than from moist slough under a dressing.

Areas suitable for exposure method. Head; neck; genitalia; single surface trunk; limbs, burnt area too large to dress adequately.

Antibiotic powder. May be sprayed on after cleansing and debridement. (Some surgeons object on grounds of unneccessary expense and danger if patient allergic. Others consider it protects against infection especially of patient's own resident organisms.)

Drying. Aided by high environmental temperature and low humidity; fan heater; electric hair dryer.

Immobilization. Necessary in neighbourhood of joints to prevent cracking.

Bed. Burnt area should be free of bedclothes — cradle, gallows traction for children with burnt genitalia or buttocks. Stryker or Zimmer bedframes. Ventilating bed — tubular frame with strong plastic mesh. Patient lies on sheet of sterilized polyurethane foam (porous, non-irritant, easily autoclaved, washable).

Position. Oedema reduced by aid of gravity. Limbs elevated. Patient gradually sat up into semi-upright position.

Infection. Prevented while scabs forming by barrier nursing as above. Visitors discouraged but may attend wearing cap, mask, gown.

CLOSED METHOD. *Purposes.* Mechanical barrier against infection; absorbs fluid, therefore provides dry surface; control oedema; vehicle for antimicrobial substances.

Suitable cases. Circumferential burns; hands; any single area which is not within 10 cm of an orifice (dressing must be larger than burn to be effective).

First dressing. After initial cleansing and debridement whole area covered with single layer of petroleum jelly or paraffin gauze, or antimicrobial cream. e.g. silver sulpadiazine 1% with chlorhexidine digluconate 2% (Silvazine). Gauze and cotton wool applied at least 1 in beyond margins of burn. Bandage applied firmly enough to keep dressing in firm contact with burn. Helps to limit oedema. Too much pressure avoided as it is painful.

Subsequent dressings. First dressing left in position for as long as practicable (bearing in mind that wet dressings are excellent breeding ground for bacteria). Reinforce outer layers. Change only if soaked, or evidence of infection, or if dislodged. Usually changed on third day then left for 7–10 days, then for another 5–7 days, by which time healing will generally be complete. Dressings must be performed under strict aseptic precautions in single dressing room or in theatre. General anaesthetic may be necessary.

Slough removal. Deep burns. May need assistance if area to be grafted 10–14 days after burn.

Methods. 1. Bunyan-Stannard envelope. Limbs only. Oiled silk or plastic bag with inlet and outlet. Fits over limb and sealed to healthy skin above burn. Solution, e.g. Milton 2½%, irrigated every 4 hours. Painlessly removes slough and washes it out. Oxygen blown through bag after irrigation dries area.

2. Chemical debridement with proteolytic enzymes, e.g. Trypure Nova.

3. Surgical incision.

Skin grafting. Essential in deep burns to prevent infection, scar contraction and to promote healing. Usually performed in third week after slough separated. May be done in initial treatment for small, deep, well-defined burn; occasionally, a few days after burning, when patient's condition satisfactory. Will not take in presence of infection.

Amnion dressing applied immediately after debridement and cleansing. Reduces pain, protects against infection, speeds healing.

Amnion prepared by stripping it from decidua of afterbirth,

cleansing of blood clots, jelly and meconium under running tap water. Sterilized in 2% kanamycin solution for 12 hours. May be stored in this solution up to 3 weeks at 4–10° C.

Amnion smoothed over burn eliminating bubbles. Left exposed to dry. Adheres to burnt surface. Pockets of exudate collecting under amnion aspirated with fine needle. As healing occurs edges of amnion peel up and are trimmed daily.

Warm saline or tap-water baths. (1) Necessary to ensure that area for grafting perfectly clean. (2) May be used to 'float' dressings which are stuck and would cause pain during removal. (3) May be used to remove scabs from patient treated by exposure method. (4) To treat infection.

Treatment of infection. Pockets of pus trapped under slough may be debrided. Swab taken and appropriate antibiotic started. Warm saline dressings or baths. General measures – see later. Dressings containing antibiotic cream. In exposure method, moist areas sprayed with antibiotic.

General care

Rest. Patient may be restless due to toxaemia or psychological factors. Heavy sedation necessary for first few nights.

Nourishment. Oral fluids introduced gradually. Diet rich in protein, calories, vitamins A and C to correct tissue damage, plasma loss, catabolic response to stress, and to assist in rapid granulation and epithelialization. Protein deficiency results in loss of weight, poor healing, anaemia, increasing debility, proneness to pressure sores. Protein 2–3 g per kg body weight plus ½–1 g per day for each 1% of body surface burnt. If patient finds high protein diet nauseating, it may be given by intragastric tube. High protein powders may be used, e.g. Casilan, Complan, dried skimmed milk.

Drugs. 1. Antibiotics. Prophylactic course, e.g. penicillin, started on admission. If infection occurs antibiotic given according to sensitivity of organisms.

2. Tetanus prophylaxis. Booster dose of tetanus toxoid or prophylactic tetanus antitoxin after initial skin test.

3. Vitamins and iron. Supplement diet with tablets.

4. Tranquillizers, e.g. promazine 50–100 mg, chlorpromazine 25–50 mg. Necessary for physical reasons (lack of protein) and

for anxiety of patient.

5. Sedation, e.g. chloral hydrate 1 g at night.

6. Steroids. (a) Protein sparers, e.g. Anabol, Durabolin – to increase anabolism. (b) Prednisolone sometimes advocated to speed epithelialization. Only used after prolonged period of impaired healing.

Hygiene. 1. Skin care. Sponge unburnt areas daily. Routine care of all pressure areas. Careful attention to bed making in exposure method. Sheet carefully folded with separated scabs and removed.

2. Eyes, nose, mouth. Carefully cleansed and kept free from infection. Oral sepsis or other infections make patient more prone to infection of burnt areas.

3. Hair and clothing kept clean and neat to boost morale. Nails clean and short.

4. Bladder. Catheter removed in 48 hours. Copious fluids encouraged. Patient observed for urinary infection, renal calculi.

5. Bowels. Diarrhoea may develop because of high protein intake or from oral antibiotics. Controlled by diet and/or changing antibiotic. Constipation prevented by increasing roughage, copious fluids and exercises.

Physiotherapy. 1. Chest and vascular complications prevented by: Use of semi-upright position. Deep breathing and coughing exercises (particularly important if burns involve chest). Leg exercises. Frequent changes of position.

2. Joints. All those not burnt must go through full range of movement daily. Immobilized joints gradually introduced to movement when healing is progressing satisfactorily.

3. Contractures. Exercises given to stretch scar tissue.

4. Foot and wrist drop prevented by support, elimination of pressure, and exercises.

Observations and charting. 1. Vital signs. 4-hourly observations continued until risk of infection passed, then continued twice daily.

2. Fluid balance chart. Careful and complete account until dangers of shock, paralytic ileus and renal failure passed.

3. Weight. Loss usually continues 5–6 weeks. Weekly record to determine effectiveness of diet.

4. Haemoglobin estimation. Blood transfusion may be

required later.

Morale. 1. Some reasons for patient's depression, fear and anxiety: Sight and smell of burnt flesh. Danger of disfigurement especially with facial burns. Unfamiliar surroundings and people. Pain. Painful and embarrassing procedures. Prolonged isolation, hospitalization and treatment.

2. Ways in which nurse may help: (a) Show no distaste or disgust at sight or smell of area. (b) Establish satisfactory nurse-patient relationships with a warm friendly, accepting attitude thus helping patient to voice any fears. (c) Reinforce doctor's explanations as to treatment and satisfactory end result. (d) Avoid prolonged isolation. Stop and talk to patient as often as possible. As soon as danger of infection past and patient feels able, encourage visitors, especially close relatives. Encourage diversional therapy and an interest in things around him. (e) Ensure physical comfort even if patient must adopt unusual position. See also under hygiene above.

Rehabilitation. Slow and gradual. Skin grafting and plastic surgery may go on for months or years. Patient must be assisted to take place in society, especially if disfigured.

SKIN GRAFTING

Transfer of healthy skin from one area of body to meet deficiency elsewhere. Grafts almost always autogenous. Occasionally one individual may donate skin to another if blood groups compatible. These grafts are always rejected by recipient in about 3 weeks but may be used as a temporary life-saving measure, e.g. in severe burns. Grafts may be transferred between identical twins without rejection occurring.

Indications. Replacement of lost tissue: injuries, burns, wide surgical excisions. Where rate of healing needs accelerating: ulcers, burns. Removal of contractures (scar tissue) interfering with joint function. Disfiguring facial scars and blemishes. Reconstitution of defects: hare lip, unsightly nose, ears, missing eyelid.

Types. (1) Free skin: (a) partial thickness, (b) whole thickness, (c) pinch grafts. (2) Pedicle grafts: (a) direct flap, (b) tubed pedicle.

70

FREE SKIN

Area completely removed from donor site, transferred to recipient site.

Partial thickness. (a) Thin (Thiersch) graft: epidermis only; tissue-paper thickness approximately. (b) Thick (split-skin) graft: epidermis and part of dermis (about half total thickness of skin); leaves enough behind for epithelialization of donor area. (c) Patch grafting: donor skin cut into pieces about ½ × 1 in. These are laid flat with small gaps between on raw area. (Advantages — exudate can escape and necrosis is confined to small areas instead of whole graft.)

Indications. Covering raw area where there is no stress or strain.

Contraindications. Hands, face and feet: cosmetic appearance; little resistance to trauma.

Donor sites. Anterior surface of thigh or forearm, abdominal wall, back.

Method. Skin cut with (i) flat ground razor, (ii) special knife with guarded blade and small roller to flatten graft as it is being cut (Humby), (iii) electric dermatome — knife mounted on special drum to which skin attached by adhesive; as drum rotates skin lifted and knife cuts at an even depth.

Cut skin placed with cut surface uppermost on tulle gras spread on flat surface. Wrinkles smoothed out and skin applied to recipient area. Secured with stitches.

Pressure dressing applied. Graft must be pressed firmly against recipient surface otherwise serous exudate or oedema intervenes depriving graft of nourishment and it dies.

Whole thickness. Wolfe. Epidermis and dermis free from subcutaneous tissue.

Indications. Small areas, surgically created, e.g. after excision of neoplasm or scar tissue, where even pressure can be exerted.

Contraindications. Granulating surface: risk of infection too great. Irregular surfaces where even pressure cannot be exerted.

Donor sites. Abdominal wall, back of pinna, mastoid area.

Method. Recipient area. Meticulous haemostasis. (Diathermy avoided as it damages surrounding areas.) Carefully measured. Exact pattern and size excised (fat excluded as it causes necrosis). Very fine sutures or skin hooks used to control graft (forceps

71

avoided to reduce trauma to graft). Sutured in position with fine mersilk on atraumatic needles. Very small drain tube may be left under graft to prevent haematoma formation. Pressure dressing applied.

Survival of free graft depends on early vascularization. Graft must be in complete and continuous contact with its bed.

Pinch grafts (Reverdin). Small discs with diameter of about 1–3 cm. Consist of dermis with some subcutaneous fat and blood vessels in centre, epidermis only at periphery.

Indications. Extensive area of skin lost; to accelerate healing of ulcer; may survive in presence of sepsis.

Contraindications. Cosmetic — scar formation usually excessive. Slow healing — poor quality skin of donor and recipient area.

Donor areas. Upper thigh or arm.

Method. Small cone raised with needle or small hook. Excised with scalpel held flat against skin surface. Transferred to recipient site with point of needle. Laid in rows with gaps between until whole surface covered. Islands of epithelium eventually join up to cover area completely. Covered with tulle gras and pressure dressing.

PEDICLE GRAFT

Graft remains attached to donor site by pedicle to maintain blood supply. Other end attached to recipient area or to intermediate situation until new blood supply grows into it.

Indications. Large defects. Reconstruction surgery.

Direct (approximation) flap. Donor and recipient areas close together, e.g. one leg to another, trunk to upper limb, arm to leg, abdominal wall to hand.

Method. Three-sided flap made in donor area. Consists of epidermis, dermis, subcutaneous tissue and blood vessels. Free end placed in position, anchored with fine sutures. Small drain tube may be left in as precaution against haematoma.

Pressure dressing applied. Immobilization achieved by means of bandaging or plaster fixation.

After 21 days graft severed from pedicle, trimmed as necessary, sutured in position. As much of pedicle returned to donor areas as possible. Remainder of donor site may be approximated with sutures.

Tubed pedicle. Used when donor and recipient areas are far apart.

Method. Three stages.

1. Tube made. Parallel incisions made in donor skin but ends remain attached. Cut edges turned inwards and sutured to form tube. (No raw surface exposed so danger of infection minimal.) Edges of donor area approximated by sutures under tube.

2. Six weeks later one end of tube freed, opened out, trimmed and sewn into recipient area (if near enough).

3. Three weeks later graft freed entirely from donor area, opened out and applied to recipient area. As much pedicle as possible returned to donor area.

If distance from donor to recipient area too great for one step, tube may be grown into intermediate site for 3 weeks and then rotated into final position, e.g. from abdominal wall into arm then from arm to face.

PRE-OPERATIVE PREPARATION

Recipient area. Must be: (1) free from all infection; (2) dry, i.e. free from all oedema; perfect haemostasis; (3) healing – showing healthy granulation tissue; (4) free from all antiseptics (lowers vitality of cells rendering them prone to infection); (5) free from hair.

Donor area. (1) Shaved carefully and thoroughly. (2) Washed with soap and water. (3) Swabbed with spirit, allowed to dry. (4) Cleaned with normal saline to ensure that no antiseptic remains. (5) Covered with sterile towel.

No antiseptic whatsoever applied in theatre.

POST-OPERATIVE CARE

Graft area. Graft must not move or slip on recipient area. Nurse must ensure pressure dressing and bandage checked frequently; immobility with pedicle graft – bandages, plaster or elastoplast must be undisturbed; pedicle tube checked frequently for pressure or tension.

Dressings. *Donor area.* Petroleum jelly gauze and bandage left in position 7–10 days, then removed. Epithelialization should be complete. If dry — left open.

Graft area. Dressing and sutures removed by doctor (sometimes in theatre) after 7- 21 days depending on thickness and site of graft.

Infection. Prevented by prophylactic antibiotics, leaving dressing undisturbed, and general measures (p. 26).

Observations. Four-hourly temperature, pulse and respirations. Report immediately if patient complains of pain, burning sensation, or if evidence of discharge or odour from dressings.

General measures. Avoid applications of heat, hot baths, strong antiseptics. Diversional and occupational therapy encouraged to relieve boredom in an otherwise fit individual.

Chapter 4

NEOPLASMS

Tumour, neoplasm, new growth: abnormal mass of cells serving no useful function. Rate of growth and cell division increased, not coordinated by body.

Classification. According to behaviour. Two main groups (benign and malignant), but as they do not always behave consistently there are many exceptions.

BENIGN (INNOCENT, SIMPLE)

CHARACTERISTICS
Reproduce structure and pattern of tissue of origin, i.e. appear as normal cells. Grow slowly (sometimes rapid initial growth but soon slows and may stop). Does not destroy tissue: grows by expansion (usually spherical) pushing normal tissue out of its way, sometimes compressing surrounding tissue. Does not infiltrate. Becomes encapsulated with fibrous tissue. Growth may therefore be 'shelled out' completely at operation. Does not kill host except by (1) pressure on vital organ, e.g. brain; (2) excessive hormone production, e.g. excessive insulin from adenoma of pancreas; (3) interference with function of organ, e.g. excessive bleeding from fibroma of uterus; (4) becoming malignant, e.g. papilloma.

CAUSE
Unknown.

TYPES
Derive name from tissue of origin. Suffix '-oma' denotes tumour.

75

EXAMPLES

Epithelial tissue. (1) Papilloma: cauliflower-like growth. Common sites: tongue, cheek, skin, bladder, rectum, kidney. Although originally benign, spreads by seeding, eventually becomes malignant. (2) Adenoma; glandular tissue: may secrete hormones or other material which normal gland produces, e.g. thyroxin: thyroid gland; insulin: pancreas. (3) Fibro-adenoma. Gland tissue containing fibrous tissue also, thus limiting secretory activity, e.g. fibro-adenoma of breast.

Connective tissue. (1) Lipoma: most common benign tumour. Composed of fatty tissue, therefore widespread distribution, e.g. subcutaneously especially shoulders and back; under synovial membrane of joints; under mucous membranes; in gut wall; in breast. (2) Fibroma: fibrous tissue. May be hard, small or more widespread, e.g. 'keloid' scar. (3) Osteoma: bone, mostly at end of long bones. (4) Chondroma: cartilage, commonly at epiphyses of immature bones. (5) Myoma: muscle, commonest site – uterus.

Nerve tissue. (1) Neuroma, rare, true nerve tissue. (2) Neurofibroma, most common, connective tissue of nerve sheath. May occur singly or along sheath of peripheral nerve. Considerable variation in size. (3) Meningioma, meninges, may cause increased intracranial pressure. Usually easily removed.

Blood vessels. (1) Angioma: vessel not filled with blood. (2) Haemangioma (usually congenital) purplish discolouration, birth marks. May be large involving arteries and veins. Bleed profusely if injured. May involve capillaries only (naevi), often strawberry in colour.

Reproductive system. Special cells. Dermoid cyst of ovary containing variety of embryonic tissue: hair, teeth, sebaceous material.

TREATMENT

Indications. (1) Cosmetic or psychological if in unsightly position. (2) Interference with vital structure or function. (3) Subject to constant irritation, friction or injury. (4) Known to be pre-cancerous.

Method. Complete removal by surgical excision or destruction of tumour by diathermy. Not necessary to remove capsule but incomplete removal of tumour material may result in recurrence or malignant change.

MALIGNANT (CANCER)

CHARACTERISTICS

Pattern of parent cells never reproduced exactly, i.e. new cells abnormal; the greater differentiation the more malignant the growth. Grows rapidly, continues to grow at expense of host. Destroys and replaces normal tissue, forms ulcers on surfaces, causes spontaneous fracture in bones. Produces inflammatory reaction but grows beyond and encircles fibrous tissue, therefore does not become encapsulated, has no clearly defined edge. Spreads from point of origin by (1) infiltration into surrounding tissues and adjacent organs, (2) metastases (spreading 'seeds'), i.e. small piece breaks off, carried to new site where it establishes secondary growth. Common sites: bones, liver, lungs, brain, kidneys.

Metastases may spread via: (1) Lymphatics: primary growth infiltrates lymph channel, small piece broken off, carried to gland or node where it establishes secondary growth. Piece of secondary may then break off and be carried to next node and so on until it reaches blood stream; (2) blood stream: (a) via lymphatics as above, (b) direct infiltration into blood vessel, piece breaks off and is carried to new site; (3) across coelomic spaces (i.e. envelopes of smooth fibrous tissue lining body cavities), peritoneum, pleura.

Cancer causes death of host by (1) destruction of vital function or structure, e.g. brain compression, haemorrhage; (2) obstruction of hollow tube, e.g. larynx, oesophagus; (3) progressive cachexia, i.e. by robbing body of nourishment. Patient loses weight, becomes weak, anaemic and has characteristic sallow discoloured skin.

CAUSE

Actual cause unknown.

CONTRIBUTORY FACTORS

Chemicals, e.g. those contained in tar and soot (chimney-sweep's carcinoma of prostate gland due to irritation from soot). Certain food-colouring agents and drugs known to produce tumours in animals but inconclusive in humans.

Injuries. Known to develop from simple injury, or multiple, or repeated injury to an area.

Chronic irritation, e.g. lips or tongue affected by septic or broken teeth, ill-fitting dentures or prolonged contact with clay or foul pipe.

Inhalation. Excessive cigarette smoking, air pollution from factory waste, particularly radioactive fallout.

Radiation. Radium, X-rays, excessive ultraviolet light. Skin (rodent) ulcers common where sunlight is abundant.

Viruses. Much research being done on this aspect and cancers have been produced in animals.

Sex hormones. 'Hormone dependent cancer.' Produced by upset in hormone balance, e.g. breast and prostatic carcinoma.

Pre-cancerous benign tumours.

TYPES

1. Epithelial tissues. (a) Carcinoma. Further classified according to type of tissue, e.g. squamous cell, basal cell, columnar cell, transitional cell, etc. (b) Adenocarcinoma of glandular tissue. (c) Melanoma. Pigmented cells (may also be benign).

2. Connective tissues. Named according to tissue involved: fibrosarcoma, liposarcoma, etc.

3. Nerve tissue. Glioma: brain, nerve cells and retina of eye. (May be benign.)

4. Reticulo-endothelial system. Hodgkin's disease; lymphosarcoma; leukaemia.

5. Special cells in reproductive system. (a) Teratoma (similar in structure to dermoid cyst above) of ovary or testis. (b) Chorionepithelioma. Testes or pregnant uterus. (c) Seminoma. Testes.

DESCRIPTIVE TERMINOLOGY

Scirrhous, if hard and composed of connective tissue. Encephaloid, if soft. Melanoid, black or brown due to pigments. Cauliflower or fungating, proliferates rapidly and spreads. Ulcerative, central portion breaks down due to lack of blood supply (i.e. becomes necrotic) and ulcer results. Annular, grows in circle in wall of hollow tube and tends to produce scar tissue (may result in stricture).

SIGNS AND SYMPTOMS

Vary with site (see various sections). Various warning signs — sores which do not heal; lump or thickening in breast or elsewhere; unusual bleeding or discharge; change in wart or mole; persistent indigestion, dysphagia, hoarseness, cough; change in normal bowel habits; vague ill health, loss of weight, or unusual persistent tiredness.

AIDS TO DIAGNOSIS

X-rays. Shadows and filling defects shown by plain X-ray or contrast media.

Radio-isotope scanning. Lesions take up isotope, differentially.

Blood tests. No known test to detect cancer directly (except leukaemia) but various specific tests indicate malfunction of organ or structure involved.

Endoscopy. Demonstration of lesion under direct vision, e.g. oesophagoscopy, sigmoidoscopy, gastroscopy.

Biopsy. Small piece of tissue removed from tumour, examined under microscope, abnormal growth patterns may be recognized. (Histology.)

Cytology. Examination of smears of various body secretions and excretions for cancer or pre-cancerous cells shed from epithelial surfaces with normal exfoliative process. Sputum may contain cells from carcinoma of bronchus; urine from bladder; vaginal aspirate (or cervical smear) from cervix.

TREATMENT
SURGICAL

Principles: complete excision of tumour with wide margin of surrounding tissue and any involved draining lymphatics. For details see separate sections.

Radical surgery. i.e. aimed at complete cure. Impossible if (1) growth in an inaccessible position, e.g. brain; (2) too extensive for safe removal; (3) metastases are widespread.

Surgery combined with radiotherapy. Breast cancer: simple mastectomy, radiation of all draining lymphatics and muscle wall.

Cancer of tongue: block resection of all draining lymphatics, irradiation of primary growth in tongue.

Palliative surgery. Relief of symptoms but no attempt to remove tumour, e.g. colostomy for bowel obstruction, gastro-enterostomy for carcinoma head of pancreas.

RADIOTHERAPY

Use of radiation, i.e. energy emission by atoms carried through space as alpha or beta particles or as electromagnetic waves such as X- or gamma-rays.

Effects. Main action: to damage nucleus and block mitosis. Kills cells but those undergoing rapid mitosis more readily destroyed than others. Very small doses may produce mutation of nuclear genes without destruction of cell. Aim is to direct the narrowest possible beam of radiation for the minimum time so that malignant cells, which are dividing more rapidly, are killed and there is minimal damage to normal cells.

Depending on rate of mitosis, some types of tumour are highly sensitive to irradiation, e.g. lymphosarcoma, carcinoma of tongue and skin, while others such as malignant melanoma are un-affected. Some tumours disappear with irradiation but tend to recur. Others become resistant in a similar way to micro-organisms becoming resistant to antibiotics.

Side effects. As all rapidly dividing cells are easily affected widespread damage may occur to skin, bone-forming tissue (marrow) and gastro-intestinal tract (radiation sickness).

Skin. Inflammation of surrounding tissues, ulceration, impaired healing, hair falls out.

Alimentary tract. Nausea, vomiting, diarrhoea. May cause dehydration.

Blood. Destruction of red blood cells: anaemia, platelets; impaired clotting, white cells reduced: lower resistance to infection. Normal body flora may gain entry to deeper tissues and overwhelming infection result.

Types of treatment

Deep X-rays (short-wave length). Capable of penetrating deeper tissues by use of higher voltage (½–1 megavolt. Mega = million) than used for X-ray photography; higher voltage, deeper penetration; more penetrating rays, less superficial damage to skin but more lethal damage to tumour. For deep penetration of rays radioactive cobalt is being used in a special machine. Said to be less skin reaction and greater degree of accuracy. Higher voltage (6–15 megavolts) is reached by using radio waves in production of beam in special machine: linear accelerator.

Whichever method used, growth irradiated from several angles to reduce damage to overlying structures through which rays must pass. Depth, time, site and dosage of radiation carefully and accurately determined. Treatments usually extend over several weeks. Care must be taken to protect skin not directly concerned with area from contact with rays by using lead screens.

SPECIAL POINTS IN NURSING CARE. *Psychological aspects.* Nurse must endeavour to understand individual differences in reaction to cancer. Patient may feel generally unwell (due to radiation sickness) as well as apprehensive and depressed about his condition. Nurse can help by: (1) establishing satisfactory nurse-patient relationships so that patient will trust nurse and feel free to discuss any fears or anxieties; (2) taking every opportunity to increase patient's confidence in doctor and treatment; (3) fostering patient's interest by encouraging visits from relatives and friends, encouraging patient to mix with other occupants of ward, especially more cheerful ones undergoing similar treatment, watching television, listening to radio, reading, engaging in occupational therapy, handicrafts, painting, etc.

Skin care. Treated area should be left exposed unless broken or infected. Light application of zinc cream may be ordered following treatment. Kept dry. Bathing or washing in hot water not recommended. Skin must never be rubbed or scrubbed but only cleansed lightly. If skin becomes moist after desquamation, single layer of petroleum jelly gauze may be applied, bandaged lightly to keep skin as dry as possible.

Minor injuries to area may result in severe ulceration, delayed healing, so patient warned of danger. On no account must adhesive plaster be used, pressure and chafing from wrinkles in bandages avoided at all costs.

Nausea and vomiting. Early symptom of radiation sickness, accompanied by anorexia. Patient encouraged to eat and various anti-emetics tried – chlorpromazine 25–50 mg, promethazine

25–50 mg, Dramamine 50–100 mg, Torecan 6.5 mg, Cyclizine 50–100 mg.

Mouth and throat. Mucous membranes become dry. Frequent mouth washes necessary and glycerine may be left on tongue to encourage salivation. Because of lowered resistance mouth must be kept scrupulously clean and free from infection.

Diarrhoea. Often distressing and may persist for 3–6 weeks after treatment. Stools pale and loose. May contain mucus and blood. Diet regulated accordingly – frequent small meals, high protein, high calorie, vitamin supplements.

Blood. Frequent examination. If anaemia present: iron administration and/or blood transfusion may be necessary (often improves morale as well as condition).

Radium. Element first isolated by Marie and Pierre Curie from pitchblende. Alpha and beta particles and gamma-rays given off.

Types. Minute particles of radium 1–5 mg may be placed in hollow needles or casings of platinum, gold or silver which prevent escape of alpha and beta particles but permit passage of gamma rays.

Radon gas given off by radium when acted upon by hydrochloric acid; radioactive for limited time. Gas placed in seeds or tiny beads of platinum, gold or silver. (Because of short time of activity, radon seeds may be left in situ indefinitely whereas radium needles must be removed after a specified time to prevent overdosage and damage to healthy tissues.)

Methods of use. (1) Interstitial irradiation: needles, seeds or tubes are embedded directly into tumour. Each container has long silk thread attached which is anchored to skin. Extreme care taken to ensure that they do not become dislodged or lost in dressings. When not in use, radium-containing appliances must be stored in lead-lined box. (2) Surface irradiation: specially moulded appliances may be used to hold needles, seeds or tubes so that they are carefully spaced. Mould applied to surface or area to be treated. May be held in situ for hours or days depending on the dosage required.

Special precautions. (1) Patient confined to bed while radium in situ. (2) Safe storage in lead-lined box before and after use, speedy return of box to special radiotherapy centre after use. (3)

Careful checking to ensure radium is in correct position, especially before disposal of dressings.

Radioactive isotopes. Elements which have been exposed to powerful source of atomic energy and have themselves become radioactive, but the atomic weight has not been altered and their chemical properties are unchanged. Radium remains radioactive for thousands of years but isotopes may remain so only for hours, days or weeks.

Examples. (1) Gold or tantalum made into wires which can be implanted directly into tumour. (2) Chemicals, e.g. iodine, phosphorus, when given in small quantities orally are taken by blood stream to specific parts of body (e.g. iodine to thyroid gland, phosphorus to bone); by placing Geiger counter over area information can be gained as to degree of activity (diagnostic). In larger quantities these irradiated chemicals will be taken up by specific tissues and will destroy the rapidly dividing malignant cells including metastases (therapeutic). (3) Colloid preparations, e.g. radioactive gold salts may be injected directly into body cavities and because of their large molecular size will remain localized and thus produce far greater local irradiation than could be provided by external application of deep X-rays or radium, e.g. pleural and peritoneal cavities.

Precautions. Those in contact with patient must take every precaution to ensure that they are exposed to rays for minimum time and that their body does not become contaminated. Most radioactive isotopes are in liquid form and are excreted in all excreta — urine, faeces, sputum and in any secretions, e.g. ascitic fluid. (1) Minimal time spent with patient by visitors and staff. (2) Confine patient to single ward. (3) Gloves and gown worn by nurse when handling patient or any article likely to be contaminated by secretions or excretions. (4) Provide patient with special urinal, bedpan, linen container. (5) Retain excreta and linen in special containers until period of radioactivity has elapsed — may then be treated as normal. (6) Frequent checks with Geiger counter to detect degree of radioactivity. (7) Photographic film to be worn by staff to measure degree of exposure.

Cytotoxic drugs. Produce an effect similar to that of X-rays. Also called radio-mimetic drugs.

Action is to poison (toxic) cells (cyto-). Two main groups: (1)

83

alkylating agents which poison cell directly, e.g. nitrogen mustards, thio-tepa, Endoxan, Melphalan; (2) antimetabolites which block action of an enzyme system, e.g. Methotrexate. 5-fluouracil, Mercaptan.

Effects. Variable: some tumours respond to single course. Others need repeated courses. Most valuable effect is to reduce activity of growth and thus reduce pain.

Side effects. Radiation sickness (p. 80, 81).

Methods of administration. Oral; intravenous; intra-arterial infusion; intrapleural injection; regional or isolation perfusion – method of administering high concentrations of drug to a particular segment or organ which is temporarily isolated from systemic circulation so that body does not receive maximum toxic effect. Totally occlusive tourniquet applied to limb, main artery and vein cannulated. Oxygenated blood pumped in via artery and out through vein where it is reoxygenated and recirculated. At end of treatment cannulae removed, artery and vein closed and tourniquet released. Nursing care. As for radiotherapy.

Hormones. Some tumours grow if there is an excess of hormone in the blood, others if there is a deficiency, and some when there is a change in hormonal balance.

Prostate gland carcinoma. Controlled by administration of female hormone – oestrogen (stilboestrol). Primary growth slowed down, metastases regress thus relieving pain and eliminating incapacity. After initial setback malignant cells adjust to change in hormone balance and recurrence as extensive as before. Ever-increasing amounts of stilboestrol required. However, as this state may be delayed for several years it is a worthwhile form of treatment.

Carcinoma of breast. Some are controlled by increase in stilboestrol, others by increase in male hormone – testosterone. Surgical removal of ovaries (oophorectomy), adrenal glands (adrenalectomy) and pituitary gland (hypophysectomy) have been advocated as palliative measures to temporarily defer pain and incapacitation in advanced breast cancer, especially in younger age-group women who still have family responsibilities.

84

Chapter 5

ALIMENTARY TRACT

MOUTH AND THROAT

CLEFT LIP (HARE LIP)

Failure of fusion between maxillary and/or medial nasal processes which normally occurs by tenth week of gestation.

CAUSE

(1) Heredity. (2) Maternal malnutrition especially mineral and vitamins (3) Hormonal imbalance seems to be contributory factor.

TYPES

Incomplete or complete, i.e. from small notch at border of lip to complete separation involving floor of nose and nostril which is depressed and broadened.

TREATMENT

Surgical repair, aims at repairing defect, restoring normal symmetry of lip and normal nasal contours.

Time. Some advocate 48 hours after birth (newborn babe able to withstand considerable trauma), ensures better cosmetic result, facilitates sucking. Others advocate operation at 3 weeks old when babe gaining weight satisfactorily, or when 6.5 kg (12 lb) body weight reached.

Method. Cleft due to displacement rather than deficiency. Lip mobilized, joined without tension. Tension prevented by Logan's bow — bridge of spring metal strapped to each cheek.

CLEFT PALATE

Failure of palatal processes of maxillae to fuse together.

CAUSES

As for hare lip. The two conditions often co-exist.

TYPES

Varies from small cleft involving uvula and soft palate only to extensive cleft involving hard palate and alveolar ridge.

TREATMENT

Surgical repair aims closing cleft and elongating soft palate which is usually shortened.

Time. 9–18 months, i.e. before child learns to speak.

Method. Various techniques. Bony union not necessary but palatal mucoperiosteum must be shifted to midline to ensure satisfactory length of soft palate.

PRE-OPERATIVE PREPARATION, SPECIFIC

Admitted to hospital several days pre-operatively to familiarize baby with surroundings and to establish feeding regime.

Investigations. Upper respiratory tract infection — nasal and/or throat swabs taken.

POST-OPERATIVE CARE

Child must not put fingers or objects in mouth. Various forms of restraint used. Crying minimized by good nursing care and use of hypnotics, e.g. rectal paraldehyde or chloral.

Feeding. After lip repair — gavage for first week then bottle feeding. Cleft palate without lip involvement — spoon feeding well back in mouth. Feeds preceded and followed by water.

Mouth. Occasional syringing with antiseptics. Swabbing forbidden as it may break down stitches. Lips smeared with petroleum jelly or peppermint ointment as dribbling usually excessive.

Nose. Drops used to relieve nasal congestion and improve airway.

Infections. Prone to streptococcal infections. No staff or visitors with signs of cold or sore throat allowed to approach.

Speech training by therapist when child 3 years old or co-operative. Dental plate or obdurator may be necessary to fill gap left in palate.

TONSILLITIS
Inflammation of palatine tonsils.

CAUSE
Commonly staphylococci and streptococci. Gain entry through nose or mouth.

SIGNS AND SYMPTOMS
Dysphagia; sore throat; tonsil area red and swollen; cervical nodes enlarged; general signs of fever and toxaemia.

TREATMENT
(1) Conservative for acute attack. (2) If attacks are frequent or tonsils chronically infected at expense of patient's general good health, tonsillectomy performed, but not advised before 5–7 years.

Pre-operative care, specific
Observations to ensure that no upper respiratory tract infection present. (If so, operation postponed.) Pre-operative medication. Children: some surgeons prefer barbiturates, e.g. quinalbarbitone or, more recently, trimeprazine (Vallergan), and oral atropine so that child will be asleep or drowsy when he comes to theatre. Others prefer no premedication, to avoid unnecessary injections. Usually given 'umbrella' of antibiotic, e.g. penicillin, starting pre-operatively.

Operation
Tonsils removed by dividing mucous membrane of anterior and posterior pillars of fauces. Tonsil capsule identified, divided out from upper pole to tongue. Lower end removed with scissors or snare. Haemostasis achieved by (1) packing bed with gauze or, (2) ligation with thread or catgut or (3) if bleeding particularly troublesome, pillars may be sutured with catgut, (4) diathermy.

Guillotine method sometimes used. Tonsil enucleated from bed with wrenching movement in special cutting instrument which encircles tonsil. Much quicker operation but bleeding often more profuse.

Post-operative care, specific

Nurses' principal duty during unconsciousness is to maintain free airway and prevent inhalation of blood. Position: prone with head lower than shoulders to allow free drainage of blood and mucus. When consciousness regained: elevated to semi-upright as condition allows.

Observations. Immediate: haemorrhage. Any bright blood from mouth reported at once. ¼-hourly pulse for first 2 hours, then ½- to 1- to 2-hourly for next 12 hours, then 2- to 4-hourly for next 48 hours. Evidence of increased swallowing while patient unconscious may indicate bleeding. Vomiting of swallowed blood.

Later: observe temperature, pulse and respirations for evidence of infection. Inspect throat and ears.

Fluids. Sips encouraged as soon as conscious to prevent stiffness of pharyngeal muscles. Also improves blood supply to area, promotes healing.

Diet. Light diet for first 48 hours because of dysphagia and possibility of disturbing organized blood clot in tonsil bed. Most children can manage normal diet.

Pain and restlessness. Relieved with initial injections, e.g. pethidine on return to consciousness. Helps to prevent haemorrhage by allowing clot to organize in tonsil bed. Later — calcium aspirin gargles 0.5 g before meals.

Mouth care. Teeth cleaned after meals, frequent mouthwashes given to reduce possibility of infection.

Physiotherapy. Deep breathing exercises started on awakening and continued until discharge.

Ambulation. Out of bed on first post-operative day. Discharged 3–4 days (adults 6–7 days). Advise parents: (1) may need analgesia before meals; (2) normal diet; (3) observe for and report to doctor immediately any coughing, spitting or vomiting blood; any pallor or restlessness; persistent sore throat; earache; cough, dyspnoea or chest pain; if skin feels hot.

Complications

HAEMORRHAGE. (1) Reactionary within first 24 hours; (2) secondary 7–10 days after operation due to infection.

Treatment. May cease if clot removed from tonsil bed and pressure applied with swab to bleeding area. If persistent — return to theatre for ligation or insertion of pack. Blood transfusion may be necessary.

THROAT INFECTION. Slough forms on tonsil bed and breath becomes foetid. Enlarged cervical lymph nodes.

Treatment. Irrigations and/or gargles of antiseptic. Antibiotics orally and systematically.

OTITIS MEDIA. Spread of infection along Eustachian tube.

Treatment. Antibiotics locally and systematically. If drum red and bulging — myringotomy.

PERITONSILLAR ABSCESS (QUINSY)

Localized collection of pus in potential space between tonsil and soft tissues of palate.

CAUSE

Complication of tonsillitis.

SIGNS AND SYMPTOMS

Unilateral sore throat. Pain increases on swallowing. Trismus may be present. Swelling extending into soft palate forces tonsil toward or across midline. Uvula displaced. Cervical adenitis usually present.

TREATMENT

Symptomatic, antibiotics. Incision and drainage after 3—5 days when swelling fluctuant. Tonsillectomy advised 1 month after abscess clears.

CARCINOMA OF TONGUE

Incidence. Most common area of oral malignant disease. Men over 60 years more commonly affected than women.

Site. May occur anywhere but most commonly occurs as ulcer on lateral border of middle third.

Pre-cancerous lesions. Traumatic ulcer from jagged tooth, badly fitting denture. Papilloma. Chronic superficial glossitis. Syphilitic lesions.

SIGNS AND SYMPTOMS

Lump. May resemble blister, wart, pimple, plaque or a definite ulcer may appear. Pain may or may not be present in early stages;

intermittent, aggravated by food or alcohol, later becomes constant, may radiate to ear or mandible.

Increased salivation. Tongue movements painful and limited.

Later symptoms. Loss of taste, foetid breath, inability to speak clearly; dysphagia, haemorrhage resulting in secondary anaemia. Severe oedema may develop, dyspnoea and stridor ensue. Cervical lymph nodes — enlargement may be first sign especially in carcinoma of posterior third of tongue. Nodes may become inflamed and tender if secondary infection occurs.

TREATMENT

Simple. Tip of tongue: wedge resection, reconstruction of tongue. Middle third: irradiation with interstitial radium needles. If this fails to cure, hemiglossectomy if on lateral border or sub-total glossectomy if in body of tongue. Posterior third: deep X-ray; posterior portion of tongue and larynx removed, pharynx reconstructed. Inferior aspect: deep X-ray, subtotal glossectomy if necessary.

Radical. When surrounding tissue and lymphatic nodes involved. Deep X-ray followed by total or subtotal glossectomy, excision of floor of mouth, excision of affected portion of mandible, block dissection of cervical lymph nodes (p. 80). Usually unilateral but if metastases have spread to contralateral side — block dissection on side where nodes are larger and removal of lymph nodes on other side conserving jugular vein.

Palliative. Treatment of oral sepsis. Deep X-ray to lymph nodes if ulceration threatens. Ligation of external carotid artery to control haemorrhage. If pain unrelieved by analgesics — trigeminal neurectomy. Tracheostomy for severe dyspnoea. Intragastric feeding if dysphagia makes swallowing impossible.

Pre-operative care, specific

Oral hygiene. Decayed teeth removed or filled, mouthwashes, irrigations or toilets 2- to 4-hourly.

Diet. High calorie, added vitamins. Nutritious and tasty. Purées | necessary. Avoid pips, seeds, hot foods. Methods — fluids with straw, feeding cup, tube attached to plastic bottle. Intragastric feeding in severe cases.

Associated conditions. e.g. chest infections, anaemia, treated.

Physiotherapy. Chest exercises especially taught and practised for post-operative period. Moustache shaved off or clipped short.

Post-operative care

Position. Semi-prone while unconscious to prevent asphyxiation from tongue, blood, mucus, saliva. Foot of bed raised to aid drainage. Ligature may be passed through tongue. Forceps attached so that tongue can be easily pulled forward. Removed when consciousness regained. When conscious — gradually elevated to upright with head well forward for drainage of saliva. Frequent gentle suction essential to clear saliva, vomitus, etc. Provide patient with ample tissues to wipe away excess saliva when conscious.

Fluids. If dysphagia marked, intravenous or rectal fluids necessary. If prolonged beyond second day intragastric feeding started, copious nourishing fluids given.

Diet. Started as soon as patient can swallow without extreme difficulty. Mild analgesia, e.g. asprin, Panadol, anaesthetic lozenge may be given before feeding. Bland thickened fluid feeds at first. High calorie and protein. Graduate to more solid foods as tolerated.

Oral care. Irrigated under gentle pressure 2-hourly before and after feeds, using normal saline or weak antiseptics, e.g. Milton 2½% or hydrogen peroxide 1 in 4 until patient able to wash out own mouth.

Sutures. Usually slough out but may be removed on seventh to tenth day.

Bowels. Should open second to third day to rid body of swallowed blood and discharge.

Physiotherapy. Chest and leg exercises started as soon as patient conscious, continued at regular intervals.

Ambulation. If possible should sit out on second day to reduce risk of complications from prolonged immobilization, especially in elderly.

Antibiotics. Mouth wounds prone to infection. Antibiotic cover to prevent oral sepsis and spread to ears or chest.

Communication. Pencil and pad or slate provided while talking difficult. Speech therapy after healing has occurred.

Complications

(1) *Asphyxia*. Tracheostomy may be performed pre-operatively as precautionary measure. (2) *Haemorrhage*. Mouth extremely vascular. Greatest danger is secondary haemorrhage due to infection. May be preceded by 2 or 3 minor oozings. Any bleeding, however slight, must be reported immediately. (3) *Infections*. Prevented by strict oral hygiene and antibiotics. Chest infection, especially atelectasis and pneumonia. Prevented by posture to avoid inhalation of infected material, blood, etc. (4) *Recurrence*. Incidence low if adequately treated in early stages.

Radium therapy

Preparation for interstitial irradiation as for pre-operative preparation above.

Special post-operative care

Unconsciousness. Nurse must remain beside patient until fully conscious and aware that object in mouth must not be ejected. Salivation may be inhibited especially if salivary glands irradiated. Dry foods avoided. Small pellets of butter may be given to keep mouth lubricated thus helping to reduce risk of infection.

Ambulation. Patient remains in bed, except perhaps to use commode, until needles removed because of danger of accidental loss. Stress vigorous breathing, leg exercises.

Needles. Frequent checking of needles especially at hand-over of staff. Removal, usually after 6–10 days depending on dosage ordered. Not painful as tract of needle insensitive. Sloughs not forcibly removed, allowed to separate spontaneously.

Communication. Talking forbidden while needles in situ. Provide pencil and pad or slate.

DENTAL EXTRACTION

Indications. (1) Alveolar abscess. (2) Caries, when unsuitable for conservation. (3) Pain which cannot be relieved by conservative measures. (4) Prosthesis where better cosmetic result obtained by extraction. (5) Impaction. (6) Orthodontics: misplaced teeth, or to provide more spaces. May be performed under general anaesthetic often as outpatient procedure. Patient accompanied by responsible person who will take patient home afterwards. Fasts overnight. Pre-operative medication given on arrival, patient prepared for theatre.

Aftercare
Patient sent home when bleeding has ceased. Advise to avoid for 24 hours — mouthwashes, very hot food and fluids, strenous exercise, alcohol. Next day — mild analgesia, e.g. aspirin, and hot saline mouthwashes (teaspoon salt to glass of water). Relieves pain and soreness in gums. Return to dentist if bleeding persists.

Complications
Bleeding. Treatment, pressure pack (haemostatic drug may be added, e.g. adrenaline) held on bleeding socket, patient instructed to bite on it for 10 minutes. May need suture to draw socket edges together thus compressing damaged blood vessel. Blood transfusion may be necessary in severe cases.

Dry socket. Inflammation of lining of socket. Treatment — syringing of socket with antiseptic lotion. Sedative dressing to prevent food entering and to relieve pain. Mouth rinses to keep mouth clean and increase blood flow to area thus assisting healing.

OESOPHAGUS (GULLET)

TRACHEO-OESOPHAGEAL FISTULA
Abnormal communication. between oesophagus and trachea. Most common form: upper portion of oesophagus ends in blind pouch. Lower portion connects stomach to trachea near its bifurcation.

CAUSE
Congenital. During normal embryonic development trachea and oesophagus formed from same primitive tube. Occasionally separation into two tubes incomplete.

SIGNS AND SYMPTOMS
Recognized in first 24 hours of life. Drooling of excessive, frothy saliva (cannot be swallowed). Transient cyanosis as trachea obstructed by saliva. First feeding accompanied by gagging,

coughing, regurgitation, cyanosis. Abdominal distension may be present (air passing from trachea to stomach).

DIAGNOSIS

Confirmed by passing fine catheter (10–12 F) which stops 10 cm from lips. 1–2 ml radio-opaque dye passed down catheter and X-ray taken. Plain abdominal X-ray shows gas in stomach and intestines.

COMPLICATIONS

Pneumonia from spillage of saliva and milk from full blind pouch into lungs. Dehydration.

TREATMENT

Corrective surgery.

Pre-operative. Cease oral feedings as soon as condition suspected. Suction continuous or intermittent every 10 minutes with fine catheter in upper oesophagus. Position: head of cot lowered to prevent inhalation of mucus. Insulcot – ideal, as temperature and humidity can be controlled; child left unclothed to observe respirations; barrier nursing easier; oxygen may be easily introduced. Crying avoided, blows air down trachea into stomach; distension causes pressure on diaphragm, impairs breathing. Antibiotic therapy, prevent infection. Intravenous fluid: amount and type carefully estimated.

Surgery. Incision right side of chest. Lower end of oesophagus freed from trachea and anastomosed to upper end. Gastrostomy may be done as oedema with temporary obstruction of oesophagus may occur during healing stage.

Post-operative. *Insulcot.* Controls temperature (babe loses heat rapidly during surgery). Controls humidity (should be 100%), reduces insensible loss, prevents drying of mucous membranes.

Oxygen. 60% for first 12–24 hours then decreased according to infant's behaviour. (Not more than 40% for premature babies: danger of retrolental fibroplasia.)

Suction. As necessary for 3–5 days. Catheter must not go beyond pharynx: danger of rupture of anastomosis.

Position. Head lower than feet (allows pooling of saliva and mucus in cheek), easier aspiration.

Drainage tube. Into pleural cavity. Removed 3—5 days.

Intravenous infusion. Continued 48—72 hours.

Feedings. Commenced 48—72 hours via gastrostomy opening. 10—15 ml, 10% glucose in water 2-hourly, added milk according to formula until normal feeding achieved on fourth to fifth post-operative day. Oral feedings commenced when babe swallowing saliva, about eighth day. Feedings increased as tolerated. Gastrostomy tube removed in 4 weeks, abdominal wall closes spontaneously.

Drugs. Antibiotics continued 5—7 days post-operatively. Analgesics as required, dosage according to weight.

Sutures. Removed after 7—10 days. Discharged in 10 days. Breast feeding may be re-established.

Complications. Pneumonia. Disruption of anastomosis. Stricture of oesophagus.

OESOPHAGEAL STRICTURE
Narrowing of oesophageal lumen.

CAUSE
Congenital. Acquired (1) following ingestion of corrosives, (2) secondary to surgery or penetrating injuries; fibrous tissue replaces mucosal lining.

SIGNS AND SYMPTOMS
(1) Congenital: regurgitation most marked when changing from liquid to semisolid food (oesophagus capable of dilating enough to accommodate moderate quantities of liquid); respiratory distress: if dilatation above stricture presses on trachea. (2) Acquired: dysphagia; inability to swallow (solids rather than liquids); weight loss; poor development; mild anaemia.

TREATMENT
Aim is to keep lumen open. (1) Regular passage of bougies (rubber dilators). At first twice weekly, later, monthly. Patient taught how to manage these himself. Oral feedings may be continued. (2) Gastrostomy. Small pouch of stomach brought on to abdominal surface, sutured in position. Tube passed into stoma, patient fed through this. Fluids only given. Nurse must endeavour

to make meal times pleasurable for patient by ensuring that sight and smell of food will not only stimulate appetite but also encourage flow of saliva to keep mouth moist and clean. (If patient unable to swallow saliva paper tissues and kidney dish may be provided.) May be temporary measure until bougies have dilated oesophagus sufficiently to allow passage of oral fluids. Careful oral hygiene needed to prevent dirty mouth and consequent spread of infection. (3) Oesophageal replacement. Only considered when oesophagus cannot be dilated. Extensive intrathoracic surgery where new oesophagus reconstructed from jejunum or colon (pp. 96–97).

CARCINOMA OF OESOPHAGUS

Not uncommon. Prognosis poor because of early spread to regional lymph nodes.

Incidence. Males over 45 years.

Type. Epithelioma which grows around and obstructs oesophageal lumen.

SIGNS AND SYMPTOMS

Steadily increasing dysphagia, first with solids, later with fluids, eventually even with saliva. Patient can usually indicate accurately where food sticks. Loss of energy. Weight loss.

Spread. Trachea, forming fistula; recurrent laryngeal nerve, hoarseness; surrounding tissues, pain radiating between scapulae; metastases via blood stream.

DIAGNOSIS

Confirmed by barium swallow, oesophagoscopy and biopsy.

TREATMENT

1. **Radical surgery**. Only possible if diagnosed early. Five-year survival rate: 30%. Growth removed and surrounding healthy tissue for 3 cm or more above and down to stomach below. All surrounding lymph nodes removed.

Restoration of continuity. Anastomosis of both remaining ends of oesophagus or upper end to stomach (palliative measure to relieve obstruction).

Roux-en-Y anastomosis. Jejunum divided from duodenum,

joined to stump of oesophagus; cardiac end of stomach oversewn, duodenum implanted into jejunum further down. Thus food bypasses stomach, pancreatic enzymes and bile come in contact with food in jejunum via duodenum.

POST-OPERATIVE CARE. (a) Re-expansion of lung — upright position; deep breathing exercises; chest X-ray. (b) Drain tube in pleural cavity connected to underwater seal; removed 24—48 hours if lungs re-expanded. (c) Analgesics and moist inhalations necessary before secretions can be coughed up. (d) Antibiotics continued 10 days. (e) Fluids: intravenous infusions for 2—3 days. Ryle's tube to prevent paralytic ileus. Oral fluids commenced third day — clear at first, later, milk and egg drinks, gradually increasing from 30 to 120 ml hourly, semisolid diet introduced as tolerated.

POST-OPERATIVE COMPLICATIONS. Atelectasis (thoracic incision); paralytic ileus (from handling of gut); pylorospasm (if vagus nerve divided); leakage from anastomosis.

2. **Intubation.** Oesophagus dilated with bougies, flexible tube made of coiled wire spring (Souttar's) or plastic (Mouseau-Barbin's) passed, under general anaesthetic. The tubes have wide mouths to prevent them slipping past the obstruction (though they sometimes do). They keep lumen open and form a limited passageway for fluids and semisolids. Patient should be warned against swallowing large lumps of food as these block tube. Recommended to sip 30 ml hydrogen peroxide nightly to cleanse tube of debris. Warned to inspect stools for passage of tube.

3. **Radiotherapy.** Not of much value. Deep X-ray, radium implants may be attempted as palliative measures.

4. **Palliative gastrostomy.** May be justified when patient unable to swallow and general condition good. Patient learns how to cope with unswallowed saliva. Taught to manage his own feedings. He should: (a) precede feed with 15 ml water to ensure patency, follow with 15 ml water to prevent blockage; (b) care for skin around gastrostomy by applying waterproof paste or cream; (c) never leave catheter out unless replaced by gastro-stomy plug; (d) care for mouth — frequent mouthwashes, chewing gum, fruit, e.g. apple or pineapple chewed and expectorated.

ACHALASIA OR CARDIOSPASM

Spasm of cardiac sphincter associated with dilatation and hypertrophy of oesophagus.

CAUSE

Unknown. Principal theories: (1) Incoordination of nerve impulses, cardiac sphincter fails to open during swallowing. (2) Spasm of cardiac sphincter fibres. (3) Kinking of lower end of oesophagus.

Although all ages are affected, more common in early adult life. May be additional psychological factors.

SIGNS AND SYMPTOMS

Epigastric or substernal discomfort; progresive dysphagia; regurgitation of food after meals without nausea or effort — often relieves discomfort; weight loss, rapid at first.

DIAGNOSIS

Confirmed by barium swallow. Shows dilated and often tortuous oesophagus which narrows at level of diaphragm. Differentiated from carcinoma by oesophagoscopy and biopsy.

TREATMENT

(1) Octyl nitrite inhaled from small ampoule broken into cloth dilates sphincter. (Also a general vasodilator causing flushing, later headache.) (2) Dilatation: (a) mercury-loaded bougies passed daily or before meals; (b) more lasting relief if, following early diagnosis, passage of a Negus hydrostatic bag, which, when filled, exerts pressure on circular muscles so that they are evenly and fully dilated. (3) Surgery: Heller's operation. Thoracic or abdominal approach. Similar to Ramstedt's operation (p. 101). Muscle layer of lower 5 cm of oesophagus and upper 5 cm of stomach divided so that mucosa can bulge through. Closed without drainage. Fluids for 24 hours, then light diet, graduation on to normal diet within few days.

HIATUS HERNIA

Protrusion of cardia and sometimes part of stomach through oesophageal opening (hiatus) of diaphragm.

CAUSE

A competent hiatus and cardia prevents regurgitation of stomach contents into oesophagus. Competence maintained by crura of diaphragm, angle of entry of oesophagus into stomach, intrinsic muscles and rugae of stomach. Incompetence aggravated by: (1) raised intra-abdominal pressure — pregnancy, obesity, ovarian cysts, tight corsets; (2) muscular weakness — poliomyelitis, pregnancy.

SIGNS AND SYMPTOMS

Substernal soreness and burning; later — pain radiating between shoulder blades; 'heartburn': acid regurgitation, especially on stooping or lying down at night; haematemesis if ulceration severe.

DIAGNOSIS

Confirmed by barium meal: shows regurgitation when patient stoops or placed in head down position. Oesophagoscopy reveals reddened mucous membrane at lower end of oesophagus.

TREATMENT

Usually *Medical.* Aims: prevent regurgitation; avoid overfilling of stomach; neutralize acids. (1) Reduce weight. (2) Avoid stooping, tight corsets. (3) Sleep in upright position. (4) Antacids. (5) Small, frequent meals. *Surgical.* Abdominal or thoracic approach. Any herniating stomach returned to abdomen. Hiatus tightened by approximating muscle margins, fascia sutured to diaphragm.

OESOPHAGEAL VARICES

Abnormal dilatation of veins in submucous layer of lower oesophagus and cardiac end of stomach.

CAUSES

Circulatory disturbance (1) Portal: cirrhosis, portal hypertension. (2) Splenic vein. (3) Superior vena cava.

Factors contributing to rupture. Muscular effort, e.g. coughing, straining, retching. Trauma, e.g. foreign objects. Oesophagitis from regurgitation of acid contents of stomach. Lowered resistance of mucosa due to poor nutrition.

SIGNS AND SYMPTOMS

Usually unrecognized until bleeding occurs. Occasionally diagnosed because barium meal or swallow or oesophagoscopy done. May be small haemorrhage (melaena) but usually massive haematemesis.

DIAGNOSIS

Barium swallow and meal.

TREATMENT

Conservative. (1) SENGSTAKEN TUBE. Stiff rubber tube with 3 lumen and 2 latex balloons; smaller one when inflated with air anchors tube to cardiac end of stomach and compresses any varices in that area; larger one when inflated with air or mercury acts as a tamponade against bleeding varices in oesophagus. Traction is applied and maintained by pulley system. Third lumen communicates with stomach, suction applied as necessary, if emptying satisfactorily, feeding commenced. Bags may be kept inflated for 24 hours. On deflation bag kept in place; if bleeding resumes re-inflated but deflated at frequent intervals to prevent complications. Finally removed when bleeding has ceased for 72 hours.

Complications. Ulceration of pharynx, oesophagus; aspiration pneumonia; laryngeal obstruction; severe epistaxis; rupture of balloon. Bleeding controlled by conservative measures in 70% cases.

2. BLOOD REPLACEMENT. According to loss, haematocrit and haemoglobin levels.

3. VITAMIN K INTRAVENOUSLY. Where liver damage present and prothrombin time prolonged.

4. ANTIBIOTICS. To prevent pneumonia.

5. NUTRITION. Intravenous infusion or intragastric via Sengstaken tube while bleeding continues. When bleeding stops, bland diet increasing to normal but non-irritating foods, to prevent further bleeding.

Surgical treatment. Direct ligation. Distal oesophagectomy. (Both of these not now recommended as efficacy uncertain.) Various 'shunt' operations have been tried, portocaval, splenorenal (p. 160). Not done during emergency but only when bleeding has ceased and underlying cause treated.

STOMACH AND DUODENUM

CONGENITAL PYLORIC STENOSIS

Hypertrophy and spasm of pyloric sphincter. Obstructs onward passage of food from stomach to duodenum.

CAUSE

Congenital, unknown aetiology. More common in males (4:1); 2—10 weeks of age.

SIGNS AND SYMPTOMS

Babe normal at birth. At 2—10 weeks regurgitates after feeds. Vomiting becomes increasingly more projectile as reverse peristalsis becomes more violent. Dehydration, electrolyte imbalance, weight loss, constipation. (Occasionally diarrhoea occurs due to starvation.) Visible peristaltic wave may be seen passing from left to right of epigastrium. Hard smooth lump may be felt at pylorus.

DIAGNOSIS

Confirmed by barium meal.

TREATMENT

Conservative. Antispasmodic drugs, e.g. methyl atropine nitrate (Eumydrin) given with meals.

Surgical. *Pre-operative preparation.* Correct dehydration, electrolyte imbalance by intravenous or subcutaneous infusion. In some cases stomach washed out with normal saline via a fine Jaques catheter. Not more than 20 ml instilled at a time (water or sodium bicarbonate contraindicated as may further deplete salt).

Ramstedt's operation. Local or general anaesthesia. Transrectus incision. Peritoneum and superficial fibres of circular muscle incised along anterior aspect of pylorus from duodenum to stomach. Incision split so that mucous lining bulges between muscle fibres but remains intact.

Post-operative care. Feeding — oral — may commence 4—6 hours after surgery. 30 ml 5% glucose in water 2-hourly for 4 feeds then regular feedings (either formula or breast milk) gradually substituted in increasing amounts until normal feeds are resumed.

101

COMPLICATIONS

Persistent vomiting from gastritis.

PEPTIC ULCERATION

Ulcer (p. 58) occurring at (1) lesser curvature of stomach (gastric ulcer); (2) first part duodenum (duodenal ulcer); (3) stoma following partial gastrectomy (stomal ulcer); (4) Meckel's diverticulum (rare).

CAUSE

Unknown. Thought to be due to increased hydrochloric acid, and mucous membrane deficiencies. Associated with nervous stress, e.g. worry, overconscientious in work; excessive smoking; excessive alcohol especially spirits; irregular eating habits; highly spiced foods; certain drugs, e.g. cortico-steroids, salicylates. More common in people of group O blood.

SIGNS AND SYMPTOMS

Chronic dyspepsia. Pain — gastric ulcer — after eating, relieved by antacids and vomiting; duodenal — 'gnawing' hunger pains relieved by eating.

DIAGNOSIS

Confirmed by fractional test meal (p. 152); barium meal (p. 149); gastroscopy (p. 150); occult blood (p. 153).

MEDICAL MANAGEMENT

Diet. Bland, non-irritating, small meals frequently.

Drugs. Antacids, anticholinergins, sedatives. Rest — physical and mental. Elimination of stress as far as possible. Histamine H_2 receptor antagonist cimetidine (Tagemet) 200 mg orally t.i.d., p.c. and 400 mg h.s. for one month.

INDICATIONS FOR SURGICAL TREATMENT
Failure of medical treatment
Complications

1. **Haemorrhage**. Ulcer erodes large blood vessel — sudden weakness or fainting associated with or following haematemesis and/or melaena. May be merely pale and weak or exhibit definite signs and symptoms of shock.

TREATMENT. *Medical.* Rest; nil orally except ice to suck;

gastric aspiration via gastric tube ½ − 1 hourly; analgesics − morphia 15 mg; blood transfusion; observations of vital signs; diet commenced when bleeding stops; drugs: antacids, anticholinergics, sedatives.

Surgical. Subtotal gastrectomy if (a) bleeding persists for more than 48 hours; (b) known chronic ulcer; (c) patient over 50 years of age.

2. **Perforation.** Eats through into peritoneal cavity allowing escape of gastric contents, causing peritonitis. Signs and symptoms: may or may not be history of ulcer. Sudden severe epigastric pain, may be referred to tip of shoulder. Pain persists, spreads downwards towards lower abdomen and out on to flanks. Board-like abdominal rigidity, epigastric or generalized tenderness. Absence of bowel sounds on auscultation. Signs and symptoms of shock: pallor, cold, clammy skin, rapid thready pulse, falling blood pressure.

DIAGNOSIS. Confirmed by straight abdominal X-ray which shows gas under diaphragm when patient in upright position.

TREATMENT. Emergency laparotomy after shock treatment has been commenced. Either oversewing of ulcer or partial gastrectomy.

3. **Penetration.** Ulcer eats into adjacent organs, e.g. pancreas, gall bladder, colon. Signs and symptoms of peritonitis or acute pancreatitis.

TREATMENT. Laparotomy and repair if necessary.

4. **Contractions.** Result from excessive scar tissue formation. (a) *Hour-glass* stomach results from healing of large gastric ulcer in centre of stomach dividing it into two separate cavities with narrow opening between. (b) *Pyloric stenosis:* narrowing of pylorus as duodenal ulcer heals. Signs and symptoms: past history of ulcer; increasing pain; vomiting increases in frequency and amount, often effortless, copious and may contain food taken a day or more previously; weight loss; anorexia; later dehydration and electrolyte imbalance.

DIAGNOSIS. Confirmed by fractional test meal and barium meal.

TREATMENT. Correction of dehydration and electrolyte imbalance. Gastric aspiration, stomach washouts if gastritis present. Subtotal gastrectomy.

5. **Malignancy**. May occur in patient with long-standing gastric ulcer but also occurs spontaneously. Most common in males over 45 years. Signs and symptoms. Early: vague, slight dyspepsia. Advanced: weight loss, anaemia, palpable abdominal mass.

DIAGNOSIS. Confirmed by fractional test meal, barium meal, gastroscopy.

TREATMENT. Total gastrectomy — curative. Short circuit operations — palliative.

TYPES OF GASTRIC AND DUODENAL SURGERY

1. **Oversewing of perforated ulcer**. Quickest and simplest method of repair but danger of recurrence.

2. **Partial gastrectomy**. *Billroth 1*. ⅔ stomach, i.e. wide area around ulcer-bearing curvature down to pylorus removed. Remaining ⅓ closed except for area anastomosed to duodenal stump. Disadvantages — danger of stenosis and recurrence of ulcer.

Billroth 2 or Polya. ⅔ of stomach including pylorus and most of first part of duodenum removed. Duodenum closed thus creating blind loop into which bile and pancreatic juice received. Remainder of stomach closed except for small area anastomosed to loop of jejunum. Thus gastric contents bypass the duodenum but still come in contact with pancreatic enzymes and bile. Disadvantages: duodenal stump may leak causing peritonitis. Ryle's tube may pass through anastomosis into jejunum giving false impression of amount of fluid aspirated from stomach.

3. **Vagotomy and pyloroplasty**. Most effective treatment for peptic ulceration. Less complications, more permanent results. Division of both vagus nerves on anterior and posterior aspects of oesophagus just before they reach the stomach. Inhibits gastric secretions and mobility. To ensure adequate drainage of stomach pylorus incised longitudinally down to mucosa then sewn up vertically thus making pylorus shorter and wider.

4. **Gastro-enterostomy**. Duodenum short circuited. Loop of jejunum attached to lower border of stomach so that gastric contents pass into jejunum but pancreatic juice and bile may still mix with them. Indications: inoperable pyloric stenosis, duodenal ulcer, cancer — as palliative measure only. Originally done in conjunction with vagotomy.

5. **Total gastrectomy**. Radical excision of stomach, and duodenum and associated lymph nodes. For carcinoma. Roux-en-Y anastomosis may be performed – small intestine divided 15 cm or more below stump of jejunum and anastomosed to oesophagus. Other end of stump joined into side of this. Transverse colon may be used to replace stomach. Dangers – paralytic ileus, peritonitis, mechanical kinking.

PRE-OPERATIVE PREPARATION

See p. 1–4. SPECIAL FEATURES. *Diet.* Light, bland, non-irritating. Added iron if patient anaemic.

Oral sepsis treated. Decayed teeth removed. Efficient dentures.

Alimentary tract preparation. Nil orally for 12 hours. Stomach may be washed out if there is any suggestion of pyloric stenosis. Ryle's tube passed on morning of operation, remains in situ throughout operation.

POST-OPERATIVE CARE

See p. 4–12. SPECIAL FEATURES. Tray for intermittent gastric aspiration, essential to prevent gastric dilatation; ensures quick healing of suture line. Intermittent at ½ – 1 hourly intervals. Time between aspirations increased as amount of aspirate decreased. Time and amount of gastric aspirate recorded as output on fluid balance chart.

Nutrition. Intravenous replacement continues until adequate oral fluids tolerated. Small sips of water may be permitted from onset, but indications for commencement of oral fluids are: (1) decrease in amount of aspirate; (2) bowel sounds on auscultation; (3) passage of flatus per rectum.

Feeding regime (varies according to surgeon): 30 ml water hourly, each drink being preceded by gastric aspiration to determine amount being absorbed. Drink increased accordingly: 60 ml water or citrated milk alternating with fruit juice. Ryle's tube removed 2–3 days later, semisolids introduced. Gradual introduction of bland, easily digested foods – egg flip, lightly boiled or poached eggs, steamed fish, chicken, custards. Balance of carbohydrates, fats, proteins, vitamins. Gradual introduction of small meals (gastric capacity reduced), otherwise normal meals every 2 to 3 hours.

Position. Semi-upright or upright.

Physiotherapy. Patient may be afraid to breathe deeply because of pain; analgesics given before breathing exercises.

Drain tube. Occasionally inserted as precautionary measure, e.g. from duodenal stump. Removed in 48–72 hours after shortening daily.

Socio-emotional needs. Patient advised to avoid constant anxiety and 'high pressure' living. Eliminate contributing factors as far as possible.

COMPLICATIONS

Immediate. *Shock.* Determined by age, pre-operative condition, length of operation.

Haemorrhage. Slight bleeding is usual. Gross bleeding indicated by haematemesis, melaena, signs and symptoms of internal haemorrhage.

Peritonitis. Caused by (1) contamination at time of operation as stomach, small bowel opened for anastomosis; (2) leak from anastomotic line; (3) leak from duodenal stump. Suspected if pain persists more than 36 hours or if sudden severe pain occurs 3–7 days post-operatively. May lead to paralytic ileus or subphrenic abscess.

Pulmonary complications. More likely if diaphragm damaged, patient afraid of pain on deep breathing.

Gastric retention. May occur if stomach cannot empty adequately following gastro-enterostomy. Treatment aims at prevention by aspiration and avoidance of distension for 24–48 hours. If conservative measures fail re-operation may be necessary.

Later. *Recurrence.* More likely to occur at site of anastomosis. Signs and symptoms similar to original ulcer. Treatment – medical at first. If this fails – further surgery – vagotomy and pyloroplasty.

Intestinal hurry. Diarrhoea due to rapid passage of food. Usually not serious. Controlled by tabs codeine co.

Dumping syndrome. Rare complication of unknown aetiology. Theories: acute reduction of plasma volume; distension of duodenal loop instead of food passing into jejunum; accumulation of bile in proximal loop; excess insulin production in response to sudden entry of carbohydrates into intestine. Signs and symptoms: 1—2 hours after eating — nausea, sweating, pallor, fainting. Diarrhoea may or may not occur. Treatment. Low residue feedings. Avoidance of high carbohydrate foods. Restriction of fluid intake during meals. Lying down before and after meals.

Anaemia. Iron absorption may be inhibited when acid formation reduced leading to microcytic anaemia. Pernicious anaemia may develop if large portion of acid secreting cells removed as intrinsic factor may also be absent. Iron and vitamin B preparations given if necessary.

Intestinal obstruction may occur (p. 114).

PERITONEUM

PERITONITIS
Inflammation of peritoneum, localized or generalized.

CAUSES
1. *Injuries.* Penetrating, e.g. stab wound, gunshot wound, through abdominal wall. Or penetrating intestines, e.g. fish bone, swallowed pin, enema nozzle, sigmoidoscope. Or penetrating vagina or uterus, e.g. instrument in criminal abortion. Or internal injuries, e.g. ruptured liver or spleen.

2. *Perforations.* Peptic ulceration; ulcerative colitis; carcinoma; typhoid ulceration; gangrene from strangulated hernia, volvulus, mesenteric thrombosis; cysts, e.g. ovarian, hydatid.

3. *Extension of infection.* Appendicitis; Meckel's diverticulum; diverticulitis; cholecystitis; Crohn's disease (regional ileitis); salpingitis.

4. *Blood borne.* Tuberculosis; gonococcal; pneumococcal.

5. *Surgical.* Blood, bile, stomach, urine, duodenal or intestinal juices, escaping during or after surgery. Formerly-minute traces of glove powder liberated during surgery.

PATHOLOGY
Local or focal peritonitis: small source of infection sealed in by peritoneal adhesions. Allows body to overcome infection without further spread. The small 'abscess' thus produced may or may not contain pus.

Generalized or diffuse peritonitis. If there is no time, or if too much irritating material present, peritoneum unable to 'wall in' infection. Local peritonitis may become generalized if defence inadequate.

As result of widespread irritation, peritoneum exudes thick serous fluid. Provides a medium for microbial growth therefore pus forms quickly. Fluid becomes sticky, glues loops of intestines together in attempt to localize infection (adhesions are formed which may later obstruct bowel). Further attempts at localization occur as body overcomes infection. Fluid and pus gravitate to places where intestinal movement reduced, form pockets of pus — known as residual abscesses (p. 29) — pelvic, subphrenic, iliac.

SIGNS AND SYMPTOMS

Pain: local over area of irritation and generalized; severe and constant; aggravated by movement and deep breathing hence respirations shallow and rapid. May be so severe that patient is restless but usually lies on side with knees drawn up. Tenderness over area: sudden release of pressure causes acute increase of pain (rebound tenderness). Muscle rigidity: muscles overlying area become spastic thus 'guarding' the area; later rigidity diminishes if condition untreated. Diminished peristalsis, absence of bowel sounds. Vomiting: due to (1) pain and (2) paralytic ileus (p. 28). Pulse: rate increased, wiry; as condition deteriorates becomes weak, rate increases further. Pyrexia if infection present; later temperature subnormal from toxic shock. Dehydration, electrolyte imbalance and toxaemia from paralytic ileus.

TREATMENT

1. *Remove cause.* Surgery or drain abscess.

2. *Control infection.* (a) Antibiotics — penicillin and/or intravenous infusion of broad spectrum antibiotics, e.g. Reverin, Bristacin. (b) Copious fluids intravenously.

3. *Prevention or treatment of paralytic ileus.* (a) Rest and deflation of alimentary tract: (i) Nil orally; (ii) Nasogastric suction by either Ryle's tube (76–107 cm in length, usually rubber, diameter 4–10 E or 9–18 F gauge with weighted end). Suction may be either intermittent by means of syringe — every ½ to 1 hour — time interval increasing as amount decreases or

108

continuous by means of low pressure suction apparatus or by hydraulic pressure with Wangensteen's apparatus. Three bottles used. Bottle 1 suspended above bed, fluid allowed to drip at a controlled rate to bottle 2 on floor. This creates suction in bottle 1. Bottle 3 connected to bottle 1 by tubing so that suction transmitted to bottle 3 which is connected by Ryle's or Levin tube to patient's stomach, Bottle 3 placed at lower level than patient's stomach. Combination of higher pressure in stomach and lower pressure in bottle 3 causes constant aspiration of stomach. When all water in bottle 1 has transferred to bottle 2, tubing to bottle 3 and the Ryle's tube are clamped off, 1 and 2 reversed, tubing from 3 transferred to hanging bottle and clamps removed. Miller-Abbott's tube: Up to 312 cm in length with double lumen. One lumen connects to inflatable rubber balloon, the wider one used for suction. With balloon deflated tube passed into stomach (analgesic spraying of mouth and pharynx may facilitate this if patient conscious). Balloon distended with water and withdrawn against sphincter. Balloon then collapsed and tube inserted a further 25 cm. Stomach aspirated (should be acid in reaction). Patient lies on right side for ½ hour and tube should enter duodenum. Half-hourly aspirations performed and when alkaline, or contains bile, balloon re-distended; it will be carried by peristalsis to paralyzed site. Tube then affixed to cheek and continuous suction applied. (b) Intravenous infusion. Fluids, calories and electrolytes replaced according to daily requirements, gastro-intestinal loss and serum electrolyte estimations.

4. *Prevention of complications* (p. 14). (a) Residual abscess: drain tube post-operatively; pelvic abscess easier to treat than others hence — upright position. (b) Unpleasant, dry mouth: keep lips moist — petroleum jelly or peppermint ointment. (c) Abdominal distension: flatus tube.

5. *Commencement of oral feedings.* Indicated when (a) amount of aspirate diminishes, (b) bowel sounds present; flatus passed per rectum. 30 ml of water given, 1 hour later stomach aspirated. If amount less than 30 ml a further 30 ml given. Amount and time interval gradually increased if fluids tolerated as shown by decreasing aspirate preceding each feed. Ryle's and intravenous tubes removed, patient graduated on to light diet, then normal diet as tolerated.

6. *Observations for detection of complications.* Vital signs; full blood count; particular observation of stools for presence of blood and mucus denoting onset of pelvic abscess; bowel sounds.

COMPLICATIONS

Paralytic ileus; residual abscess; faecal fistula; adhesions with later bowel obstruction.

APPENDIX

APPENDICITIS

1. Acute

Inflammation of appendix which often comes on suddenly and may go on to suppuration.

Incidence. All age groups affected but occurs most commonly between 10 and 40 years.

Cause. Obstruction. (a) Peristalsis occurs in appendix, anything which enters appendix usually returned to caecum. If contents retained, there is absorption of water and a hard mass of faeces results (faecolith). (b) Lymph nodes may swell and block lumen — more likely to occur in conjunction with mesenteric adenitis. (c) Adhesions from previous infections. (d) Threadworms.

Infection. (a) Blood borne (catarrhal) associated with history of sore throat, measles or other infection 3 weeks before onset. (b) Result of stasis in appendix.

Pathology. In obstructive type — peristalsis increases in an effort to overcome obstruction. Infection and oedema may result in early mural necrosis and perforation, ending in peritonitis.

Signs and symptoms. 'Classical' epigastric or para-umbilical pain, usually associated with reflex vomiting. Empties alimentary tract, puts it to rest thus assisting arrest of inflammatory process. Within 2–3 hours pain settles in right lower quadrant (right iliac fossa) as persistent soreness aggravated by coughing and walking. Cessation of pain may indicate subsidence of inflammation or may signify destruction of nerve endings preceding stage of perforation. Anorexia; furred tongue; halitosis; malaise; slight pyrexia 37°–38°C. Constipation usual but occasionally diarrhoea. Tenderness on rectal examination.

If perforation: peritonitis, muscle guarding, localized tenderness, rebound tenderness; later generalized abdominal pain and rigidity; leucocytosis.

Depending on location of appendix, other variations may occur, diagnosis differentiated from other conditions such as pyelitis, gastro-enteritis, pain or ovulation (mittelschmerz), Crohn's disease, Meckel's diverticulum.

Complications. Perforation resulting in (a) general peritonitis and its complications (p. 107); (b) appendix abscess (p. 112); (c) pylephlebitis — suppurative thrombophlebitis of portal system with resultant liver abscesses.

Treatment. SURGICAL. Method of choice to prevent above complications.

Pre-operative preparation. Routine as for emergency operations (p. 2–4). Aperients and/or enema not given unless specifically instructed as may cause perforation of tense appendix.

Surgery. McBurney's (grid-iron) incision. Oblique incision through McBurney's point, muscle layers split (blunt dissection), fascia and peritoneum incised. Base of appendix located by following taenia coli down to caecum. Appendix and blood supply clamped, removed, purse-string suture applied to caecum. Peritoneum repaired. Skin sutures only may be inserted at closure, as muscle fibres come together and form strong closure.

Post-operative care (p. 4–12). Usually uncomplicated; normal activities resumed 2–3 weeks after surgery.

MEDICAL (OCHSNER-SHERREN) TREATMENT. Used when surgical facilities not available or where condition of more than 48 hours' duration and localized swelling palpable. Patient must be in hospital where he can receive skilled and continuous attention. (a) Upright position. If pus forms it gravitates to pouch of Douglas: easier to treat. (b) Observations. (i) Vital signs, ½ to 1 hourly. Most important sign: increasing pulse rate. Indicates need for surgical intervention. (ii) Fluid balance chart; copious fluids, oral if possible, otherwise rectal tap water. Intravenous therapy if patient very ill. Observe especially for vomitus. (c) Drugs. Morphia 4–6 hourly to prevent pain. Antibiotics. (d) Bowels. Mucus in stools denotes pelvic abscess. Purgation and enemata contraindicated for 3 days. Suppositories may be given after 3 days.

Under this treatment peritonitis should resolve. Rising pulse rate, increasing pain indicative of need for surgical intervention.

2. Appendix abscess

Pathology. To prevent generalized peritonitis, omentum and loops of small bowel become matted around inflamed appendix, collection of pus forms in centre.

Signs and symptoms. Noticeable 2–6 days after onset but may be masked by antibiotic therapy – malaise, pallor, swinging pyrexia, leucocytosis, tender mass palpable in right iliac fossa.

Treatment. *Conservative.* Ochsner-Sherren regime as above. If abscess resolves in 4–5 days appendicectomy 6–12 weeks later.

Immediate surgical treatment. Indicated if above treatment unsuccessful and signs of spread occur. Abscess drained and post-operative care aimed at prevention of paralytic ileus.

3. Chronic appendicitis

Name given to various inflammatory and non-inflammatory conditions of appendix which do not cause acute signs and symptoms.

Pathology. Wall of appendix may be normal or fibrosed. Lumen may contain faecoliths or worms. May be associated hyperplasia of lymphoid tissue and even generalized lymph node enlargement.

Cause. Result of previous acute or subacute inflammation. Adhesions from past episodes may cause obstruction.

Signs and symptoms. Pain: recurrent lasting minutes, hours or days; may be colicky, central abdominal and/or constant in right iliac fossa. Appetite: anorexia, nausea when pain present. Vomiting may occur with pain. Constipation or diarrhoea. Weight loss, patient does not feel well. Examination reveals only slight pain over right iliac fossa and usually only during attack.

Diagnosis. Made only when differentiated from other conditions. Barium enema may sometimes show abnormal appendix.

Treatment. Appendicectomy.

Appendicostomy

Appendix brought through abdominal wall, fistula formed through which colon can drain and be irrigated.

112

Indication. Originally used in intractable cases of ulcerative colitis. Now replaced by ileostomy and colectomy.

SMALL AND LARGE BOWEL

CROHN'S DISEASE

Inflammatory condition affecting patches of small and large bowel; more common in terminal ileum. Also called regional ileitis, regional enteritis.

CAUSE

Unknown. Thought to be tuberculous in origin but extensive investigations have failed to show any connection. Affects both sexes and all age groups but most common in 20—40 year group.

PATHOLOGY

Usually chronic but may appear in acute form. Inflammatory process involves whole thickness of intestinal wall. Usually begins beneath mucosa and spreads through muscle coat to peritoneum. Ulcerates mucosa. Initial lesion in 6—12 in of terminal ileum may spread back up small intestine or on into caecum and colon. May 'skip' a distance and begin another lesion several segments away. The affected parts become thickened, lumen narrowed.

SIGNS AND SYMPTOMS

Pain in right iliac fossa similar to appendicitis; diarrhoea; history of intestinal colic; abdominal mass may be felt; weight loss; pyrexia; anaemia; occult blood in stools. Anal fistula occurs in high percentage of cases.

DIAGNOSIS

Barium meal or enema shows narrowed segments, in advanced cases strictures, fistulae.

COMPLICATIONS

Intestinal obstruction; fistulae; abscess; perforation; steatorrhoea; ankylosing spondylitis (reason unknown).

TREATMENT

No cure. May 'burn' itself out, recurrence with or without treatment common.

Medical. (1) Diet: maintain nutrition, high calorie, low residue, bland, vitamin and iron supplements. (2) Rest, prolonged; fever tends to settle. (3) Drugs: cortico-steroids usually reserved for seriously ill patient pre-operatively; antibiotics of doubtful value.

Surgical. Three reasons: (1) severe ill health, (2) complications, e.g. bleeding, fistulae, obstruction, (3) mistaken diagnosis of acute appendicitis.

Ileum above lesion anastomosed to transverse colon as short circuit. Right hemicolectomy may be performed (p. 126). Recurrence following surgery 20–60%.

INTESTINAL OBSTRUCTION

Anything which interferes with onward flow of bowel contents.

TYPES

Paralytic (adynamic): motility of bowel diminished or absent.

Mechanical (dynamic): lumen of bowel may be actually blocked. May be acute or chronic.

CAUSES

Paralytic. Paralytic ileus (p. 28); megacolon (Hirchsprung's disease) (p. 117).

Mechanical. *Intraluminal.* (Inside lumen of bowel.) Impaction of: (1) foreign objects accidentally swallowed, e.g. food improperly digested aggregates to form solid mass; (2) gall stones: fistula forms between gall bladder and duodenum, large stone passes into bowel, becomes wedged in narrower ileum; (3) faeces: frequently occurs in large bowel of elderly; (4) meconium ileus: occurs in babies with fibrocystic disease of pancreas, meconium not liquefied because pancreatic secretions are deficient, hence blocks bowel; (5) large intestinal parasites may occasionally block bowel, more common in children under 10 years.

Mural. (Wall of bowel.) (1) Congenital abnormalities: (a) atresia: failure of development of portion of bowel, may be gap between two blind ends or joined by a section of fibrous tissue with no lumen, (b) malrotation: midgut, on its return from umbilical cord into abdomen, fails to rotate thus causing

114

obstruction. (2) Intussusception. (3) Volvulus. (4) Inflammation: (a) Crohn's disease; (b) tuberculosis (usually secondary to pulmonary tuberculosis – implantation of sputum in intestinal wall; (c) diverticulitis. In acute phase obstruction due to oedema and inflammatory process; later narrowing of lumen due to fibrosis. (5) Neoplasm: benign or malignant. May obstruct by protruding into lumen or causing ring of constriction.

Extramural. (Outside wall of bowel.) (1) Strangulated hernia: most common cause of bowel obstruction. (2) Adhesions – bands of fibrous tissue resulting from (a) inflammation: peritonitis, (b) abdominal surgery, (c) pelvic surgery. Adhesion – obstruction due to sharp angulation, or actual strangulation of bowel, or may produce volvulus. Post-operative adhesions may obstruct any time from a few weeks after surgery to several years after. (3) Meckel's diverticulum. (4) Mesenteric thrombosis. (5) Neoplasm from other organs, e.g. ovarian cyst.

ACUTE MECHANICAL OBSTRUCTION. Strangulation; intussusception; volvulus; gall stones.

CHRONIC MECHANICAL OBSTRUCTION. Neoplasms; adhesions; impaction; diverticulitis.

CHRONIC WHICH BECOMES ACUTE. Neoplasms; adhesions; strangulation; inflammation; mesenteric thrombosis.

PATHOLOGY

Eight litres of fluid (saliva, gastric juice, bile, pancreatic juice, intestinal juice) poured into gut daily; 90% of this reabsorbed when it reaches lower ileum. Area above obstruction becomes distended with fluid and swallowed air. In high intestinal obstruction there is copious vomiting and little opportunity for fluid absorption; dehydration rapidly follows. In low intestinal and colonic obstruction vomiting and dehydration not as marked, most of distension is gaseous.

In mechanical obstruction increased peristalsis above obstruction occurs at first, but in later stages, and in paralytic obstruction no peristalsis audible.

Simple obstruction may lead to dehydration, electrolyte imbalance and toxaemia (stagnant fluid in bowel quickly becomes infected – toxic products absorbed) but blood supply to part remains adequate. If strangulation occurs (i.e. nipping and occlusion of blood supply to area), infarction, gangrene, perforation and peritonitis may result if obstruction not relieved.

SIGNS AND SYMPTOMS

Paralytic. See p. 28.

Acute mechanical. 1. Acute colicky pain associated with loud rushing peristalsis on auscultation, or occasionally visible peristalsis. Later no audible peristalsis when bowel grossly distended.

2. Vomiting. At first stomach contents, then bile stained, increasing in amount to copious brown faecal fluid. (Not as marked in low intestinal and colonic obstruction.)

3. Abdominal distension — tympanic abdomen (due to interference with blood supply not to blockage of lumen).

4. Absolute constipation of flatus and faeces.

5. May be associated with signs and symptoms of shock, dehydration, toxaemia, peritonitis.

Chronic mechanical. May last for months or years, severity varies but gradually increases.

1. Pain, intermittent attacks of colic.

2. Vomiting, usually absent, not faecal, may follow ingestion of food.

3. Abdominal distension, occasionally visible peristalsis may be present or palpable tumour.

4. Change in bowel habits: constipation, or alternating constipation with diarrhoea, solid faeces decompose and so liquefy and are then easily evacuated. Rectal examination may reveal ballooning if obstruction below splenic flexure of colon.

TREATMENT

Paralytic. See p. 28.

Acute mechanical. In doubtful cases gentle enema may be given followed by a second to prove absolute constipation (first enema may only clear faecal content below obstruction).

CONSERVATIVE. (1) Decompression of bowel by gastric or intestinal suction may be sufficient to relieve obstruction in small bowel. (2) Intravenous fluid replacement. (3) Antibiotics.

SURGICAL. Essential if likelihood of strangulation and must be undertaken with minimal delay.

Pre-operative preparation. Emergency routine. Analgesics to

116

relieve pain, minimize shock. Correction of dehydration by intravenous route. Blood taken for serum electrolytes. Urine tested for specific gravity, chlorides. Intragastric tube to remove stomach contents, prevent vomiting, inhalation pneumonia during surgery. If abdomen painful, washing, shaving may be deferred until patient anaesthetized.

Operation. Incision: paramedian which may be extended up or down if necessary. Examination: to find obstructed area. Often difficult to distinguish between distended small bowel and large intestine. Decompression of bowel where necessary. Relief of obstruction: freeing of adhesions; untwisting of bowel; enlarging of window in strangulated hernia; in inoperable cases — temporary colostomy until patient's general condition improves, or bypass surgery, e.g. gastro-enterostomy; resection of gangrenous portion or tumour. Restoration of continuity: end-to-end anastomosis; temporary colostomy until swelling subsides then anastomosis; permanent colostomy or ileostomy.

Post-operative care. Specific: aimed at prevention of peritonitis and its complications — paralytic ileus, residual abscess, faecal fistula. Colostomy care (pp. 132—134).

Chronic mechanical. Immediate surgery — resection of obstructed area, anastomosis or colostomy to restore continuity. If chronic becomes acute: colostomy performed, bowel sterilized prior to later anastomosis.

Contraindication to surgery. Faecal impaction. Danger of peritonitis when faeces removed via incised gut. Soften faeces with warm olive oil, remove with enemata or manually.

HIRSCHSPRUNG'S DISEASE AND MEGACOLON
Dilatation and hypertrophy of colon occurring without organic obstruction.

CAUSE
Hirschsprung's disease. Usually confined to children. Congenital absence of ganglion cells in nerve supply to sigmoid colon and rectum.

Megacolon. Constipation and ignoring urge to defaecate. Rectum and colon become dilated. Anal spasm thought to be contributory cause.

PATHOLOGY

Coordinated peristalsis cannot pass beyond aganglionic area and chronic partial obstruction results, with mass of faeces in rectum. Accumulation of faecal material causes hypertrophy and dilatation of proximal colon and abdominal distension. In severe cases colon so dilated that haustral markings are entirely absent. Erosion of mucosa may occur.

SIGNS AND SYMPTOMS

Constipation: days, weeks or even months. Progressive abdominal distension, in severe cases causing respiratory and cardiac embarrassment. Pelvic 'tumour' — faecal mass may be palpated. Pain due to partial obstruction, increases with distension.

DIAGNOSIS

Confirmed by barium enema. Doubtful cases — rectal biopsy to establish presence or absence of ganglion cells.

TREATMENT

Medical. Mild cases: low residue diet; bowel evacuation (colon emptied with enema and washout continued daily as necessary). Encourage regular habits. Keep faeces soft with liquid paraffin. Avoid aperients. Abdominal exercises. Parasympathomimetic drugs.

Surgical. Resection of inert bowel. Temporary caecostomy or colostomy may be necessary in seriously ill patients to relieve obstruction. Later resection, anastomosis. Satisfactory result in 80% cases.

INTUSSUSCEPTION

Telescoping or invagination of one part of bowel into next segment (usually proximal into distal loop). Bowel literally 'swallows' itself.

CAUSE

In children: unknown. Common between ages of 6 months–2 years. Often associated with such factors as change of diet, increase in lymphoid tissue, viral disease.

118

In adults may be associated with Meckel's diverticulum, neoplasm.

PATHOLOGY
Occurs in segment of small intestine or at ileo-caecal junction in infants. Invaginating loop consists of two layers but distal portion one layer. As the invaginating loop moves down lumen it takes mesentery with it. Blood vessels in mesentery become nipped; veins compressed first. Bowel becomes congested, swollen. Blood may fill lumen and mix with faeces. Later, arteries compressed, blood supply cut off, bowel gangrenous, perforates.

In adults, intraluminal profusion of tumour or Meckel's diverticulum moved along by peristalsis taking attached bowel with it thus initiating intussusception. Blood vessels obstruct as above. In rare cases intussusception may present at rectum.

SIGNS AND SYMPTOMS
Sudden onset. Pain severe, paroxysmal. Child doubles over, draws up legs, goes pale. Between spasms child relaxes, is normal colour, appears healthy. Vomiting common, increases in severity. Bowels: tenesmus. After 8–16 hours blood and mucus passed per rectum ('red-currant jelly' stools). Mass sausage-shaped, may be felt in right upper abdomen; left upper abdomen feels 'empty'. Shock and dehydration develop later.

TREATMENT
Conservative. Reversible if no appreciable swelling. Barium enema, under X-ray control, may force small bowel back through ileo-caecal valve by hydrostatic pressure.

Surgical. Simple reduction. Loop decompressed and slowly ejected. If grossly swollen or gangrenous: resection with end-to-end anastomosis. Occasionally temporary ileostomy or colostomy if patient critically ill.

VOLVULUS
Twist of a viscus on its mesentery to such a degree as to patially or completely occlude its blood supply.

119

CAUSES

(1) Congenital. Small bowel: mesentery fails to attach. Caecum: may be unusually mobile or undescended. (2) Adhesions. Rotation of loop around a fixed point. (3) Constipation. Sigmoid colon commonest area: long redundant area twists around a faecal mass.

PATHOLOGY

Twist more commonly clockwise than anticlockwise. Rotation may occur through 360° or more. More common in males (4:1). Infarction, gangrene, perforation may result if blood supply occluded.

SIGNS AND SYMPTOMS

As for acute intestinal obstruction above.

DIVERTICULITIS

Inflammation of pouch-like diverticula. (Protrusions or pockets of mucous membrane through muscle layer of colon.)

PATHOLOGY

Diverticula occur more commonly in descending colon and sigmoid flexure, but may also localize in other sites, e.g. caecum, small bowel. Most frequently arise opposite appendices epiploicae into which they penetrate. Age group commonly over 35. More common in males than females, and in overweight and constipated people.

Small diverticula have all layers of colon but as they grow muscle layer disappears, mucous membrane atrophies. In larger diverticula absence of muscle causes retention of bowel contents. Stagnation and water absorption occurs, these small hard masses can become infected, may lead to other complications.

SIGNS AND SYMPTOMS

Diverticulosis (presence of diverticula with few or vague symptoms); diverticulitis (inflammation of diverticula). Similar to acute appendicitis but more common in left iliac fossa.

COMPLICATIONS

Perforation (see peritonitis, p. 107). Stenosis: Due to oedema and inflammatory process, or to healing with fibrosis, leading to acute or chronic bowel obstruction. Vesico-colic fistula. Patient passes faeces and flatus via urethra. Ascending infection of bladder and kidneys may occur. Massive haemorrhage: signs and symptoms of peritonitis and internal haemorrhage.

DIAGNOSIS
Confirmed by barium enema.

TREATMENT
Inflammation. Medical. Rest; copious fluids; combined antibiotics penicillin and streptomycin or tetracyclines; high fibre diet instituted early — bran in any form, fresh vegetables, fruits; liquid paraffin; avoid aperients; bulk forming agents — psyllium, methylcellulose, sterculia (Normaclol).

Surgical. Treatment of complications as above. Temporary colostomy, ileostomy may be necessary to treat inflammation by resting bowel Later, resection and anastomosis. Occasionally total colectomy and ileostomy.

MECKEL'S DIVERTICULUM
DESCRIPTION
Pouch usually located approximately 2 ft from ileo-caecal valve on ileum. Varies in length, 25–130 mm, and shape, sausage, saccular, conical, vermiform, filiform, hemspherical, vestigial. May have its own mesentery. Lumen usually as large as ileum so that it empties readily by peristalsis.

CAUSE
Congenital malformation. In early embryonic life duct connects yolk sac to intestine. This usually closes, often a remnant remains as cord from intestine to umbilicus. Meckel's diverticulum is this sac which has failed to close.

PATHOLOGY
Intestinal obstruction (1) diverticulum acts as spear head to form intussusception, (2) strangulation of loop of intestine. Occasionally contains aberrant gastric tissue and is site of ulcer due to acid secretion. May perforate or bleed. May become infected in same way as appendix and produce similar signs and symptoms.

TREATMENT

Surgical removal.

MESENTERIC THROMBOSIS

Occlusion of superior or inferior mesenteric arteries or veins.

CAUSES

(1) Embolus from vegetations on heart valves in bacterial endocarditis. (2) Arteriosclerosis. (3) Cardiac disease. (4) Liver disease and acute abdominal infections (from portal vein drainage). (5) May follow splenectomy.

PATHOLOGY

Whether obstruction is arterial or venous a short-lived pallor of bowel may be seen at laparotomy but infarction soon occurs. Intestine and mesentery become swollen and oedematous. Demarcation between healthy and infarct tissue gradual. Blood-stained fluid fills bowel lumen and is exuded into peritoneal cavity. Area of infarction becomes gangrenous and perforation causes peritonitis.

SIGNS AND SYMPTOMS

Acute onset with profound shock, severe abdominal pain, abdominal distension, vomiting, often blood stained, bloody diarrhoea. Occasionally indefinite palpable lump in thin patients.

TREATMENT

Immediate laparotomy, resection of infarct area, anastomosis. Anticoagulants — heparin and Dindevan occasionally used as conservative treatment and in post-operative stage.

ULCERATIVE COLITIS

Inflammation and ulceration of part of colon.

CAUSE

Unknown. Stress plays a part at onset.

SIGNS AND SYMPTOMS

Diarrhoea frequently containing blood, mucus and pus. Desire to defaecate urgent, often accompanied or preceded by colicky abdominal pain. Hurry of food through bowel causes malabsorption, malnutrition, weight loss, dehydration and electrolyte imbalance. Pyrexia and prostration may accompany acute attacks.

COMPLICATIONS

(1) Perforation of bowel during acute attack. (2) Haemorrhage: ulcer eats through vessel in large bowel wall. Secondary infection leading to severe toxaemia. (3) Stricture: scar tissue forms during healing, later contracts. (4) Carcinoma: 10–30% of cases over 10 years' duration. (5) Anaemia: chronic blood loss or sudden severe haemorrhage. Lost iron not readily replaced due to poor absorption from gut. (6) Other rare complications: nonsuppurative arthritis, iritis, anorectal abscess causing fistula.

DIAGNOSIS

Confirmed by (1) Sigmoidoscopy. In early cases mucosa oedematous, reddened, submucosal blood vessel pattern not visible. Mucosa bleeds easily – so-called 'contact bleeding' – when area lightly swabbed. Irregular superficial ulceration may be seen in later stages. Bowel lumen may be filled with fluid stools containing blood, mucus and pus. Overgrowth of mucosa may form warty outgrowths termed pseudopolypi. (2) Stool culture, to differentiate from other causes of diarrhoea, e.g. amoebiasis, dysentry, sprue, Crohn's disease. (3) Barium enema: often difficult and even harmful during an acute attack. In early stages reveals typical ulcerations; later, tube-like colon with loss of haustrations due to oedema and scarring. Pseudopolypi, strictures and carcinoma may be detected.

TREATMENT

Medical. Aimed at rest of body, mind and gastro-intestinal tract. Bedrest during acute attacks. Psychological reassurance, sympathetic understanding, occupational therapy. Fluid and electrolyte imbalance corrected with intravenous infusions. Blood transfusion to correct anaemia if necessary. Diet – high calorie, high protein, low residue, vitamin and iron supplements.

Drugs – Symptomatic. Control pain, diarrhoea, anaemia – codeine, kaolin, belladonna, phenobarbitone, amylobarbitone,

123

iron orally or by intramuscular injection.

Treat infections promptly — sulphaguanadine, Sulfasuxidine, broad spectrum antibiotics.

Curative. Sulphas and steroids — either orally or by retention enema. Dramatic results have been obtained by steroids (e.g. ACTH, prednisolone), but may sometimes mask symptoms of perforation and infection. Sulphasalazoline (Salazopyrine) 1 g q.i.d. orally.

Surgical. *Indications.* (1) Chronic invalidism from frequent relapses unresponsive to medical treatment. (2) Complications, e.g. anorectal abscess of fistula, arthritis, iritis, skin lesions. (3) Acute stages, as life-saving measure when general condition deteriorating. (4) Suspicion of malignancy.

Types of surgery. Originally appendicostomy, frequent irrigation; or temporary ileostomy to rest colon, rectum. Both now superseded by more radical surgery — proctocolectomy and permanent ileostomy. (Rectum usually involved, anastomosis of ileum to rectum contraindicated. If rectum not involved result may be satisfactory.)

Results. Elective surgery: mortality 1—2%. Emergency surgery: mortality 20% or higher.

NEOPLASMS OF THE BOWEL

Benign

Adenoma, papilloma, fibroma, myoma, lipoma, rarely dermoids and cysts. (Rare in small intestine.)

Adenomatous polypi most common. Vary in shape and size. May be pedunculated.

Cause. Generalized polyposis: (1) familial predisposition; (2) chronic ulcerative colitis due to 'tabs' of mucosa spared in destructive process; (3) parasitic infection (rare).

Signs and symptoms. Bright blood in stools. Abdominal pain. Diarrhoea resulting from irregular peristalsis or secondary infection. Any of these may be the only presenting symptom.

Diagnosis. Confirmed by sigmoidoscopy, barium enema, aerogram (air introduced into bowel after barium evacuated. Thin film of barium may be left covering polypi).

Complications. Malignant change (unsettled question), malignant cells found in superficial specimens but rarely in deeper layers. Intussusception. Anaemia. Malnutrition.

Treatment. (1) Complete removal by cautery or excision if within reach of sigmoidoscope (after biopsy for malignancy). (2) If beyond sigmoidoscope — laparotomy and (a) colotomy and excision of polyps; (b) partial colectomy; (c) total colectomy and ileostomy.

Because of high incidence of recurrence — endoscopy every 3 months for first 6 months and then every 6–12 months thereafter.

Malignant

Carcinoma: common. Less common: lymphoma, melanoma, fibrosarcoma.

Predisposing causes. Familial multiple polyposis. Chronic ulcerative colitis. More common in over-40 age group. Males more than females (3:2), but can occur in younger age group, occasionally in infancy.

Types of carcinoma. Ulcer; 'cauliflower' type; annular; metastatic (late stages only).

May cause (1) increased peristalsis and diarrhoea from irritant action; (2) mucus, blood and pus from ulceration; (3) obstruction: constriction from annular growth, blockage from cauliflower growth; (4) constipation: faeces have difficulty passing narrowed lumen; (5) intussusception.

Spread. From all areas except rectum. Slow spread because of poor lymph drainage. May spread to other organs, e.g. bladder, but usually late spread.

Signs and symptoms. Vary according to site and size. Onset insidious. Bowels: passage of blood and mucus; change in habits — increasing constipation or loose stools in previously constipated patient, or alternating periods of constipation and diarrhoea ('spurious' diarrhoea). Pain uncommon unless partial or complete obstruction or intussusception. Colicky pain sometimes due to increased peristalsis. Distension results from obstruction. Anaemia: secondary, with associated weakness and weight loss. Palpable tumour. Occasionally liver enlargement and ascites due to secondary growths.

Special sites. *Small bowel.* Relatively rare. Younger age group (e.g. lymphosarcoma of distal end of ileum common in infancy).

Caecum. Cauliflower growth. Main signs and symptoms: palpable tumour, diarrhoea, occult blood but not visible blood, discomfort (mainly flatulence).

Hepatic flexure. As caecum but obvious blood may be present in stools.

Transverse colon. Cauliflower or annular growth. Main presenting symptoms — obstruction, diarrhoea or constipation, palpable tumour.

Splenic flexure. Early obstruction. No palpable tumour. Pain on right side. Alternating diarrhoea and constipation.

Pelvic colon and rectum. Tenesmus, obvious blood and mucus in stools. Severe pain if anal sphincter involved and spasm occurs.

SURGERY OF BOWEL
Colectomy
Removal of colon.

TOTAL COLECTOMY. Rare. May be performed for ulcerative colitis and occasionally for carcinoma with spread to aorta or superior mesenteric artery. Permanent ileostomy.

PARTIAL COLECTOMY. Large amounts of colon may be removed because of relatively poor blood supply, except for transverse and pelvic colons. In carcinoma amount removed also depends on lymph spread (channels follow same course as arteries).

1. *Right hemicolectomy.* Terminal 10 in of ileum, caecum, ascending colon, proximal third of transverse colon. Ileo-transverse colic anastomosis.

2. *Transverse colectomy.* If growth localized to nodes around middle colic artery, 3 in healthy bowel on each side of tumour. Hepatic and splenic flexures mobilized and anastomosed.

3. *Left hemicolectomy.* Distal third of transverse colon, descending colon and upper part of pelvic colon. Transverse and sigmoid colon anastomosed.

4. *Pelvic colectomy.* Growth and 3 in healthy bowel on each side removed. Colon anastomosed to rectum.

These operations may be performed in one stage if patient fit and no acute obstruction present. A two-stage operation may be needed — temporary relief obtained by bringing portion of gut above obstruction out on to skin, e.g. ileostomy, caecostomy, colostomy. Two to three weeks after these temporary measures, suitable partial colectomy performed.

Pre-operative preparation — elective surgery.

SPECIFIC (in addition to routine preparation).

1. Explanation careful and adequate by doctor, reinforced by nurse if patient to have permanent colostomy (p. 130), ileostomy or caecostomy.

2. Ambulation encouraged.

3. Diet. High protein and vitamin. Copious fluids.

4. Blood transfusion, correction of electrolyte imbalance.

5. Bowel preparation. Aims — to empty of faeces and sterilize. (a) Low residue diet 2–5 days pre-operatively. (b) Aperients (if no obstruction or diarrhoea) for 3–5 days, but none given 48 hours pre-operatively. (c) Enema if necessary and bowel washouts 2 days but must cease 12 hours pre-operatively. (d) Sterilization of bowel — phthalylsulphathiazole (Sulphathalidine) 4 g, 6-hourly for 5 days pre-operatively; 2 days pre-operatively: oral streptomycin 1 g, twice daily or neomycin 1 g, hourly for 4 hours then 4-hourly.

5. Skin preparation: abdomen, pubic and perineal areas.

6. Bladder must be emptied before patient leaves ward, if not, surgeon must be warned because of danger of perforation of bladder during surgery.

7. Nasogastric tube may be needed if patient vomiting or as a preventive measure for paralytic ileus.

Post-operative care. See pp. 4–12.

COMPLICATIONS. (1) Shock (from inadequate preparation in emergency surgery, prolonged anaesthesia, excessive handling of gut during surgery). (2) Haemorrhage. (3) Peritonitis from (a) perforation pre-operatively, (b) contamination with faecal contents during surgery, (c) leakage from anastomosis post-operatively. (4) Paralytic ileus from peritonitis as above, excessive handling of gut, prolonged anaesthesia, electrolyte imbalance. (5) Following peritonitis: residual abscess, faecal fistula, adhesions.

DRAIN TUBES into area of anastomosis in case of leakage. When drainage minimal gradually shortened and removed to prevent fistula formation.

Abdominoperineal resection of rectum

Indications. Carcinoma of rectum. Ulcerative colitis in conjunction with total colectomy.

Method. Two phases; 2 surgeons working together.

1. *Abdominal incision.* Liver, peritoneum and lymph drainage examined; sigmoid colon and rectum freed down to pelvic floor; colostomy or ileostomy established.

2. *Perineal incision.* Anus closed to prevent leakage (in females, posterior wall of vagina may be removed when perineal incision made). Draining lymph channels and nodes examined; anal canal and rectum freed and removed. Peritoneal floor closed by surgeon working from above. Perineal wound may be only partly closed in some cases to ensure free drainage. Wound packed with gauze rolls or strip of tubing.

Pre-operative preparation. As for colectomy. Catheter (indwelling Foley's bag) to ensure empty bladder before operation; to prevent soiling of perineal wound post-operatively; to overcome disturbances of micturition due to damage to pelvic floor.

Post-operative care. As for colectomy. Bed elevated at foot to minimize ooze from raw surface of perineum. Pain severe — give morphia 15 mg, 4-hourly for 24 hours, then reduce as indicated.

Position. Alternating sides with increasing number of pillows — patient unable to sit upright. May sit out on fourth day and graduated exercises encouraged.

Diet. See colostomy or ileostomy care (pp. 132, 135).

WOUND CARE. *Abdominal.* Sealed off with waterproof adhesive tape, left undisturbed for 7−10 days when sutures removed.

Colostomy or ileostomy (pp. 129, 134).

Perineal. Dry dressing held in place with 'T' binder. Drainage: underwater drainage has two advantages — keeps dressing dry and facilitates easy, accurate measurement of blood-stained fluid. According to amount of drainage — tube shortened ½−1 in daily until removed — seventh day.

Packing may be inserted and left in situ for 3−4 days. Anaesthetic may be required prior to its removal. Sutures removed eighth day, after which patient has daily baths. If infection present: daily irrigations with antiseptics which are harmless to tissues, e.g. Milton 1 in 40, Eusol 1 in 8, hydrogen peroxide 1 in 50. Patient may need to continue with such packs after discharge until healing is complete.

CARE OF BLADDER. Continuous drainage necessary 2–3 days as nerve supply to bladder may be impaired. Fine, non-irritating catheter used, e.g. Gibbon's. Tidal drainage may be used to establish rhythmic filling and emptying of bladder until it regains normal habits. Alternatively, patient may be catheterized twice daily until he regains sensation of filling and desire to micturate. After removal of catheter, residual urine measured twice daily. If more than 150 ml, catheter replaced.

Complications. Shock; haemorrhage; infection (especially perineum); damage to bladder (nerve damage causing retention; fistula from perineum); peritonitis (paralytic ileus); pulmonary and vascular complications.

Caecostomy

Opening into caecum for purposes of drainage.

Indications. (1) Temporary initial treatment for bowel obstruction to allow decompression of bowel especially in poor-risk patients. (2) Divert bowel contents to allow healing of anastomosis at higher level in ascending colon.

Method. Tube inserted into caecum through stab wound (fluid nature of caecal contents enables drainage through narrow opening), secured with purse-string suture. Tube brought through abdominal wall in right iliac fossa, drained into bedside bag or bottle. A satisfactory seal quickly established in peritoneal cavity as caecum becomes adherent to peritoneum of anterior abdominal wall. When tube removed (after obstruction relieved) opening in caecum closes without further surgery.

Disadvantages. (1) Damage to skin. Leakage of intestinal fluid difficult to avoid. Powerful enzymes present which digest skin unless protected with barrier cream. (2) Adhesion of caecum to anterior abdominal wall which encourages fistula formation.

Colostomy

Artificial opening of colon which is brought on to skin surface for purpose of drainage (artificial anus).

Indications. 1. Relieve obstruction of bowel either temporarily (acute dynamic bowel obstruction) or permanently (inoperable carcinoma).

129

2. Defunction portion of bowel as temporary measure by bypassing diseased section: (a) inflammation, e.g. diverticulitis, ulcerative colitis; (b) repair of vesico- or recto-vaginal fistulae; (c) prior to resection of inflamed or oedematous portion of bowel where immediate anastomosis would break down.

3. Rectal conditions: (a) trauma, usually temporary; (b) congenital abnormalities, temporary or permanent; (c) carcinoma — removal — permanent.

4. Anal injury or abnormality resulting in incontinence — colostomy is more manageable.

5. Spinal cord injuries, occasionally when paralysis of anal sphincter and incontinence occur.

Types. 1. PERMANENT. (a) Terminal. Should be in left iliac fossa in pelvic colon (faeces more solid and manageable). Single barrel — cut end of colon brought out on to skin, mucosa everted, sewn to skin to prevent retraction. Colon distal to colostomy removed. (b) Loop of colon brought out and V-shaped flap of skin passed under it. Loop may be opened immediately if evacuation of contents urgent, or opened 24—48 hours later.

2. TEMPORARY. (a) Loop. Simplest way of relieving obstruction. Loop of colon above obstruction brought out on to skin. Opening made at apex of loop. Glass rod passed under loop through mesentery and kept in position by 'bucket handle' effect of rubber tube attached to both ends of rod. This prevents retraction of loop. (b) Defunctioning colostomy. Similar to loop above but loop completely divided 24—48 hours later. This prevents spill of faecal contents from proximal to distal end. Disadvantages of both these operations — laparotomy required to close colostomy. (c) Spur (Paul-Mikulicz operation). Involved section of bowel either resected immediately or brought out on to surface (exteriorization) and resected after abdomen has been closed (to prevent contaminating peritoneal cavity). Base of loop (or two arms of remaining bowel) sutured together side by side for several inches within the abdomen thus making a double-barrelled colostomy. A crushing clamp (enterotome) may be applied to close the colostomy — when spur broken, artifical opening sinks back below skin level and gradually atrophies leaving small fibrous spur. Advantages of this method are that closure is extraperitoneal (peritoneal wound healed after 24—48

hours thus sealing off peritoneal cavity), thus eliminating risk of peritonitis and perforation.

Pre-operative preparation. As for colectomy (p. 127). Special psychological preparation is necessary: (1) careful explanation of reasons for colostomy; (2) emphasis on and explanation of how patient may continue to live normal life and learn how to control colostomy; (3) introduction to patient who has successfully managed his own colostomy. Natural antipathy to thought of faecal contamination of skin overcome by nurse's sensible reassurance.

Post-operative care. As for colectomy. Oral fluids may be commenced on demand when there is audible peristalsis, sips at first then gradually increasing amounts. If vomiting occurs nasogastric tube passed, stomach contents aspirated otherwise risk of paralytic ileus, peritonitis.

Management. AIM. To make patient comfortable and, by nurse's attitude and efficiency, to teach patient to manage his own colostomy so that he can lead a normal life of work, sport and social entertainment without fear of embarrassment. Normally when rectum full, usually once a day, there is desire to defaecate. Patient with colostomy receives no such warning.

OPENING OF COLOSTOMY. *Immediate:* at time of operation to allow escape of gas and faecal material to relieve obstruction. Danger is that peritoneal cavity takes 24–48 hours to seal and may become contaminated during this time. To prevent this a bent glass tube (Paul's tube) is sewn into opening and drained into bedside underwater drainage via some thin wide latex tubing (Paul's tubing). Tube may be removed in 2–3 days or may allowed to slough out in 5–8 days.

Delayed: when bowel action not expected for 2–3 days. This obviates risk of peritoneal contamination or excoriation of skin.

Method of opening. May be done in ward without anaesthesia (no sensory nerve endings in colon). For aesthetic reasons may be opened in theatre under general anaesthesia. May be incised with scalpel or electric cautery. Latter method gives better control over haemorrhage.

BOWEL ACTIONS. Should be expected within 3–4 days. Aperients seldom needed. May be necessary to remove obstruction with gloved finger. Occasionally small colonic washout may be needed to initiate defaecation.

131

DRESSINGS. Frequent dressings for first few days until regular habit established. Nurse must avoid showing any distaste or disgust and perform dressing in an efficient 'matter of fact' manner, using minimum equipment without fuss. This helps patient to accept colostomy, and that its dressing is well within his capabilities. Patient encouraged to play active part as soon as he is willing but never forced to do so.

Method. Bulky faeces removed with dressing. Area around colostomy stoma cleansed with detergent lotion, e.g. cetrimide 1%. Stoma gently cleansed. Skin may need protection until it becomes accustomed to faeces – barrier cream, silicone cream, aluminium paste. Stoma may be protected with layer of petroleum jelly gauze. Several thicknesses of cotton wool applied, kept in place with binder.

CARE OF WOUNDS. (1) Glass rod: removed in 10 days after formation of adhesions which prevent retraction of colostomy. (2) Abdominal wound: covered with adhesive waterproof tape, left undisturbed until sutures removed 7–10 days. (3) Colostomy wound: sutures removed 7–10 days.

Observations for complications. (1) Haemorrhage. (2) Strangulation of loop, colour should be pink. Report pallor, cyanosis or hyperaemia. (3) Obstruction – stenosis – report if no flatus or faeces passed within 3–4 days. (4) Retraction of loop. Glass rod prevents this; report immediately if it slips out. (5) Prolapse. Causes: weakness of abdominal wall, premature removal of sutures, increasing obesity. Loop 'slips' forward. Surgical treatment necessary. (6) Wound infection: tenderness, inflammation, pyrexia. Skin excoriation.

Continuing care. REGULAR CONVENIENT BOWEL ACTIONS. Depends on temperament of patient, some adjust easily, others take some time, a few never manage.

Establishment of regular habits. May be acquired by 'leaving it to nature' and patient may train colostomy to empty at convenient time, e.g. after breakfast and again in the evening. May need to be initiated by colonic washout at these times for a few days or weeks. Patient either wears pad over stoma before expected bowel action or goes to toilet and sits with receptacle under colostomy until action is complete. Afterwards he cleans area with soap and water, wears thin square of cotton wool covered with shield and belt, no further leakage anticipated.

·*Control of consistency of stools.* 1. Diet. Mainly trial and error for each individual patient. Aim is to produce a formed soft stool. In early post-operative period after fluids are being tolerated, light easily digested diet commenced with increasing protein and vitamin C to aid healing. Roughage gradually introduced — sufficient to stimulate peristalsis without causing diarrhoea. Foods and fluids which cause gas and odours should be eliminated. Depending on personal choice and experimentation, patient encouraged to eat foods rich in proteins — meat, fish, dairy products — and 'constipating' foods — potatoes, macaroni, spaghetti — but to avoid carbonated drinks, raw fruits and vegetables, especially those with skins and pips.

2. Drugs. May be needed to increase or decrease bulk of stool. (a) Methyl cellulose preparations increase bulk (granules taken with water, swell in alimentary tract). (b) Codeine, diphenoxylate (Lomotil), 'Kaomagma', may be necessary if diarrhoea becomes troublesome — usually due to dietary indiscretion, elimination of cause better than treatment. (c) Suppositories or small enema if constipation unrelieved by diet or methyl cellulose. Use of aperients avoided as control of bowel action uncertain. (d) Colostomy washouts. Not advocated as routine because of excess water absorption from colon and damage to bowel. May be used in hospital to initiate regular bowel actions. Some patients, unable to adjust to a regular routine, may need them daily to ensure security.

Method: Special irrigating tubes or fine 10–12 E Jaques catheter inserted about 15 cm into opening and 300–400 ml of water or normal saline allowed to flow slowly into bowel. Tube removed, return of fluid directed into a kidney dish. May be necessary to use up to 1 litre of fluid to ensure efficient evacuation. Patient learns this procedure 10–14 days post-operatively.

CARE OF SKIN. Skin gradually adjusts to ̇faeces but prolonged contact or diarrhoea may cause excoriation. Skin protected by: (1) Solid faeces — delay opening colostomy until 48 hours post-operatively or drain contents into bedside bag via Paul's tube and tubing. Maintain formed soft stool as above. (2) Barrier creams — silicone, zinc or aluminium cream. (3) Dressing

133

changed frequently until belt and bags worn, may be on second day or delayed until sutures removed. (4) Treatment of skin excoriation — leave bag off, temporarily cover skin with barrier cream, apply pad and bandage. (5) Skin cleaned thoroughly with soap and water after bowel action. Patient encouraged to have daily bath or shower.

APPLIANCES. 1. If patient able to control colostomy: during day cotton wool pad covered with plastic disc kept in place with specially designed and measured belt, or two-way stretch bandage, or type of corset; at night pad of cotton wool and bandage.

2. If patient unable to control colostomy: will need to wear bag and belt continuously except at night. Several varieties available: one-piece rubber bag and belt; two-piece: belt with disposable plastic bag. Patient must not use those which tend to produce suction — danger of prolapse. (Use of colostomy bag should be avoided if possible.)

ACTIVITIES. Patient encouraged to resume normal work, sport and general activities. Advise to join Colostomy Association soon after discharge. Members help each other to adjust.

Testing patency of distal loop. May be necessary when obstruction has subsided. (1) Colostomy washout through distal loop; patient sits on bedpan, or rectal tube passed to allow fluid to discharge through rectum. (2) Methyl cellulose preparations may be inserted into distal loop and patient should have bowel action. (3) Barium enema.

Closure of colostomy. (1) Enterotome (spur colostomy). Jaws of clamp placed in each limb, colon ('spur') crushed by screwing jaws together. Takes 2–3 days. Enterotome drops off when spur breaks down. (2) Laparotomy, anastomosis of limbs of colostomy which may be done in conjunction with resection of obstruction.

Ileostomy

Artificial opening in terminal portion of ileum which is brought out on to skin for purposes of drainage.

Indications. *Temporary.* To rest bowel by diverting faecal stream.

Permanent. Following total colectomy, e.g. in ulcerative colitis, Crohn's disease. As these two conditions involve a younger age group a great deal of psychological support is required from nurse to help patient adjust to the idea of discharging fluid faeces on to skin for rest of life.

Pre-operative preparation. Patient should be in best possible physical condition for elective surgery. As patient will have to wear bag continuously site for ileostomy carefully chosen; patient may be measured for appliance before going to theatre. Ideal site — below girdle line at 'hipster' level and in area where it neither impinges on hip nor becomes dislodged by flexion of thigh.

Post-operative care. Stoma is long (1½–2 in) so that its discharge does not come in contact with skin (juices very rich in digestive enzymes). May have Paul's tube and tubing in situ and bag applied 4–5 days later, or bag may be attached immediately in theatre.

Fluids. Accurate fluid balance chart essential as patient loses copious fluid and electrolytes via ileostomy. Intravenous fluid replacements determined by serum electrolyte estimations and urinary chloride loss. Discontinued when patient tolerating copious oral fluids. Electrolyte balance and copious fluids must continue until patient's metabolism adjusts to new situation.

Oral feedings commenced first post-operative day. No intra-gastric feeding is needed unless patient is nauseated and/or vomiting. Fifteen ml water hourly on first day, gradual increase until by third day patient tolerating 90 ml of any clear fluid hourly. Fourth day free fluids should be tolerated, light diet gradually introduced. By eleventh day full, low residue diet may be tolerated. Fruit and vegetables gradually introduced until by time of discharge patient is having normal diet. Diet is unrestricted but should be high in protein and fluids.

Appliances. Various. Should not be so bulky that women cannot wear straight skirts and slacks. Three main varieties but patient may choose combination of each.

1. One piece: bag and flange joined. Worn with narrow belt. Flange adheres to skin with special cement solution or with double-side adhesive plaster.

2. Two piece. Similar method of application but bag and flange separate.

3. Non-adhesive. Increasingly used. Plastic bag (disposable) and perspex flange with protective foam rubber ring. Worn with

belt. Must be changed frequently whereas adhesive types need be changed only once a week. (They have outlet at bottom of bag to allow discharge of contents whenever necessary.)

Method of application (of two-piece adhesive type – others similar). Skin thoroughly cleansed with soap and water, any previous adhesive removed with carbon tetrachloride. Tincture of benzoin compound or nobecutane may be sprayed on skin to prevent excoriation. Hole cut in two-sided adhesive to size and shape of stoma. Flange applied to adhesive, gently but firmly pressed to skin – ileostomy protrudes through hole. Thin roll of cotton wool inserted around ileostomy and inside wall of flange to protect skin. Bag then applied to flange, belt adjusted carefully. Stopper in bag checked to prevent leakage.

Problems of management of ileostomy. Unlike colostomy, faecal contents of ileostomy are fluid and cannot be trained to act 1–2 times daily. Bag has to be worn continuously but ileal washouts are not necessary.

SKIN IRRITATION AND EXCORIATION. Causes: too frequent removal of adhesive; incorrect application of appliances; stoma too short.

Treatment. (1) Use Karaya gum instead of adhesive. (2) Thick layer of barrier cream spread around stoma and large piece of lint with hole cut in middle placed over it. This is covered with waterproof adhesive and flange placed over this. Skin must heal before adhesive used again.

ULCERATION OF STOMA. Cause: because stoma is insensitive to all but distension a carelessly applied flange can press on stoma resulting in necrosis. Patient will feel no pain until there is reactionary swelling. In severe cases stoma may slough leaving a fistula at skin level.

Treatment. Laparotomy and formation of new ileostomy.

FOOD OBSTRUCTION. Cause: oedema of ileal stoma due to infection.

Pathology. Accumulation of food and fluid in loop of bowel behind stoma becomes infected. Ileostomy continues to function in passing small amounts of foul-smelling fluid frequently.

Treatment. Wide bore catheter passed through stomal opening and bowel washed out with water or normal saline. Usually condition subsides after several days. Patient advised not to eat high residue foods for a few weeks as this predisposes to food obstruction.

PROLAPSE OF ILEAL STUMP. Late complication. Causes: inadequate internal fixation of ileum; relaxation of abdominal opening, e.g. patient becomes obese.

Treatment. (1) Deeper flange may be adequate in mild cases. (2) Laparotomy with revision of ileostomy and adequate internal fixation.

EXCESSIVE FLUID LOSS. Copious fluid stools may occur at any time from dietary indiscretions or partial obstruction of lumen. Patient warned of possibility and advised to seek medical aid should it persist.

Treatment. Codeine or methyl cellulose in attempt to make stool more solid and bulky; high residue diet; prompt correction of electrolyte imbalance.

MECHANICAL OBSTRUCTION. Early or late complication. Cause: adhesions either to pelvic floor or between loops.

Treatment. Gloved finger inserted into stoma may release gas and thus decompress bowel and relieve obstruction; surgical correction.

PSYCHOLOGICAL ADJUSTMENT. As for colostomy except for (1) younger age group; (2) no control ever achieved but patient able to engage in full active life. Even dancing and swimming are possible with aid of modern appliances. There is also an Ileostomy Association in each country and a panel of members visit others who have to have an ileostomy. Meetings are held which surgeons and appliance manufacturers attend to discuss problems with members.

RECTAL PROLAPSE
Protrusion of rectal mucous membrane through anus.

Types
1. Complete: involving all layers of rectal wall and considerable amount of bowel presenting through anal canal.

2. Concealed: intussusception of rectum not protruding through anal sphincter.

Cause
Weakness of supporting structures, e.g. ischiorectal fat in

debilitation. Occurs most commonly in infants who are allowed to sit on 'pottie' for long periods; following attack of diarrhoea in which weight loss marked. In adults — associated with haemorrhoids, vaginal prolapse or trauma to perineal area. (Differentiation: mucosal ridges arranged concentrically in rectal prolapse, radically in haemorrhoidal prolapse.) Rarely becomes strangulated.

Signs and symptoms

Pain. Mucopurulent discharge occasionally blood stained. Symptoms intensified if constipation and straining at stool occur.

Treatment

Conservative. Improve general health by diet, extra fluids, exercises. Children — gently push back rectum and then strap buttocks together, or apply pad and 'T' bandage. Train child to defaecate on side until general condition improved then gradually elevate to sitting position.

Partial prolapse — may respond to injections with sclerosing agent, e.g. 5% phenol in oil or quinine in hydrochloride (5% solution). Injected into submucous coat at base and apex of prolapse, results in aseptic inflammation forming adhesions thus anchoring mucous membrane to muscle layer.

Surgical. 1. Excision of prolapsed mucosa. Operation similar in technique to haemorrhoidectomy (p. 141), may be curative in partial prolapse providing sphincter tone is satisfactory.

2. Thiersch's operation. When sphincter tone poor and patient in poor general condition: circumanal ring of silver wire acts as substitute for anal sphincter.

3. Amputation: rectosigmoidectomy. Performed for complete prolapse. Patient lies in lithotomy position, prolapse drawn down as far as possible. Circular incision made through mucous membrane, various techniques employed to support remaining rectum which is resutured on to remaining anus.

4. Abdominal repair of perineal floor. Strengthens and narrows opening through which rectum passes, e.g. by suturing, either anteriorly or posteriorly, the puborectales together.

5. Recent technique. Polyvinyl alcohol sponge introduced around lower rectum before it passes through pelvic opening.

Granulation tissue invades its interstices and sponge becomes incorporated into body tissue, thus forming a strong fibrous band which will prevent rectum from sliding through.

Post-operative care

Bowels confined for 5 days. Paraffin oil 15 ml daily to keep stools soft. Suppository on fifth day (enema not advised because of danger of vigorous peristalsis). Sphincter exercises.

HAEMORRHOIDS

Varicosity of lower rectal and anal branches of superior haemorrhoidal veins.

Causes

Unknown. May be familial — congenital weakness of vein wall or abnormally large arterial supply to haemorrhoidal plexus.

Main contributory factors

1. Increase in intra-abdominal pressure: pregnancy, fibroids, ovarian cyst.

2. Straining associated with constipation, diarrhoea, enlarged prostate or other causes of bladder neck obstruction.

3. Draining blood vessels, e.g. portal vein hypertension, intra-venous congestion: congestive cardiac failure or pulmonary conditions, superior haemorrhoidal veins compressed by carcinoma of rectum.

Physiology

In lower rectum, communication between veins of portal and systemic circulation (superior haemorrhoidal vein drains into portal vein, middle and inferior haemorrhoidal veins drain into iliac vein). Superior haemorrhoidal vein has no valves and has to support pressure of both circulations. Dilation common. Veins situated deep in submucosal layer.

Types

1st degree. Dilation protruding into anal canal only. Bleeds readily: streaks of bright blood seen in stools.

2nd degree. Veins dilated, elongated and tortuous. Prolapse out of anus on straining but return when straining ceases. Do not bleed freely. Visible as pink lump when straining only. Pain may occur during defaecation due to stretching of anal sphincter.

3rd degree. Remain prolapsed. May bleed easily. Mucus may leak from anus and irritate skin producing prilitis (often the most irritating symptom). Pain may occur with defaecation.

Strangulated haemorrhoids

Results from spasm of anal sphincter surrounding haemorrhoids and occluding blood supply. Results in thrombosis, oedema, ulceration, ending in gangrene if not relieved. Pain severe due to swelling.

Signs and symptoms. Bleeding: bright streaks of blood in stools. Prolapse: soft lump presenting at anus. Prilitis. Pain during defaecation or due to strangulation. Chronic anaemia may result from loss of iron due to bleeding over long period.

Diagnosis. Of 1st and 2nd degree: manual or proctoscopic examination.

Sites. Right anterior, right posterior and left lateral. On clock face with patient in lithotomy position: 3, 7 and 11 o'clock.

Treatment. CONSERVATIVE. Low residue diet. Non-irritating aperients (paraffin, mild agar) to keep stool soft. Warm saline baths. Soothing suppositories (Anusol) 2—3 times daily to relieve prilitis.

INJECTIONS. 1st degree where bleeding, 2nd degree if patient poor risk for surgery. Contra-indicated if infection present or haemorrhoids thrombosed, strangulated, prolapsed.

Preparation. Rectum should be empty but no special preparation.

Method. Special syringe (Gabriel's). Needles with a bayonet-type attachment (to prevent needle perforating rectum), either angulated or straight with special locking device to prevent needle being forced off syringe. Patient in left lateral or knee-chest position. Haemorrhoids identified. Injection of 1 ml 5% phenol in almond oil into submucous layer (not into haemorrhoid) just above vein. Resultant aseptic inflammation causes fibrosis which slowly strangulates the haemorrhoid. Injections at weekly intervals.

Complications (minimal). (1) Pain if solution seeps beneath skin. Relieved by heat or patient lying down for ½ hour. (2) Haemorrhage, due to ulceration or puncture of haemorrhoid. (3) Necrosis of mucosa – injection too superficial.

Thrombosed or strangulated haemorrhoids. Relieve pain with morphia 10–15 mg, 4-hourly, hot bath, evaporating lotions, e.g. lotio plumbi, icepack. Keep faeces soft: liquid paraffin.

SURGICAL. Haemorrhoidectomy.

Pre-operative preparation (specific). Low residue diet 48 hours. Enema evening before operation to ensure empty lower bowel, then nil orally. Pubic and perineal areas shaved carefully. Correction of chronic anaemia.

Operation. Lithotomy position. Proctoscope inserted. Vein dissected off muscle wall of anal canal. Suture attached to pedicle. Haemorrhoid and surrounding tissue excised. Raw surface left (occasionally, may be sutured). Small drain tube surrounded with petroleum jelly pack inserted to prevent and detect early haemorrhage. Haemorrhage can be very severe if ligature slips; risk slight, tube often omitted. Drain tube also allows escape of flatus.

Three raw areas after operation; care taken to prevent anal stricture.

Post-operative care. Position of comfort. May find relief if sitting on air-ring. Pain usually severe. Give morphia 10–15 mg, 4-hourly if required. Drain tube removed in 48 hours. Dressings left undisturbed for 48 hours; after removal of drain tube petroleum jelly gauze placed over raw areas, pad and 'T' bandage applied to keep skin edges separated. Diet. Low residue until bowels open on fourth to fifth day then normal diet. Bowels. First action expected fourth to fifth day. Mild aperient to keep faeces soft, e.g. paraffin given on third day. If no bowel action on fifth day – small olive oil enema 180–200 ml. When patient about to have first bowel action analgesic given (usually morphia 10–15 mg). Patient may go to lavatory. (He may be allowed to sit out of bed on first post-operative day.) After each bowel action warm bath and fresh dressing applied. Digital dilatation. Essential until canal heals – from third day onwards. Done by surgeon; patient taught importance of continuing this at home; prevents anal stricture.

Complications. Shock: minimal. Haemorrhage: reactionary, secondary (patient warned of possibility of latter when discharged). Infection: because of contamination by faeces; area usually contaminated but heals well in spite of this. Stricture (anal) prevented by digital dilatation as above. Retention of urine. Common with any anal surgery, may sometimes precipitate acute urinary retention in patients with enlarged prostate gland.

Outpatient treatment. Haemarrhoid encircled with elastic band causing it to slough off in 4—7 days.

PERI-ANAL HAEMATOMA

Rupture of one vein of external haemorrhoidal plexus (often called external haemorrhoids).

Cause
Straining at stool.

Signs and symptoms
Pain at anus, sudden, severe. Lump (bluish) varying in size from pea to almond — almost always immediately after straining.

Treatment
Conservative. Small haematoma or one that has been present for more than 48 hours — codeine for pain, paraffin to soften faeces. Pain and swelling gradually subside until after 1—2 weeks only small nodule remains.

Surgical. Large haematoma seen less than 48 hours after formation — local anaesthetic infiltrated around swelling, elliptical piece of skin removed and blood clot expressed.

FISSURE-IN-ANO

Small crack or break in skin of anal canal.

Cause
Injury when passing constipated stool. Vitamin B deficiency.

Pathology
At first simple linear tear, becoming deeper with indurated margins and 'sentinel tag' forms at lower end. As fibrosis occurs anal sphincter involved.

Signs and symptoms
Intense pain on defaecation. Occasionally small amounts of

blood passed. Associated with constipation and also tends to cause it as patient afraid to defaecate because of pain.

Treatment.

Acute attack. Pain causes anal spasm, healing will not take place while this persists. Application of local anaesthetic cream. Liquid paraffin to soften faeces.

Subacute attack. (More than 48 hours but less than 3 weeks). Relaxation of anal sphincter by dilatation under general anaesthesia. 10 ml proctocaine in oil injected round anus.

Chronic. Surgical excision of crack, allow to heal by granulation. Sphincterotomy: incision made into floor of fissure to divide part of fibrotic sphincter.

ISCHIORECTAL ABSCESS

Abscess in fatty tissue of ischiorectal fossa (space between rectum and ischial tuberosity).

Cause

Micro-organic invasion: (1) blood borne; (2) penetrating wound of perineum; (3) perforation of rectal wall, e.g. fissure, ulcerated haemorrhoids.

Signs and symptoms

General signs and symptoms of abscess formation. Dull throbbing pain, patient unable to sit in comfort. Perineal skin becomes red and oedematous to one side of anus.

Treatment

(1) Local heat: Sitz baths. (2) Antibiotics. (3) Incision and drainage when localized: cruciate incision and flaps of skin resected making saucer-like cavity which heals by granulation to prevent fistula formation.

ANAL FISTULA

Abnormal epithelial tract leading from rectum or anal canal to skin.

Cause

Ischiorectal or anal gland abscess.

143

Signs and symptoms

Chronic purulent discharge on skin near anus. Pruritis. Tenderness or pain on defaecation.

Treatment

Surgical. Incision or excision of fistula, either closing rectal or anal opening or allowing wound to heal by granulation (as for ischiorectal abscess). If sphincter involved (i.e. high anal fistula) two-stage operation necessary. First stage: silk thread remains in fistula for 3 weeks causing inflammation and thrombosis. Second stage: tract excised but sphincter muscle cannot now retract because of fibrosis, thus sphincter control retained.

HERNIA

Protrusion of part of contents of a cavity through a weakness in its containing wall. Abdominal herniae most common but can occur elsewhere, e.g. brain, muscle sheath.

Abdominal hernia. Protrusion of a sac of peritoneum which may contain an organ or part of an organ, through a weakness in abdominal musculature.

Causes

Congenital, e.g. persistence of opening where umbilical cord was attached (true umbilical hernia), persistence of pouch of peritoneum through inguinal canal.

Acquired. (1) Develops through natural weaknesses in muscle wall as a result of injury or strain (see common sites below), e.g. perpetual coughing, heavy lifting, multiparity, straining to micturate when bladder neck obstructed, straining at stool in chronic constipation, following surgery. (2) Loss of muscle tone through disuse, illness, stretching and obesity.

General signs and symptoms

(1) Lump. At first may only appear on straining, later may be persistent. (2) Impulse in lump on coughing (contents of sac momentarily increased) unless hernia is irreducible or strangulated.

Pathology

Abdominal hernia: pouch of peritoneum (hernial sac) pushed

through opening. Inside of pouch is continuous with abdominal cavity therefore abdominal contents (omenta, small or large bowel) can pass into sac. Mesentery and blood vessels accompany bowel into sac. Orifice may enlarge so that it is never too tight. Sometimes sac enlarges as it lies beneath the skin but the orifice remains the same size. Neck of hernia becomes tighter, may constrict (1) lumen of gut, causing obstruction, and (2) blood vessels, causing strangulation, gangrene, perforation. Immediate surgical correction needed to prevent latter results.

Types of abdominal herniae

Reducible. Contents of sac may be returned to abdominal cavity by manipulation.

Irreducible. Contents cannot be returned due to adhesions or narrowing at neck of hernia. Incarceration occurs when oedema results and viscera cannot be replaced.

Strangulated. May quickly follow above when arterial blood supply to sac occluded.

Common sites of abdominal herniae

Inguinal. Most common site is inguinal canal. More common in men than women.

Anatomy. Inguinal canal: oblique tube-like canal through anterior abdominal musculature 1½ in long, superior to medial half of inguinal ligament. Formed by: external oblique muscle, anterior wall; inguinal ligament, floor; conjoint tendon of transversus and internal oblique, roof; internal oblique, posterior wall. Inlet to canal from abdominal cavity − internal abdominal ring through transversalis fascia and internal oblique muscle. Outlet − external abdominal ring through aponeurosis of external oblique muscle. Transmits ilio-inguinal nerve and spermatic cord in males, round ligament in females.

TYPES. *Direct (acquired)*. Sac passes through inguinal canal, emerges beneath skin. Rarely passes into scrotum.

Indirect (congenital). Sac passes through inguinal canal inside spermatic cord and enters scrotum. Such herniae are often 'sliding', i.e. a viscus (commonly colon) actually forms part of wall of sac. Usually large herniae and difficult to reduce.

Femoral. Most common type in females. Occurs through femoral canal.

145

ANATOMY. Funnel-shaped tube of fascia (femoral sheath) passes between inguinal ligament and innominate bone. Divided into 3 compartments by septa of fibrous tissue. Lateral and middle compartments occupied by femoral artery and vein. Medial compartment usually empty or contains lymph nodes. Compartment known as femoral canal — conical in shape, ¾ in long, mouth (femoral ring) wider in women than in men, forms weak spot in abdominal wall.

Sac forced through femoral ring, down femoral canal. Becomes superficial by passing through gap in fascia through which long saphenous vein joins femoral vein and then turns up and back on itself in front of inguinal ligament.

SPECIAL SIGNS AND SYMPTOMS. Urinary symptoms — dysuria, frequency, haematuria — may precede palpable evidence of hernia.

Umbilical. *Congenital.* Failure of closure of fascial ring at umbilicus. More common in dark-skinned races, more often female than male (2:1). Often spontaneous closure at about 3 years, neither helped nor hindered by treatment (reduction and pressure applied — sponge rubber pad strapped to umbilicus or special belt worn). Adhesions and strangulation rare hence surgical treatment uncommon.

Acquired (para-umbilical hernia). Adults. Weakness in wall below umbilicus. Occurs most commonly in elderly obese females with a history of multiparity and/or chronic cough. This type of hernia usually large, more prone to incarceration, strangulation.

Epigastric. Rare; occurs almost entirely in linea alba between xiphoid and umbilicus. Mainly contains small fatty mass from falciform ligament of liver. Pain may sometimes be confused with peptic ulcer or cholelithiasis. Majority — irreducible and require surgery.

Ventral (incisional) hernia. (p. 27.)

Diaphragmatic hernia. May result from trauma or from wide oesophageal opening.

Treatment

Conservative. If patient poor operative risk, obese, has incurable cough, or umbilical hernia in children: (1) Reduce hernia by position and manipulation; place foot of bed on blocks;

icebag may be suspended over swelling. In inguinal and femoral herniae hip slightly abducted, slightly flexed. Doctor attempts to return contents of sac to abdomen with gentle pressure. (2) Truss (surgical appliance which supports weakness in abdominal wall to prevent further escape of contents). Can only be applied if hernia reducible otherwise may compress and damage contents. Ineffective in femoral hernia as contents are trapped by inguinal ligament.

Surgical. Treatment of choice. Essential if hernia obstructed or strangulated. Strongly advised if hernia irreducible.

PRE-OPERATIVE PREPARATION. Correction of cough, obesity or prostatomegaly.

Physiotherapy. Deep breathing and abdominal exercises — to correct existing weakness and prepare patient for post-operative period. Patient discouraged from smoking for several days before and after operation.

Bowels. Bowel action before going to theatre — suppository or small enema if necessary.

Skin preparation. Prepare whole abdomen. Shave pubic hair. Prepare donor area of thigh if fascia to be taken for repair.

OPERATIONS. *Herniotomy.* Hernial sac exposed and opened, contents returned to abdominal cavity, sac removed. Inguinal hernia in babies.

Herniorrhaphy. Herniotomy plus repair and strengthening of muscular weakness by 'darning' with nylon or braided silk, or by inserting patch of nylon tricot, or by sewing with steel wire.

Hernioplasty. Herniotomy and herniorrhaphy but repair effected by means of 'living sutures' — strips of fascia from thigh.

POST-OPERATIVE CARE. Specific.

Position. Semi-upright to prevent strain on wound.

Scrotal support. Supported with either cotton wool or suspensory bandage to reduce oedema.

Dressings. Support wound. Undisturbed until sutures removed 8—14 days.

Exercises. As well as leg and chest exercises special abdominal exercises to strengthen without putting strain on operation area.

Ambulation. Patient may sit out of bed on first day of herniotomy only. After herniorrhaphy — opinions vary — patient may have to stay in bed 1—2 weeks.

147

Retention of urine. Common complication. If ordinary nursing measures fail subcutaneous injection carbachol 0.25—0.5 mg or catheterization under strict aseptic conditions.

Bowels. Full diet as soon as possible. Mild aperient, suppository or small enema if bowels not opened 3 days after diet commenced. Patient must not become constipated and strain at stool.

Activity. Patient must avoid all straining such as lifting, pushing or jerky movements for at least 2 months. Normal activity, e.g. walking, beneficial — increases tone of muscle wall.

COMPLICATIONS. (1) Retention of urine. (2) Vomiting (due to increased abdominal pressure with return of contents to abdominal cavity). (3) Haematoma amd oedema of scrotum. (4) Orchitis. (5) Recurrence. (6) Haematuria due to rare complication of suture needle penetrating bladder.

Strangulated hernia. As for acute intestinal obstruction (p. 115).

SPECIAL INVESTIGATIONS

X-Rays
PLAIN ABDOMINAL (STRAIGHT ABDOMINAL)
To demonstrate air and fluid levels in bowel and presence of radio-opaque calculi or foreign objects.

INDICATIONS. Bowel obstruction. Biliary or renal calculi.

PREPARATION. Usually none necessary. Done as an emergency. Bowel clearance if calculi suspected (see barium enema below).

BARIUM
Contrast medium of high atomic weight. Absorbs X-rays, therefore radio-opaque. Given as barium sulphate in water. Patient assured that taste is not unpalatable (chalky with faint vanilla flavour).

PREPARATION. All medicines containing heavy elements stopped 6—12 hours before, e.g. bismuth, magnesium trisilicate (appear as opacities on radiograph, may give false picture).

ACTION. Pass through bowel unchanged showing filling defects and irregularities of outline, e.g. from ulcer, neoplasm, diverticula, hour-glass stomach.

CONTRA-INDICATIONS. (1) Perforation of gut. (2) Bowel obstruction (water will be absorbed and inspissation of barium may turn obstruction from incomplete to complete. (Gastrografin, a water-soluble iodine salt, may be used if obstruction present.)

Barium swallow. X-ray of oesophagus.

INDICATIONS. Oesophageal stricture, neoplasm, achalasia, foreign objects, diverticula.

PREPARATION. Nil specific. Patient should be able to stand (ensure he has slippers before going to X-ray department). Occasionally an oesophageal washout required if oesophagus dilated above an obstruction and contains stagnant food.

METHOD. Patient stands in front of X-ray machine and swallows barium sulphate. Its passage down oesophagus is seen on screen. Permanent X-rays taken from time to time.

Barium meal. X-ray of stomach and intestines.

INDICATIONS. Peptic ulcer, neoplasm, stricture, pyloric stenosis.

PREPARATIONS. Mixtures containing heavy metals stopped 12 hours before. Nothing to eat or drink for 6 hours.

METHOD. Similar to barium swallow. If follow-through needed X-rays are taken at intervals throughout day and sometimes 24, 48 and 72 hours later.

Barium enema. X-Ray of colon.

INDICATIONS. Ulceration, neoplasm, stricture, diverticula.

PREPARATION. Aim is to ensure colon free from faeces and gas. Methods vary. Low residue diet 48 hours. Aperient, e.g. castor oil 15 ml, Duralax 2–4 tablets for 2 days. Cleansing of lower bowel – suppositories, enema, bowel washout (last 2 may leave bowel in spastic state with pockets of unexpelled gas and fluid). Elimination of flatus. Encourage ordinary activity during previous 24 hours. Occasionally injection of pituitrin 30 minutes before. Restrict food, fluids and heavy metals for 9 hours before.

METHOD. Patient lies on screening table. Barium sulphate instilled by enema. Watched on screen and permanent X-rays taken at intervals. Catheter removed. (Patient may complain of feeling of fullness but procedure takes only few minutes, patient can then go to lavatory.) Plain film may be taken afterwards.

AFTERCARE. (All barium X-rays.) Bowel actions observed

to ensure clearance of barium sulphate. Aperient, e.g. liquid paraffin, or small enema or suppository may be needed.

ENDOSCOPY

Oesophagoscopy. Direct examination of oesophagus through oesophagoscope.

INDICATIONS. *Diagnostic.* Stricture (may show retained food, fluid, size and signs of inflammation); neoplasm, biopsy may be taken; oesophageal reflux, especially due to hiatus hernia; varices; cardiospasm. Removal of foreign body.

Treatment. Insertion of Souttar's tube; implantation of radium.

CONTRA-INDICATIONS. Inflammatory lesions of mouth, pharynx or oesophagus. Aortic aneurysm. Spinal deformities.

PREPARATION. Fast 3–6 hours. Aspirate stomach contents only if (1) severe dysphagia, (2) vomiting, to prevent regurgitation of stomach contents and inhalation of same.

METHOD. General anaesthetic usual. Muscle relaxants given to prevent spasm. Endotracheal tube passed. Position: shoulders brought to edge of table. Head rests on special attachment so that neck extended to straighten oesophagus. Oesophagoscope tested and inserted gently. Force never used as oesophagus easily damaged. Forceps passed for biopsy specimen or removal of foreign body.

AFTERCARE Routine post-anaesthetic care. Nil specific. If local anaesthetic used: nil orally for 2–3 hours. Observations for complications: perforation of oesophagus; haemorrhage, especially following biopsy; aspiration pneumonia; oedema causing stricture, e.g. after biopsy or removal of foreign body; oesophagitis. Report – persistent sore throat, dysphagia, chest pain, dyspnoea, cough, pyrexia, signs and symptoms of shock or haemorrhage.

Gastroscopy. Direct examination of gastric mucosa with gastroscope.

INDICATIONS. *Diagnostic.* Peptic ulceration; gastritis; neoplasm; pyloric stenosis; strictures.

Investigations. Size of ulcer or neoplasm; rate of healing of ulcer; type of gastrectomy to be performed.

CONTRA-INDICATIONS. As for oesophagoscopy.

PREPARATION. Nothing by mouth 6 hours before. Intra-gastric tube may be passed and stomach contents aspirated. Pre-operative medication, e.g. Omnopon 10–20 mg or morphia 10–15 mg (to allay anxiety, promote relaxation), atropine 0.25–1 mg (to minimize flow of saliva). Local anaesthetic either sprayed or swallowed. (Occasionally done under general anaes-thetic if operation contemplated following gastroscopy.) Procedure carefully explained – may be uncomfortable and unpleasant but not painful.

METHOD. Position: lies on left side with arms in front and knees drawn up. Back support provided for added comfort. Head supported in straight line and patient requested to protrude chin. Tongue held forward.

Gastroscope lubricated with water-soluble jelly. Light tested. Swallowed by patient with surgeon directing passage. Air pumped into stomach to separate rugae. Walls of stomach examined. May take 15–30 minutes.

AFTERCARE. No food or fluid for 2–3 hours then sips of water. Observe for damage to oesophagus (p. |150)| or onset of infection.

Proctoscopy. Direct examination of mucosa of rectum with proctoscope.

INDICATIONS. *Diagnostic.* Neoplasm (biopsy may be taken); infection; sinus; fistula; fissure; haemorrhoids.

Treatment. Injection of haemorrhoids; removal of rectal polyp.

PREPARATION. Usually performed in ward. Bowel prepara-tion may be ordered. Screen bed, close adjacent doors and windows. Offer patient bedpan and/or urinal; bowels and bladder empty if possible. Explain procedure (may be embarrassing for patient). Warn patient that he may feel desire to defaecate but that there will be no involuntary emptying. Drape patient with small blanket for warmth.

METHOD. Position – Sims', left lateral or knee-chest. (Lithotomy in theatre.) Proctoscope warmed, lubricated and inserted into rectum with obdurator in position. Obdurator removed. Illumination may be provided with a light incorporated into the proctoscope or by doctor wearing a headlamp or by an adjustable spotlight. Cleansing of rectum may be necessary with swabs held in long forceps. Examination made, treatments performed, proctoscope removed.

AFTERCARE. Cleanse anus of lubricant or faecal matter and dry thoroughly. Leave patient clean, dry and comfortable.

Sigmoidoscopy. Direct examination of mucosa of upper rectum and pelvic colon with sigmoidoscope.

INDICATIONS. *Diagnostic.* Neoplasm (biopsy); diverticulitis; ulcerative colitis.

Treatment. Removal of polyp.

PREPARATION. Usually none necessary. Desirable that patient should have bowel action. (Doctor may order enema and bowel washout in some cases. Ensure that all faeces and fluid removed before sigmoidoscope inserted.) Codeine may be given to reduce peristalsis. May be performed in theatre under general anaesthetic.

METHOD. Position: left lateral or Sims' with pillow under buttock. Knee-chest or lithotomy (used less). Sigmoidoscope tested, lubricated and inserted through anal canal with obdurator in place. Obdurator removed and eye-piece attached. Air blown into bowel via attached bellows to dilate area immediately in front of instrument.

Examination made. Faeces, mucus, pus removed using special long swab-holding forceps ('alligator'). Biopsy may be performed. Sigmoidoscope removed gently.

AFTERCARE. Clean anal area. Observe for possible complications. (1) Perforation of bowel wall resulting in peritonitis (more likely to occur if bowel wall diseased or weakened). (2) Haemorrhage (after biopsy).

OTHER SPECIAL INVESTIGATIONS

Test meal. Examination of gastric contents before, during and after administration of gastric stimulant.

INDICATIONS. Peptic ulceration (increased hydrochloric acid secretion. May also show red blood cells). Carcinoma of stomach (reduced or absent hydrochloric acid. Cancer cells may be detected by special staining technique). Achlorhydria: congenital or acquired, e.g. pernicious anaemia. Pyloric stenosis (increased resting juice and delayed emptying).

SUBSTANCES. Stimulate gastric secretion. Carbohydrate

meal: gruel (30 g oatmeal in 1 litre of water boiled to half volume and strained); alcohol (7%, 50 ml). Histamine: 0.25 mg by hypodermic injection.

PREPARATION. No food or fluids for at least 6 hours.

METHOD. Procedure carefully explained to patient. Intra-gastric tube passed. Water not given to assist passage of tube. Patient asked to expectorate saliva, not swallow it. Fasting contents of stomach aspirated and saved. Meal given and/or injection of histamine. 5 ml aspirated ½-hourly for 2 hours. Last specimen — completely empty stomach. Label specimens serially and take to laboratory at once.

AFTERCARE. Remove intragastric tube and give patient a meal.

Diagnex blue test. Exchange of hydrogen ions from hydro-chloric acid using a blue ion-exchange resin — Diagnex, which is then excreted in urine. If there is no hydrochloric acid there is no exchange — negative test.

METHOD. Early morning urine specimen discarded. Two tablets of caffeine sodium benzoate given to stimulate acid secretion. One hour later urine passed and discarded. Diagnex granules given with 60 ml water. Two hours later specimen of urine collected, labelled and sent to laboratory.

AFTERCARE. Give patient a meal.

Occult blood. Examination of stools with chemicals to determine presence of microscopic amounts of blood.

INDICATIONS. Peptic ulceration. Gastric neoplasm.

PREPARATION. To ensure accurate result patient should abstain from all red meat and green vegetables for 3 days (some controversy over need for this). Three consecutive specimens collected on 3 consecutive days if possible.

THE LIVER

RUPTURE
Cause

Crush injuries to lower chest and upper abdomen, severe blow to right side, penetrating injuries.

Signs and symptoms

With mild haemorrhage may be no signs and symptoms. Pain

153

made worse on breathing, tenderness, muscle rigidity in right upper abdomen, referred pain from diaphragm to top of right shoulder. Shock if haemorrhage severe. Peritoneal irritation and infection from blood and bile. Slight jaundice often appears in first few days but is transitory.

Treatment

With small laceration and no other injuries: conservative, rest in bed, warmth without overheating. Record vital signs ¼-hourly, report deterioration. Rest alimentary tract — nil orally, intra-gastric suction, intravenous replacement of fluids and electro-lytes. Accurate record of fluid intake and output. Prepare blood for transfusion when necessary. Blood tests: haemoglobin, haematocrit, white cell count.

Small wounds will cease bleeding (spontaneous haemostasis) in 6–8 hours.

Surgery. Indicated if other injuries sustained, e.g. rupture of right kidney, fractured ribs, or evidence of severe bleeding. Exploratory laparotomy and haemostasis achieved by either pressure, sutures or packing (usually absorbable). To prevent peritonitis drain tube usually left in situ, brought out through stab wound.

Post-operative care. Careful observations to detect early signs of haemorrhage or peritonitis.

ABSCESS

Causes

(1) Secondary spread from intraperitoneal sepsis, e.g. appendix abscess. (2) Amoebic abscess following amoebiasis.

Secondary spread

SIGNS AND SYMPTOMS. Malaise. Pain in right upper abdomen referred to top of right shoulder. Swinging temperature. Pallor. Leucocytosis. Jaundice, late sign.

DIAGNOSIS. May be confirmed by chest X-ray showing elevation of diaphragm.

TREATMENT. Aspiration and injection of antibiotics. Incision and drainage with care to avoid contaminating pleural or peritoneal cavities.

Amoebic abscess

SIGNS AND SYMPTOMS. Similar to above but usually preceded by history of dysentery.

DIAGNOSIS. Confirmed by amoebiasis complement fixation test. Proctoscopy necessary to determine if ulceration present.

TREATMENT. Conservative. Intramuscular injection Emetine 30–60 mg. Antibiotics. If no improvement — aspiration and if reddish-brown pus withdrawn trocar (14–16 gauge) inserted and abscess completely drained. Incision and drainage indicated only if this treatment unsatisfactory.

Complications of both types

1. Spread to pleura. Narrow space between chest wall and diaphragm becomes obliterated. This seals off pleural cavity and makes it safe for insertion of needle for aspiration.

2. Rupture into pleural cavity, pericardium, lungs, peritoneum.

HYDATID CYST

Cyst formed in liver following infestation with dog tapeworm (*Echinococcus granulosus*).

Source of infection

Echinococcus granulosus needs two hosts for life cycle. Dog to produce worm (about 5 mm long). Ova stage in domestic animals — sheep usually, or cow — or in man. Dog becomes infected by eating offal of infected animals. Man, sheep and cows infected by faeces of dog containing ova — pasture, infected water or vegetables.

Pathology

Ovum develops in intestines, penetrates intestinal wall; carried to liver via portal circulation. (70% stay in liver, remainder carried to lungs, heart, spleen, kidneys, bones or brain.) Embryo settles in tissues, becomes enclosed in layer of fibrous tissue. Cyst made of two layers — outer laminated membrane, inner germinating layer, centre contains clear fluid. Daughter cysts having similar structure may develop within mother cyst. Cysts contain immature heads of new tapeworms which may escape by spontaneous rupture of mother cyst or accidental rupture during surgery or trauma setting up widespread secondary cyst formation.

Growth of hydatid cyst very slow; may grow to size of tennis ball without producing symptoms. Evidence of infestation may not occur for several years after original infection.

Signs and symptoms

Usually indefinite. Symptomless swelling may be first manifestation. Aching pain in side referred to shoulder. Dyspepsia. Biliary colic and jaundice may develop if cyst ruptures into biliary passages. Leakage of hydatid fluid may cause allergic reactions — urticaria, gastro-intestinal disturbances, rarely anaphylactic shock. Rupture of large cyst into peritoneal cavity causes peritonitis.

Diagnosis

Confirmed by eosinophilia and positive Casoni test. Normal eosinophil level is 2–3% of white cells. May be raised to 20–30% because of allergic reaction. Casoni test — injection of sterilized hydatid fluid intradermally 0.1–0.2 ml. Local area of erythema and oedema denotes allergy to hydatid fluid and infers previous infection. 75%–95% accurate. Complement fixation test — more difficult but 100% accurate. X-ray. Calcification of cyst walls often occurs and this may be demonstrated.

Course of disease

(1) Parasite dies, fluid absorbed, walls of cyst calcify. (2) Growth of cyst, when presence noted — surgical intervention. (3) Complications: rupture into peritoneal cavity, pleural cavity, alimentary canal or biliary apparatus. Suppuration (rare) signs and symptoms of liver abscess as above.

Treatment

Only effective method — surgery. Cyst exposed, peritoneal cavity packed off with dark material so that any escaping daughter cysts may be easily seen and removed. Cyst aspirated of half its contents and incision made in liver overlying cyst. Cyst very carefully enucleated, intact if possible. Resultant cavity in liver closed completely. If fluid escapes from cyst, area may need to be drained for several days post-operatively. Exhaustive efforts made to remove all daughter cysts and scolices (immature heads).

Complications

(1) Shock: mainly anaphylactic from escape of hydatid fluid, (2) peritonitis, (3) haemorrhage.

NEOPLASM

Primary benign or malignant hepatic tumours rare.

Benign. Cavernous haemangioma. Commonest type. Presents below liver capsule as purplish, nodular, compressible mass. No treatment needed. Papilloma, adenoma and lipoma occur occasionally but do not require treatment unless causing obstruction in biliary ducts.

Malignant. Primary carcinoma.

Incidence

Rare in European countries but comparatively common in African and Oriental races. Primary in adults of 40–50 years but can occur in infancy and childhood. More common in males.

Possible contributory factors

Cirrhosis, malnutrition, parasites, chronic irritation, congenital defects.

Types

Hepatoma: liver cells. Cholangioma: intrahepatic bile ducts. Mixed: cholangiohepatoma.

Signs and symptoms

Late manifestation. Abdominal pain, enlarged liver, pyrexia.

Diagnosis

Confirmed by needle biopsy or open liver biopsy (p. 161). Should be differentiated from secondary carcinoma but sometimes difficult without exploratory surgery if primary source unknown.

157

Treatment

Exploratory laparotomy and if solitary tumour found to be firm — even if of considerable dimension — excision should be performed, i.e. partial hepatectomy. Haemostasis achieved by approximation and deep suturing of raw surfaces. Other growths usually difficult to remove.

POST-OPERATIVE CARE. Aimed at detection of early signs and symptoms of haemorrhage, peritonitis.

METASTASES
Types
Secondary carcinoma, sarcoma, melanoma. Common.

Treatment

Solitary firm tumours may be removed usually at same time as primary source, e.g. carcinoma of colon or other abdominal organ. Following partial hepatectomy liver insufficiency may result due to recurrence of growth and subsequent destruction of remaining liver tissue (7/10 destruction results in liver failure).

PORTAL HYPERTENSION

Raised venous pressure inside portal vein and its tributaries (normal pressure about 12 mm Hg).

Anatomy

Portal vein formed by union of splenic vein (which receives gastric, pancreatic and inferior mesenteric veins) and superior mesenteric vein.

Causes

1. Intrahepatic: cirrhosis (especially nutritional, alcoholic, posthepatic types). Infiltrating lesions: carcinoma (primary and secondary).

2. Extrahepatic, i.e. in portal vein or its tributaries — thrombosis, pressure from glands or tumour, atresia, right heart failure.

Pathology

When blockage develops body compensates by raising portal

pressure to overcome obstruction and developing collateral venous circulation. (1) Small vessels in vicinity of blockage dilate and carry blood to liver. (2) Other venous channels dilate to divert blood from portal to general circulation, commonest diversions — anal canal and rectal veins (into internal iliac veins), causing haemorrhoids; oesophageal and gastric veins (into azygos drainage of thorax), causing oesophageal and gastric varices. Collateral circulation may be so effective that portal pressure subsides to normal (thus accounting for patients who have oesophageal varices but normal portal pressure). If pressure unrelieved (1) spleen enlarges due to back pressure in splenic vein, (2) ascites.

Signs and symptoms

May be history of haematemesis, oesophageal varices, enlarged liver or spleen, thrombocytopenia, leucopenia, jaundice, ascites.

Investigations

Barium swallow, oesophagoscopy to detect oesophageal varices. Liver function tests. Prothrombin estimation and platelet count. Portal venography (contra-indicated if patient has bleeding tendency): splenic puncture and injection of contrast medium outlines splenic and portal veins. Portal pressure measurement: splenic pulp pressure may be measured at same time as splenic puncture and is satisfactory measure of portal pressure. Cardiac catheter may be passed via saphenous or cephalic vein, through vena cava into hepatic vein, pushed forward until it wedges; pressure within liver lobules measured. (When portal hypertension due to cirrhosis, splenic and liver pressures are equal, when due to obstruction in portal or splenic vein, splenic pressure raised and liver pressure normal.)

Treatment

Haemorrhage from ruptured oesophageal or gastric varices common presenting sign.

Conservative treatment. (1) Control haemorrhage from oesophageal varices (p. 100) and from stomach — local gastric hypothermia — circulation of 50% ethanol at $5°-15°C$, through intragastric balloon. If haemorrhage not controlled within 3–4 hours immediate surgery indicated. (2) Prevention of hepatic coma (results of absorption of breakdown products of haemoglobin from intestine). (a) Evacuate bowel by gastric suction and saline purge. (b) Sterilize bowel to prevent breakdown by intestinal bacteria — oral Neomycin 1 g hourly for 4 hours, 4-hourly for 2 days then 6-hourly as long as necessary.

Diet. Limit protein intake. High carbohydrate especially glucose.

Surgical. Indicated if conservative measures fail to arrest bleeding or if chronic ascites persists. If general condition satisfactory emergency shunt operation may be performed but mortality rate high (25—50%). Transoesophageal ligation of varices (i.e. via an oesophagoscope), followed several weeks later by elective shunt gives better results. Portal system vein anastomosis.

PRE-OPERATIVE PREPARATION (Specific).

Liver function tests: Should show acceptable hepatic reserve. Prothrombin estimation: As near normal as possible. Diet: 3,000 calories, low protein (0.5 g/Kg). Commercially available protein and amino-acid supplements may be used. Glucose fluids encouraged. Ascites: Drained as necessary. Low sodium diet — diuretics — thiazide therapy with or without Spironolactone. Therapeutic doses of vitamins C, K and B complex. Anaemia corrected as necessary with whole blood or packed cell transfusion.

SURGERY. *Portocaval anastomosis.* Most successful shunt. End-to-end or side-to-side anastomosis of portal vein and inferior vena cava. Provides a wide anastomosis with only slight risk of later obstruction by thrombosis.

Splenorenal anastomosis. End-to-side anastomosis of splenic to renal vein. Indicated if portal vein blocked. The drop in pressure resulting from this operation is less owing to smaller size of veins. Greater risk of thrombosis which will close the shunt.

Cavamesenteric anastomosis. Inferior vena cava divided as low as possible and upper end turned forward and anastomosed to side of superior mesenteric vein. Satisfactory in children when portal vein blocked as splenorenal veins too small.

POST-OPERATIVE CARE (Specific). Prevent or minimize liver failure (common complication). (1) Intranasal oxygen 6—7

1/min for 24–48 hours. (2) Minimum of 250 g glucose intravenously daily until oral intake tolerated. (3) Pre-operative vitamins continued.

Treatment of liver failure

1. Cease oral protein for short period then limit to 0.5 g/kg per day.
2. Increase glucose intake to 300 g or more daily.
3. Blood transfusion to maintain haemoglobin level.
4. Oral antibiotics as in conservative treatment to sterilize bowel.
5. Peritoneal dialysis may be used to remove blood toxins with which failing liver unable to cope.
6. Arginine therapy (hexose base amino acid which replaces ammonia in blood). Chief value – to tide patient over acute ammonia intoxication until gastro-intestinal ammonia production can be eliminated by saline catharsis, or sterilization with Neomycin. 500 ml 5% arginine hydrochloride in 10% glucose intravenously over 2 hours, repeated 8–12 hourly as necessary. Beneficial effect noted within 48 hours (usually ineffective in chronic hepatic insufficiency).

Other, more drastic, measures to control oesophageal varices

1. Obliteration of varices. Thoracotomy, with exposure of oesophagus which may be opened transversely or longitudinally. Varices sutured.
2. Obliteration of gastric varices by division of perioesophageal vessels. Thoracic incision extended to abdomen. Spleen removed. All vessels around fundus of stomach divided. Stomach divided 5 cm below oesophagus and resutured.
3. Oesophagogastrectomy. Only indicated when all other methods have failed. Lower 1/3 oesophagus and upper 2/3 stomach excised and continuity restored with anastomosis.

These are palliative procedures only as they do not remove cause of portal hypertension.

SPECIAL INVESTIGATIONS
Liver biopsy
Removal of liver tissue for microscopic examination.

Indications. Neoplasm; jaundice when diagnosis obscure after several weeks' investigation: cirrhosis, when biochemical tests normal but liver and spleen enlarged: reticulosis, 70% of patients with Hodgkin's disease have liver involvement, biopsy indicated when other routine investigations not conclusive.

Methods. OPEN TECHNIQUE. At operation. Small piece of liver removed from lower edge. Wound in liver closed with sutures and abdomen closed without drainage.

NEEDLE TECHNIQUE. *Preparation.* Patient must be co-operative and have full control of respiration so that he can hold his breath while needle in liver, otherwise liver may be torn. Prothrombin time and platelet count. If necessary vitamin K given by intramuscular injection until normal prothrombin level reached. One litre blood crossmatched and held for 24 hours after procedure. Paracentesis abdominis performed if there is free fluid in peritoneal cavity.

Position. Recumbent, right side as near edge of bed as possible. Pillow in lumbar region on left side. Hands above head.

Needle. Convex shallow bevelled tip. Short nail inside needle to prevent biopsy being fragmented by forcible aspiration into syringe. Trocar and cannula may be used instead of needle.

Puncture. Skin prepared with antiseptic. Local anaesthetic infiltrated to subcutaneous tissue, pleural diaphragm, liver capsule. Small incision made, needle connected to 10 ml syringe filled with normal saline. Needle inserted down to intercostal space and 1–2 ml saline injected to clear needle of any tissue debris. Patient instructed to hold breath. Aspiration maintained while needle rapidly inserted into liver and withdrawn perpendicular to skin surface. (Needle should cross lower portion of pleural space or miss pleura completely. It will penetrate diaphragm.)

Aftercare. Patient remains in bed for 24 hours. May require analgesics, e.g. Pethidine 25–50 mg, for ache in right hypochondrium and tip of right shoulder. May lie on right side to diminish pain on respiration. Observe for – haemorrhage; pneumothorax; haemothorax; pleural effusion; biliary peritonitis; subphrenic abscess or haematoma; accidental damage, e.g. to colon or kidney.

Paracentesis abdominis

Puncture made through abdominal wall into peritoneal cavity to drain ascites.

Indications. Relieve strain on heart and respiratory embarrassment.

Conditions causing ascites. Portal hypertension (p. 158). Heart or renal failure especially chronic nephritis. Peritoneal tuberculosis. Malignancy of any abdominal organ.

Preparation. Shave abdomen if necessary. Morphia 10–15 mg to allay anxiety. Bladder must be empty (catheterization rarely necessary). Position: one of comfort, preferably recumbent but semi-upright if orthopnoeic. Extra blanket for warmth. Binder placed under patient so that it can be tightened as soon as fluid removed.

Method. Skin antiseptic applied. Small incision made if wide bore trocar and cannula used. Trocar and cannula inserted, trocar removed. Site – midline below umbilicus or outer border of rectus abdominis muscle. Cannula connected to drainage tubing (fluid removed rapidly except in heart failure). If several litres to be removed, tubing attached to drainage bag or bottle. Incision may need suture.

Aftercare. Binder tightened at frequent intervals. Observe – amount and type of drainage, measure, record: colour, temperature, pulse, respirations, general condition: (very rapid removal of large amount of fluid may cause shock, collapse). Change dressing as necessary: cannula withdrawn when drainage ceases. With repeated drainage large amount of protein lost, hence high protein diet given. (Occasionally intravenous serum albumin necessary to replace loss.) To prevent liver damage carbohydrates, especially glucose, given. Vitamin supplements. Fats restricted. In heart and renal failure restrict salt and fluids.

BILIARY SYSTEM

CHOLELITHIASIS (GALL STONES)

Stones formed in gall bladder. Composed of normal substances carried by bile – cholesterol, bile pigments, calcium carbonate.

Incidence

More common in 'fair, fat, fertile, females of forty or fifty', but may occur at any age (occasionally even at birth) and in both sexes (females: males 4:1) and in all physical types.

CAUSES

Metabolic. Excess breakdown of red blood cells produces pigment stones (small, hard, black, multiple). Associated with haemolytic anaemias and liver damage from toxic substances or disease.

Decreased production of bile salts results in inadequate excretion of cholesterol and formation of cholesterol stones (usually large, solitary, translucent, soft). Associated with dietary indiscretion, copious cholesterol intake. Excess sucrose intake has been found to decrease bile salt formation.

Pregnancy. Cholesterol related in chemical structure to some of the sex hormones. During pregnancy blood cholesterol rises with subsequent deposition in gall bladder.

Infection. Any organism may be responsible – *E. coli,* staphylococci, streptococci, fungi – commonly *Salmonella typhi* as gall bladder is focal point of storage in typhoid carrier.

Inflammatory reaction may cause physical disturbance in bile and throw cholesterol, bile pigments and calcium carbonate out of solution. Crystals aggregate to form stones. (Mixed stones show layering when cut. Usually multiple and soft. Often faceted.)

Stasis tends to allow stones to increase in size. Caused by blockage with calculi, infection, pregnancy and old age. In latter two, gall bladder does not contract properly.

Rare causes. Foreign objects, e.g. pips, skins, worms may work their way up common bile duct and solutes may precipitate around them.

Pathology

Formed in gall bladder. Rarely in bile duct. When stone enters cystic duct strong contractions of gall bladder occur causing biliary colic. Stone may return to gall bladder or may pass on to common bile duct. If remaining impacted in cystic duct, gall bladder may become infected (cholecystitis), develop pus (empyema of gall bladder) or remain free from infection but fill with mucus (mucocele). Stone in common bile duct may obstruct anywhere along its length or at the ampulla of Vater. If obstruction complete — cholecystitis, cholangitis, distension of gall bladder, jaundice, severe pain.

Jaundice. Bile prevented from entering duodenum. Stools become clay coloured, fatty and foul smelling. Bile transported by blood stream and deposited in tissues. Excreted in small amounts in urine which becomes dark and frothy.

Signs and symptoms

May have asymptomatic ('silent' gall stones). May have background of cholecystitis with vague indefinite symptoms of dyspepsia: nausea, flatulence, 'full feeling' in epigastrium. Usually aggravated by fatty foods and heavy meals. Biliary colic: severe pain right subcostal or epigastric region lasting minutes or hours. May be accompanied by vomiting and mild shock. May terminate if stone falls back into gall bladder or moves on into duodenum. May recur at intervals over several days. Local tenderness over gall bladder area. Jaundice due to obstruction of common bile duct or, more commonly, transient jaundice due to cholangitis.

Diagnosis

Confirmed by: (1) Radiology — plain abdominal X-ray shows radio-opaque stones. Deposition of calcium salts on stones gives typical ring shadows. (2) Cholecystogram — administration of oral radio-opaque (iodine) medium which is excreted by liver with bile and stored in gall bladder 12—24 hours after administration. Radio-transparent stones show up as filling defects in the dye-filled gall bladder. Emptying defect shown by failure to get rid of dye after giving a fatty meal. If gall bladder fails to visualize even after double dose of dye, chronic cholecystitis is suspected (recurrent infection damages mucosa and destroys its power to concentrate bile). (3) Cholangiogram. Intravenous administration of radio-opaque dye (e.g. Biligraphin) which, when excreted by liver, gives shadow on X-ray and ducts themselves are visualized. Radiolucent stones show as filling defect. (Neither of these X-rays are done during jaundice as danger of liver damage.)

Treatment

No effective medical treatment. Surgical removal of gall bladder and exploration and drainage of common bile duct as soon as possible after diagnosis. Palliative measure in 'poor risk' patients — drainage of gall bladder only.

Complications (without treatment)

(1) Biliary cirrhosis — prolonged common bile duct obstruction may cause severe liver damage or liver failure or portal hypertension. (2) Cholangitis. (3) Cholecystitis — acute and complicatons of this, see later. (4) Prothrombin deficiency. Bile is essential for absorption of vitamin K from alimentary tract. Vitamin K necessary for formation of prothrombin which is essential in the clotting process. Hence patient with obstructive jaundice may bleed profusely on injury or surgery. (5) Fistula — from gall bladder into duodenum or transverse colon. (6) Bowel obstruction. Gall stone ileus (p. 114).

ACUTE CHOLECYSTITIS

Sudden and severe attack of inflammation of gall bladder.

Causes

Infection — bile or blood stream. Commonly bowel organisms Stasis: blockage from calculi, fibrosis, dysfunction of normal emptying reflex, e.g. in pregnancy and old age.

Signs and symptoms

May occur spontaneously or follow biliary colic or be superimposed on chronic cholecystitis. Pain, becoming steadily more severe (oedema and tension in gall bladder): right subcostal region radiating to right shoulder (referred pain from irritation of diaphragm). Vomiting often severe and associated with pain. Tenderness and muscle guarding on palpation in right upper abdomen. Mass may be palpable, either tensely distended gall bladder or wrap of omentum attempting to localize infection. Pyrexia, usually mild $38°-38.5°C$. Respirations rapid and shallow due to irritation of diaphragm. Mild leucocytosis.

Possible course

(1) Resolution. (2) Pus formation — empyema of gall bladder.

166

(3) Spread – cholangitis, pancreatitis, liver abscess (rare). (4) Gangrene – perforation – peritonitis. (5) Become chronic.

Treatment

Conservative. Advocated by some because inflammation makes operation technically more difficult thus increasing risk of damage to common bile duct with resultant stricture and obstructive jaundice.

Pain relief. Intramuscular Pethidine 50–100 mg as necessary. (Morphia contra-indicated; thought to produce painful spasm of sphincter of Oddi.) Antispasmodics, e.g. Buscopan. Local heat: kaolin poultice to gall bladder area. Semi-upright position relieves tension on area. Self-lifting pole, 'monkey bar' to help patient to move without strain on abdomen. Avoid fats in diet: stimulates contraction of gall bladder thus causing pain in acute stages.

Control of infection. Sulphonamides or broad spectrum antibiotics most effective. (Some forms of penicillin not excreted in bile therefore ineffective.) Rest in bed until fever subsides. Copious fluids. If patient unable to tolerate oral route, rectal or intravenous route used depending on degree of associated dehydration.

Prevention of liver damage. Glucose fluids, avoidance of drugs, e.g. barbiturates which are detoxified by liver.

Relief of nausea. Anti-emetic drugs, e.g. Dramamine, Torecan 6.5 mg. Ryle's tube and aspiration if vomiting severe.

Observations. Accurate charting of fluid intake and output. Vital signs, especially temperature which might become swinging when pus forming. Stools and urine for onset of obstructive jaundice.

Surgical. Some surgeons perform emergency operation as soon as diagnosis established; claim that it saves patient hospitalization time, provides speedier cure and protects patient from complications that may occur without intervention (see above).

Indications (other than emergency as above). 6–12 weeks after acute attack when inflammation has settled. Frequent attacks of cholecystitis while awaiting surgery.

Complications. Empyema, gangrene, perforation.

Operations. Removal of gall bladder, exploration and drainage of common bile duct or drainage of gall bladder.

CHOLANGITIS
Inflammation of bile ducts.

Cause
Infection via bile or blood stream. Ascending from common bile duct obstruction.

Complications
Spread — liver ducts — liver — rarely liver abscess; gall bladder. Stone formation — desquamated epithelial cells, fibrin exudate, pigment and cholesterol sludge, may accumulate in ducts and predispose to stone formation.

Signs and symptoms
Constant nagging pain under right costal margin. Intermittent pyrexia and chills.

Treatment
As for cholecystitis.

CARCINOMA OF BILIARY APPARATUS
Gall bladder. Not uncommon. Associated with acute infection and gall stones. May spread into liver and duodenum. Invades and obstructs common bile duct.

Bile ducts. May arise in lining epithelium or in ampulla of Vater.

Signs and symptoms
Those of obstruction.

SURGERY
Types
Cholecystectomy. Removal of gall bladder. Kocher's incision. Cystic artery (usually a branch of the hepatic artery) and cystic duct must be ligated and divided. Because of numerous congenital anomalies in biliary tract great care taken to avoid damage to common bile duct or right hepatic artery. Gall bladder dissected from fundus downwards avoiding damage to liver. Gall bladder bed may be oversewn. Drain tube extends from gall bladder bed via stab wound in flank to drain into dressing.

168

Choledochostomy. Exploration and drainage of common bile duct.

INDICATIONS. (1) Definite stone in common bile duct as shown by cholangiogram or palpated during surgery. (2) Obstructive jaundice or episodes of transient jaundice. (3) History of recurrent biliary colic. (4) Dilatations or thickenings in wall of common bile duct. (5) Thickening of head of pancreas.

Choledochogram. Injection of radio-opaque material into common bile duct at operation before duct is opened, if there is doubt.

METHOD. Small incision made in duct and small sound or malleable probe passed to duodenum and up to liver. Stones removed.

Common bile duct is a fine tube and oedema and inflammation easily blocks it, hence drainage needed after surgery to prevent complete obstruction. Commonest method – 'T' tube. Inserted through incision. Proximal short arm extends to bifurcation of hepatic duct and distal short arm extends to ampulla of Vater. Long arm brought out through incision lateral to abdominal wound and drains into bag.

Cholecystostomy. Drainage of gall bladder.

INDICATIONS. 'Poor risk' patients in whom immediate decompression of gall bladder is necessary to prevent perforation.

Temporary measure only and followed by later cholecystectomy when patient's condition improves. Local or general anaesthesia used. Oblique incision parallel of right rib margin. Gall bladder opened, evacuated and closed round self-retaining catheter which is brought out through abdominal incision. Wall of gall bladder sutured to peritoneum and posterior rectus fascia to prevent bile leaking into peritoneal cavity.

Short circuit operations. *Choledochoduodenostomy.* Transplantation of common bile duct to an area higher up in duodenum. Indications. Carcinoma head of pancreas. Impacted stone in ampulla of Vater. Carcinoma of ampulla of Vater.

Cholecystogastrostomy. Anastomosis between gall bladder and stomach (or jejunum) as short circuit for bile in conditions where stone or growth cannot be removed from cystic duct.

Pre-operative preparation (specific only)

INVESTIGATIONS' *Radiology.* Plain abdominal; routine

chest **X-ray**; cholecystogram; cholangiogram; percutaneous transhepatic cholangiogram – may be performed on jaundiced patient. Needle inserted into liver (bile will be aspirated), dye injected and, with television monitor, outline and filling of ducts observed. This technique permits differentiation between stones and neoplasms.

Blood. Full blood examination (anaemia must be corrected where present); serum bilirubin if liver damage present; prothrombin estimation if jaundice present; serum **albumin/globulin** ratio (normally **albumin,**| made by liver, greater than globulin, made by body cells 4½ to 5:1½ to 3, in liver damage ratio reduced or reversed).

DIET. Reduced fat intake. Increased glucose fluids (glycogen content of liver impaired). Protein intake normal, but reduced in severe liver damage to rest liver. Vitamin C given in liberal amounts to assist healing.

PHYSIOTHERAPY. Ambulation encouraged. Deep breathing exercises taught and patient warned of importance of same postoperatively to prevent pulmonary complications. (Common, because of proximity of liver to diaphragm and patient's natural desire to limit pain by shallow breathing.)

SPECIAL POINTS – jaundiced patient. (1) Prevention of haemorrhage – vitamin K 10–20 mg daily intravenously or intramuscularly – for several days until prothrombin normal; calcium gluconate 10 ml 5% solution intravenously for 3 days. (2) Observations of skin, stools and urine colour. (3) Skin itch – avoid woollen clothing and overheating; cooling lotions, e.g. calamine; antihistaminic drugs if itch severe. (4) Careful choice of pre-operative medication and anaesthetic, avoiding those which are detoxified in the liver, e.g. barbiturates, ether, chloroform. (5) Ryle's tube may be inserted if vomiting is persistent.

Post-operative care

SPECIAL FEATURES. Preparation in addition to routine – gastric aspiration tray if Ryle's tube present; suitable receptacle for 'T' tube drain. Assess drainage from 'T' tube.

POSITION. On recovery from anaesthesia gradually elevated to semi-upright to aid chest expansion and relieve tension on suture line.

FLUIDS. Small quantities tolerated within few hours. Occasionally intragastric suction continued if peritonitis suspected. Intravenous infusion for hydration if vomiting continues.

DIET. Introduce as soon as tolerated — light diet graduating to normal usually within 1 week.

DRUGS. Anti-emetic, e.g. Torecan 6.5 mg; antibiotics especially in cases of cholecystitis; vitamin K 10—20 mg usually continued for several days until prothrombin level normal.

DRESSINGS. Main wound left undisturbed until sutures removed 7—10 days, unless evidence of infection or copious discharge.

DRAIN TUBES. *Gall bladder bed.* Large tube or corrugated-sheet draining haemo-serous material or little bile into dressing. Skin may need to be protected against excoriation by bile — barrier cream, zinc or silicone cream. Dressings changed frequently. Tube shortened and removed according to drainage 48—72 hours.

Common bile duct. 'T' tube draining bile into either (1) sterile glove — cuff tied round tube with tape, ends of tape pinned to binder; (2) bedside bottle — closed sterile bottle attached by connection and tubing to 'T' tube; (3) small (110—200 ml) flat-sided bottle — 'T' tube threaded through teat with enlarged hole and bottle fixed to binder.

Nursing management of 'T' tube. 1. Tubing. Avoid tension: bottle fixed to binder; tubing looped and attached to chest with adhesive plaster; length of tubing adequate to allow patient free movement; tubing attached to drawsheet with safety pin. Prevent kinking and blockage of tubing especially where tube enters bottle.

2. Drainage bottle: ensure adequate attachment. Empty when necessary.

3. Measure and record amount and type of drainage.

4. Observe stools, urine and skin to detect relief of obstruction; pain may be due to blockage of tube; leakage of bile around tube.

REMOVAL OF 'T' TUBE. Not before eighth day but may remain for as long as 3 weeks.

Physiology. Bile is extremely irritant to peritoneum. Adhesions form around tube so that when removed any further

171

drainage will drain via fistula into dressing and not into peritoneal cavity. Fistula heals quickly after removal of tube.

Indications. Patency of common bile duct. (1) Decrease in drainage. (2) Stools and urine normal colour and jaundice fading. (3) Tube clamped for 1 hour a.m. and p.m. of first day, 2 hours a.m. and p.m. second day. If no pain experienced and there is no gush of bile when clamp removed, duct is patent. (4) Choledochogram may be done. Radio-opaque dye is injected down tube and is observed under fluorescent screen as it passes into duodenum.

Tube removed by pulling straight out. It is *never* shortened daily as the short arms in the common bile duct must flatten out to be removed and would enlarge the hole in the duct if only partially removed. Small dressing applied over wound and fistula closes in 1—2 days.

CHOLECYSTOSTOMY TUBE. Drains into receptacle as above. Usually removed in 2 weeks.

Observations. Full blood count 48—72 hours; vital signs (routine) to detect early signs of onset of complications.

Physiotherapy. Deep breathing and leg exercises commenced as soon as consciousness returns: prevention of chest and vascular complications. Ambulation encouraged — patient out of bed next day and encouraged to walk short distances. Becomes more active each day until discharge in 2—3 weeks.

Loss of bile

From 'T' tube. Bile essential for absorption of intestinal contents especially fats, also contains products from haemoglobin breakdown and resynthesis, and electrolytes. If excessive amounts are being lost it may be necessary to replace this by (1) giving patient his own bile via intragastric tube, (2) giving synthetic preparations of bile.

Complications (Specific)

(1) Haemorrhage due to deficiency of prothrombin. (2) Biliary obstruction due to accidental damage, haematoma, abscess. (3) Liver failure. (4) Persistent biliary fistula when drain tube removed, due to obstruction in common bile duct. (5) Peritonitis due to leakage of bile — complications of same, e.g. subphrenic abscess. (6) Pulmonary complications due to interference in

region of diaphragm. (7) Post-cholecystectomy syndrome — recurrent symptoms similar to those before operation. Attributed to partial blockage of common bile duct by (a) post-operative stricture, (b) undetected stone, (c) spasm of sphincter of Oddi.

SPECIAL INVESTIGATIONS
X-RAYS

Cholecystogram. Organic iodine preparation administered orally, absorbed from intestine, excreted by liver and stored in gall bladder which is outlined on X-ray. Meal containing fat administered to stimulate contraction and demonstrate emptying of gall bladder, and outline of bile ducts.

Indications. Gall stones; cholecystitis; stricture of gall bladder; neoplasm of bile ducts.

Contra-indications. Kidney failure (medium also excreted via renal tract).

Preparation. Meal containing some fat at lunchtime day before. Evening before — no fatty foods. 10—12 hours before X-ray — 6 Telepaque tablets (iopanoic acid) with at least one glass of water to ensure complete disintegration. Nothing by mouth except water after this. Breakfast — black tea or coffee with sugar, fruit juice or water. May have enema shortly before X-ray to remove gas which may obscure gall bladder. Solubiloptin (propionic acid) may be given in fruit juice (to disguise taste) 1—2 hours before X-ray. Patient lies on right side for ½—1 hour (overcomes pylorospasm).

Method. X-ray taken in various positions. Fatty meal given and further X-rays taken within 5—35 minutes.

Toxic effects of media. Occasionally occur — nausea, vomiting, diarrhoea, dysuria, urticaria.

Intravenous cholangiogram. Contrast medium (Biligrafin) injected and excreted by liver.

Indications. To show extrahepatic ducts when gall bladder not functioning or absent.

Contra-indication. In severe liver damage or jaundice — will not be excreted effectively.

Preparation. Bowel preparation as above. Meal containing some fat 2 hours before to clear bile ducts.

Method. Intravenous injection given and substance should be demonstrable in bile ducts within 10—15 minutes, in gall bladder in 30—40 minutes and in duodenum in 45 minutes.

Toxic effects. As for cholecystogram but more commonly.

Choledochogram. Operative or post-operative cholangiogram. Direct mechanical filling of biliary tree.

Indications. Detection of biliary stones in ducts during surgery; testing patency of bile duct before removing 'T' tube after choledochostomy.

Methods. (1) During surgery — before removal of gall bladder. Fine polythene catheter inserted via fundus of gall bladder into cystic duct to common bile duct. (2) After choledochostomy — via 'T' tube. (3) Fine needle inserted into liver through anterior abdominal wall. Catheter introduced over needle which is then withdrawn.

Medium used. Water-soluble radio-opaque dye, e.g. Pyelosil.

THE PANCREAS

CONGENITAL FIBROCYSTIC DISEASE OF PANCREAS

Gland does not develop correctly and digestive ferments do not pass into gut. Meconium is not liquefied, causes intestinal obstruction (p. 114). Surgical intervention needed to relieve obstruction. Temporary colostomy established and closed when babe tolerates normal feeds.

ANNULAR PANCREAS

Abnormal placement of pancreas: surrounds duodenum.

Complications. Duodenal obstruction — may be mild and not manifest until adulthood or may require urgent surgical relief in early life; peptic ulcer; acute or chronic pancreatitis; biliary obstruction.

Treatment. Surgical: pancreas left intact; duodenum divided and upper portion anastomosed to jejunum. If peptic ulceration present: partial gastrectomy performed with choledocho-duodenostomy if biliary obstruction present.

PANCREATITIS
Acute

Inflammatory reaction of pancreatic tissue to presence of bile or active proteolytic enzymes.

Cause. Unknown. Thought to be due to: (1) Blood-borne infection, e.g. mumps virus, streptococci. (2) Increased intra-ductal pressure — pancreatic duct obstruction due to (a) stone in ampulla of Vater, (b) spasm of sphincter of Oddi, (c) following gastroduodenal or biliary tract surgery with increased pancreatic secretion after heavy meal. (3) Regurgitation of bile into pan-creatic duct.

Pathology. Pancreatic juice harmless while inside duct system. Extravasation into parenchyma of organ causes digestion of same. Release of proteolytic enzymes may be due to (1) inflammation and oedema resulting from infection or irritation by bile; (2) pressure within tiny ductules causing them to rupture.

Three possible results of enzyme release — (1) acute oedematous pancreatitis usually subsides after few days; (2) haemorrhagic pancreatitis — profuse bleeding in pancreas and leak of secretions into peritoneal cavity — often fatal; (3) chronic relapsing pancreatitis (see later).

Areas of necrosis result from tissue damage. Abscesses or cysts may form with sequestration of pancreas.

Enzymes diffusing into retroperitoneal tissue, mesocolon or even mediastinum, convert fatty tissue into a 'soapy' material. This results in characteristic yellow blotches — fat necrosis. If islet cells damaged — diabetes may result.

Incidence. Any age group — more common 30–50 years.

Signs and symptoms. ACUTE OEDEMATOUS PAN-CREATITIS. Pain: sudden onset, severe. Epigastrium referred to back and lower scapular region. Nausea and vomiting may accompany pain or, in later stages, may be due to paralytic ileus from peritonitis after enzyme leak into peritoneal cavity. Abdominal signs: tenderness over pancreas, mild muscle spasm, diminished peristalsis. Jaundice — mild, transient, due to blockage of common bile duct by oedematous pancreas. Vital signs: low pyrexia, slightly increased pulse rate.

ACUTE HAEMORRHAGIC PANCREATITIS. Profound shock — may be rapidly fatal. Exaggeration of above symptoms. Hyperglycaemia often.

Investigations. Full blood examination: marked leucocytosis, increased haemoglobin and haematocrit (haemoconcentration). Serum amylase level shows marked increase within 24 hours of onset. May remain elevated for several days or may return to normal within 24 hours. Urinary diastase output should rise proportionately — determined on two 1-hour urine specimens to estimate hourly quantitative excretion. Glucose tolerance test — detect early diabetes. Radiology. Straight abdominal — radio-opaque gall stones, calcification of pancreas, gas-filled loops of intestine — paralytic ileus. Pancreatogram — radio-opaque dye injected directly into pancreatic duct at operation — guides surgeon in relieving obstruction in duct.

Differential diagnosis. Cholecystitis; cholelithiasis; peptic ulcer; mesenteric thrombosis.

Treatment. CONSERVATIVE. (1) Intragastric suction to reduce need for pancreatic juice to be secreted. (2) Intravenous fluids. (3) Anticholinergic drugs to block vagal stimulation of pancreas: atropine 0.3—0.6 mg, Probanthine 15—30 mg, 4—6 hourly. (4) Pain relief: intramuscular Pethidine 50—100 mg (morphia avoided as said to stimulate spasm of sphincter of Oddi). (5) Insulin if hyperglycaemia evident. (6) In acute hae-morrhagic pancreatitis — resuscitation measures for shock. Transfusion for blood loss. (7) Diet. After 48—72 hours, small quantities of bland, low fat, fluids. If tolerated, remove Ryle's tube, increase feedings. Increase proteins to speed healing of pancreas.

SURGICAL. Indicated if (1) diagnosis in doubt; (2) acute haemorrhagic pancreatitis to prevent further tissue destruction where supportive measures failing.

Types of surgery. (1) Cholecystectomy may cure pancreatitis when cause is gall stones. (2) Choledochoduodenostomy — may prevent bile reflux. (3) Transduodenal sphincterectomy. Pancreatic and gall bladder ducts made to enter duodenum separately. Sphincter of Oddi split to achieve this thus preventing bile reflux up pancreatic duct. (4) Partial pancreatectomy.

Chronic relapsing pancreatitis

Series of relapses, i.e. attacks of acute pancreatitis with seemingly normal health between attacks until pancreatic damage severe.

Associated contributory causes. Alcohol. Malignant disease. Penetrating peptic ulcer. Hepatobiliary disease. Generalized atherosclerosis.

176

Incidence. More common in males (6:1) and about ⅓ are alcoholics.

Pathology. Repeated attacks of acute oedematous pancreatitis lead to progressive fibrosis, varying degrees of tissue destruction and failure of function. Prognosis usually poor unless surgery can prevent progressive fibrosis.

Signs and symptoms. Repeated attacks of acute pancreatitis lasting a few hours or up to 2 weeks. Anorexia, nausea, vomiting, flatulence and constipation are common. Glycosuria may be present.

Complications. Narcotic addiction common. Diabetes mellitus. Cyst or abscess formation. Jaundice. Peptic ulcer. Malnutrition steatorrhoea.

Investigations. As above. Other conditions (see differential diagnosis above) must be eliminated or treated.

Treatment. CONSERVATIVE. (1) Remove aggravating factors when possible, e.g. biliary tract disease, penetrating peptic ulcer, alcohol. (2) Diet. Non-irritating, low fat, low protein. Predigested protein supplements may be necessary. (3) Drugs. Replacement of deficient enzymes, e.g. Pancreatin 2 g, 8-hourly; supplementary vitamins and minerals − B complex, iron, calcium gluconate, to replace those lost in stools. Narcotics are best avoided. If sedation required − phenobarbitone 15−30 mg thrice daily or sodium amytal 15−30 mg.

SURGICAL. As for acute.

NEOPLASM

Benign. Rare. Adenoma of Islet cells. Tends to produce insulin causing spontaneous hypoglycaemia. Tumour can be removed.

Pseudocyst. Collection of pancreatic fluid in retroperitoneal space or lesser sac.

CAUSE. Rupture of pancreatic duct.

SIGNS AND SYMPTOMS. Follows trauma or pancreatitis. Epigastric pain. Epigastric mass, tender and tense. Anorexia, weight loss. Pyrexia, rigors may occur.

TREATMENT. Surgical. Drainage via de Pezzer catheter. Internal − cyst joined to loop of jejunum (cystojejunostomy).

Carcinoma
    Not uncommon.

Head of pancreas. Most common site (75%).

SIGNS AND SYMPTOMS. Jaundice due to blockage of common bile duct. Pain vague and diffuse in epigastrium; severe pain radiating to back indicates spread beyond pancreas.

DIAGNOSIS. May be confirmed by increased serum amylase and urinary diastase (blockage of pancreatic duct). Barium meal may show distended duodenal loop. Diagnosis usually late.

TREATMENT. Surgery.

Pre-operative preparation. Care of jaundiced patient (p. 165).

Operation. (1) Pancreaticoduodenectomy. Stomach divided at pyloric entrance. Pylorus, duodenum, head and body of pancreas and lower part of common bile duct removed. Restoration of continuity — anastomosis of common bile duct, stomach and main pancreatic duct stump into loop of upper jejunum. Only performed if tumour small and mobile. Five-year survival rate — only 10%. (2) Palliative. To bypass duodenum. Cholecystojejunostomy (p. 169). Gastrojejunostomy.

Post-operative care. Blood transfusion and vitamin K continued for several days. Routine care of severely shocked and ill patient.

COMPLICATIONS. Leakage from common bile duct and pancreatic duct anastomosis.

Body and tail of pancreas. (25%.)

SIGNS AND SYMPTOMS. None characteristic in early stages. Generalized symptoms of late carcinoma (p. 79). Pain in epigastrium radiating through to left lumbar region indicates spread.

TREATMENT. Resection possible only if no spread, but signs and symptoms rare until spread has occurred. (Usually fatal.)

SPLEEN

TRAUMA

Cause

Because of position, violent blow, crushing or penetrating injury needed to rupture normal spleen. In certain diseases, malaria, typhoid fever, spleen enlarged, more friable, may rupture on minimal trauma.

178

Clinical types

(1) Subcapsular: tear in splenic pulp without peritoneal tear. Haematoma forms. (2) Intraperitoneal haemorrhage: more severe trauma, blood pours into peritoneal cavity. (3) Delayed rupture: variable time up to 15 days following initial injury.

Causes

(1) Greater omentum may have localized bleeding in peritoneal cavity. (2) Subcapsular haematoma bursts. (3) Blood clot digested by escaping secretions from injury to tail of pancreas.

Signs and symptoms

Subcapsular. Pain. Tenderness in left hypochondrium. Unexplained anaemia.

Diagnosis. May be confirmed by X-ray which may show (1) diffuse haziness, absence of splenic shadow in left hypochondrium; (2) elevation of left diaphragm; (3) medial, downward displacement of stomach and left colonic flexure; (4) absence of renal and left psoas shadows.

Intraperitoneal. Pain and tenderness left hypochondrium referred to left shoulder (due to irritation of diaphragm). Signs and symptoms of internal haemorrhage, severe shock (p. 13). Mild generalized peritoneal irritation, usually accompanied by paralytic ileus. If enough blood collects in abdomen — shifting dullness may be heard on percussion.

Diagnosis. If in doubt — X-ray findings as above; abdominal paracentesis will recover fresh blood in 75% of cases.

Delayed. Signs and symptoms as above. Diagnosis may be missed if history of trauma not elicited.

Treatment

Severe haemorrhage, may be fatal unless immediate splenectomy performed. Conservative measures: as for ruptured liver (p. 154).

SPLENOMEGALY

Enlargement of spleen.

179

Causes

(1) Infections — malaria, typhoid fever, glandular fever, parasitic diseases. (2) Reticulosis (diseases of blood forming and reticulo-endothelial systems) including leukaemia and Hodgkin's disease. In both these causes splenectomy only performed if spleen so large that it causes restriction of abdominal and diaphragmatic movement. (3) Haemolytic anaemias.

Types

Congenital acholuric jaundice. Hereditary condition: red blood cells more fragile than normal, rapidly destroyed by spleen, resulting in anaemia and enlarged spleen. Jaundice from excessive amounts of bilirubin from haemoglobin of broken down red cells. Gall stones also formed (p. 163). Remissions and exacerbations characteristic of this condition.

Acquired. (1) Idiopathic, possibly auto-immune condition. (2)

Secondary to poisoning by toxic agents (lead, sulphonamides) or malignancy.

Treatment

Blood transfusion in acute stage. Splenectomy usually cures symptoms.

THROMBOCYTOPENIC PURPURA

Spleen also destroys platelets (thrombocytes). Thought to be an auto-immune process in most, if not all, cases. Platelets necessary for blood clotting. Therefore patient bleeds freely on slight injury, or may have spontaneous haemorrhages. In milder cases — spontaneous bruising, petechiae (otherwise asymptomatic skin rash). Spleen not enlarged. Condition may be improved by splenectomy.

SPLENECTOMY

Removal of spleen.

Indications. Rupture. Splenomegaly. Thrombocytopenic purpura. Cysts and tumours (rare). 'Wandering' spleen — has very long pedicle, floats free in peritoneal cavity, may become twisted on its pedicle. Portal obstruction.

Contra-indications. Pernicious anaemia. Thalassaemia. Sickle cell anaemia (unless haemolytic factor prominent). Poly-cythaemia. No particular pre-operative preparation; blood transfusion may be needed.

Operation. Left paramedian or subcostal abdominal incision common but thoracic approach gives direct access via diaphragm to splenic vessels. Precautionary drain tube left in splenic bed. If thoracic incision — underwater drainage necessary.

Post-operative care. (Specific.) Recognition and prevention of complications. (1) Chest complications especially pneumonia and collapse of left lung. Breathing painful therefore patient needs adequate analgesia and continuous encouragement to do deep breathing exercises. (2) Vascular complications, especially in thrombocytopenic purpura, prevented by early ambulation. (3) Hiccoughs — irritation of left dome of diaphragm. (4) Burst abdominal wound. If tail of pancreas damaged, liberates trypsin, digests sutures, excoriates skin. Should this occur suitable barrier cream applied to skin.

CERVICAL ADENITIS

Inflammation of cervical lymph nodes.

Cause. Spread of infection from scalp, ear, nasal or oral cavities. Most frequently occurs in acute or chronic tonsillitis.

Signs and symptoms. Depends on virulence of infection, location and source and whether pus has formed. Pain, tenderness and swelling in area underneath jaw. Cellulitis of neck (Ludwig's angina) may develop. Spreads from nodes towards larynx, causing dysphagia and dyspnoea. Severe case may develop oedema of glottis causing asphyxiation and necessitating tracheostomy.

Treatment. (1) May resolve spontaneously if cause removed. (2) Conservative. General measures (p. 40). Local measures: heat, e.g. plastine poultice, local cold applications to reduce oedema. Oral hygiene, because of pain on swallowing and natural tendency to keep jaw still, frequent mouthwashes necessary. (3) Incised and drained. Glove drain 3–5 days. (4) Aspiration. May be as effective as incision.

TUBERCULOUS ADENITIS

Infection of cervical lymph nodes with *Mycobacterium tuberculosis.*

Cause. Lymph-spread from adenoids, tonsils or gums or from lungs via blood stream.

Course. Inflammation goes through stage of exudation and may then heal spontaneously by calcification, or may proceed to caseation, liquefaction, cold abscess (p. 40) and sinus formation.

Treatment. (1) General measures against tuberculosis (p. 206). (2) Rest neck between sandbags or in plastic collar. (3) Aspiration and introduction of P.A.S. (4) Excision of infected nodes (rarely necessary with antitubercular drugs).

BLOCK DISSECTION OF CERVICAL LYMPH NODES

Removal of block of neck tissue including all upper and deep cervical nodes, internal jugular vein and sternomastoid muscle.

Indications. Carcinoma of tongue with metastases. Lymphadenoma and other generalized glandular disorders. Malignancy of lung, stomach, oesophagus or pharynx. May be removed for (1) diagnostic purposes, (2) curative measure, (3) palliative measure.

Pre-operative preparation. As for carcinoma of tongue (p. 90).

Post-operative care. Additional measures: (1) Position: neck must never be hyperextended or jerked (may break vessels and cause haemorrhage). (2) Observe for: haemorrhage, causes asphyxia if pressing on trachea (p. 18); infection (tracheitis, laryngitis) weakness and hoarseness of voice, cough. Infection may spread to mediastinum because of removal of protective tissues; surgical emphysema (p. 203); lung collapse — pleura extends into root of neck and may be damaged during surgery.

Sutures or clips removed 2—4 days because of rapid healing.

SALIVARY GLAND

SALIVARY CALCULI

Incidence. More common in submandibular glands than parotids (5:1).

Types. Single or multiple. Vary in size from 1 mm to several cm. Composed mainly of inorganic salts, e.g. calcium, phosphorus and often have central core of foreign material.

Signs and symptoms. Depends on size and site. Painful swelling aggravated just before eating. May subside in 1—2 weeks but will recur. Saliva, if infected, may show flecks of pus or may be thick frank pus. Palpation of duct may show one or more stones. Bimanual palpation may disclose stones in hilum of gland.

Diagnosis. May be confirmed by X-ray, radio-opaque stones show up. Sialogram: injection of iodized oil into duct with lacrimal syringe, or radio-opaque dye, e.g. Urographin, instilled via polythene tube.

Treatment. Removal of calculi. Duct dilated and stone 'milked' out or duct slit near opening and stone removed with forceps, or gland excised through incision in neck and oral stump of duct ligated.

NEOPLASM

Incidence. More common in parotids than others (10:1).

Types. 'Mixed' cell. Not malignant at first. Encapsulated but with finger-like projections penetrating lobules. Removal must be complete to prevent recurrence.

Signs and symptoms. Painless hard swelling usually in lower pole of gland. Occasionally tumour lies in deeper parts of gland and grows towards pharynx and palate.

Diagnosis. Confirmed by sialogram. Biopsy should not be performed because of danger of seeding to other tissues.

Treatment. Surgical removal of gland and good margin of surrounding tissues. Incision in front of ear to hyoid bone. Facial nerve identified and branches carefully dissected out and preserved but if it is malignant it is sacrificed. Radical neck dissection if secondary spread present.

Complications. Nerve damage. (1) Facial. May be temporary due to stretching. Develops in 1 to 2 days and recovers within 2–3 days. Permanent facial paralysis if nerve severed. Nerve graft may be performed. If not, possible facial structures supported with graft of fascia lata. (2) Auriculotemporal nerve syndrome. Thought to be due to regrowth of nerve fibres into cutaneous tissues. Consists of area of redness and sweating in front of ear. Usually minor inconvenience but may be severe enough to cause sweat to run down and drip from chin. Treatment – division of nerve.

Salivary fistula. Saliva may leak from wound. Usually temporary. Closes spontaneously.

THYROID GLAND

GOITRE

Enlargement of whole or part of thyroid gland which may or may not be accompanied by increase in production of thyroxine.

Types. *Non-toxic (simple) goitre.* (1) Occurs in women at times of normal increase in physiological activity, e.g. puberty and pregnancy. Evidenced by visible swelling in neck. (2)

Parenchymatous — due to prolonged deficiency in dietary iodine. Gland enlarges because of presence of increased T.S.H. produced in response to reduced output of thyroxine. Some areas become nodular because of degeneration as increase in size outstrips available blood supply. Common type of goitre in parts of world where iodine deficient in soil and water supplies. Can be controlled by adding iodine to table salt.

Surgery not usually indicated in non-toxic goitre unless: (a) pressure symptoms occur (dysphagia, dyspnoea, pressure of recurrent laryngeal nerve causing hoarseness of voice); (b) 'plunging' goitre-enlargement of retrosternal section. (Removed because great danger of pressure on trachea); (c) cosmetic reasons; (d) suspicion of malignancy; (e) development of hyperthyroidism; (f) haemorrhage of nodule.

Toxic. Characterized by excessive secretion of thyroxine. May arise in previously normal gland (Primary thyrotoxicosis, Graves' disease), or in gland already enlarged, usually nodular goitre.

Signs and symptoms. Gland enlarged, diffuse and smooth: Graves' disease or nodular in toxic nodular goitre. Hyperthyroidism: nervousness, irritability, tiredness, palms of hands sweaty and warm, increased tolerance to cold but intolerant to heat, loss of weight in spite of voracious appetite, fine tremor of hands and tongue, restlessness and quick movements. Exophthalmos (i.e. prominent eyes with widening of palpebral fissures produces a staring expression) due to oedema and later cellular infiltration of orbital tissues, thought to be caused by excessive secretion of T.S.H. hence thyroidectomy does not always cure the condition. Cardiovascular signs: tachycardia, atrial fibrillation and congestive cardiac failure may occur in older patients.

Investigations. B.M.R., serum protein bound iodine (P.B.I.) hormones T3, T4 and T.S.H. all raised. Cholesterol reduced.

NEOPLASM
Adenoma

Benign growth of glandular tissue. May be single or multiple. Usually slow growing and encapsulated. May or may not produce thyroxine. Complications necessitating surgery: (1) malignant change; (2) hyperthyroidism; (3) haemorrhage; (4) pressure symptoms.

Malignancy

Incidence. All age groups. Most common over 40 years.

Onset. Primary, in previously unaffected gland or from benign nodule.

Signs and symptoms. Painless firm nodule. Pressure symptoms and recurrent laryngeal nerve paralysis may be first presenting symptoms. These indicate wide spread. Spread may be rapid depending on type of carcinoma, e.g. papillary type: slow spread and high cure rate. Follicular type rapid spread via blood stream especially to bones and brain, also via lymph channels. Undifferentiated type: rapid spread and does not take up radio-active iodine, mortality high.

THYROIDITIS
Hashimoto's disease

Rare disease confined to women over 40 years.

Cause. Unknown. Thought to be an auto-immune condition in which patient becomes sensitized to own thyroglobulin.

Signs and symptoms. Enlarged thyroid gland — diffuse, bilateral non-tender swelling. Occasionally causes pressure symptoms, mild myxoedema (p. 190).

Treatment. Thyroid therapy. Pressure symptoms — splitting of isthmus, subtotal thyroidectomy may be necessary.

Riedel's struma

Extremely rare condition of unknown aetiology. Fibrous tissue invades gland causing it to enlarge and tighten across isthmus thus producing symptoms of tracheal pressure and myxoedema. Gland feels fibrotic and hard and is slightly enlarged often unilaterally only.

THYROIDECTOMY
Pre-operative preparation for thyrotoxicosis

ANTITHYROID DRUGS. One of the following: Methyl thiouracil 0.2—0.6 gm daily. Carbimazole (Neo-mercazole) 20—40 mg daily. Potassium perchlorate 0.2—2 gm daily. Used until patient becomes euthyroid. Lugol's iodine 15—30 minims daily given to patient for 2 weeks prior to surgery. This reverses high vascularity and sponginess caused by previous antithyroid drugs and makes gland firm and hard. Beta adrenergic blockade slows tachycardia, reduces anxiety. Admission 1—2 weeks prior to surgery for (1) complete mental and physical rest, (2) familiarize patient with surroundings and staff to reduce anxiety, (3) allow time for investigations.

INVESTIGATIONS. In addition to those for thyrotoxicosis: (1) Chest X-ray to detect any intrathoracic extensions. (2) Blood grouping and crossmatching. (3) Sleeping pulse (raised in thyrotoxicosis helps determine degree of anxiety).

DIET. Increased calories (to keep up with increased metabolic rate). Avoid excess protein to keep down ammonia and urea formation. Copious fluids to reduce toxicity and prevent post-operative urinary and vascular complications.

SEDATION. Essential to ensure complete rest.

EYES. In severe exophthalmia there is danger of damage to cornea if eyes do not close completely. Care taken with bedclothes, towels, etc. Drops instilled to prevent dryness, e.g. castor oil drops.

Operation

Position. Recumbent with sandbag placed under shoulders and head extended to throw neck forward.

Infiltration. Some surgeons infiltrate skin and neck muscles with adrenaline to minimize bleeding.

Incision. Transverse 1—2 in above sternum. Follows natural crease in neck.

Removal. Gland located, blood vessels isolated, gland rolled to midline. Inferior thyroid vessels and recurrent laryngeal nerve preserved. Amount of gland removed depends on condition: 4/5 usual for thyrotoxicosis, occasionally only 1 nodule, whole gland for malignancy. Left behind: enough gland tissue to prevent myxoedema, the parathyroid glands, recurrent laryngeal nerves. Muscles loosely sutured.

Wound closure. Michel clips for skin. Drain tubes brought out at either end of wound. Laryngoscopy may be performed to ensure correct functioning of vocal cords.

Post-operative care, specific

Preparation. Bed in quiet part of ward. Pillows covered with mackintosh. 'Goitre tray' beside bed (for prompt treatment of asphyxia due to haemorrhage). Tray contains Michel clip remover, scissors, artery forceps, suture material.

Position. Neck must not be hyperextended during the unconscious stage. On recovery, patient gradually elevated to upright position with neck well supported.

Observations. Routine and special for detection of complications (see later).

Fluids. Rectal or intravenous may be necessary for first 24 hours if there is dysphagia.

Diet. Light diet as soon as dysphagia abates and patient tolerates fluids. Progress as rapidly as possible to normal diet.

Drugs. Lugol's iodine continued in decreasing amounts for 10—15 days. May be given rectally or orally (is mild gastric irritant). Routine analgesia according to severity of pain. Sedation usually continued at night.

Dressing. Observed carefully for presence of blood. Drain tubes removed 24—48 hours. Skin clips 48—72 hours.

Ambulation. Out of bed in 1—2 days.

Complications

1. **Reactionary haemorrhage.** Rare, because of dressings bleeding may not be evident until haematoma sufficiently large to cause pressure on trachea. Gland highly vascular and blood pressure high in gland owing to proximity to heart and great vessels. Haematoma may form rapidly.

Treatment. Prompt action to relieve pressure and prevent asphyxia. Doctor should be summoned at once, but if not available nurse must take action. (1) Proceed quickly and quietly without panic. Screen bed. Give morphia if this has been ordered. Sit patient in upright position. (2) Remove dressing and skin clips. This may be sufficient to relieve pressure but occasionally bleeding occurs behind infrahyoid muscle. If pressure unrelieved, remove muscle sutures and dislodge any clots. (3) Patient may require oxygen. (4) Prepare patient for return to theatre where cause of bleeding will be corrected and sutures replaced. (5) If prompt relief not forthcoming doctor may perform tracheostomy.

2. **Thyroid crisis.** Should not occur with careful pre-operative preparation. Presents within 48 hours of surgery and is due to massive release of thyroxine during surgery. Is prevented by ensuring quietness during immediate post-operative period, continuation of Lugol's iodine and ensuring adequate sedation.

Signs and symptoms. Restlessness indicating rising nervous tension, excitement even to delirium. Rising pulse rate, tachycardia, atrial fibrillation. Rising temperature, sudden onset progressing to hyperpyrexia. Sweating. Faster respirations. Unconsciousness.

Treatment. (1) Sedation to control restlessness. Morphine or chlorpromazine. (Larger than usual doses required because of increased metabolic rate.) (2) Control of hyperpyrexia — tepid sponges, electric fans, cold packs, iced fluids, copious amounts of glucose fluids. (3) Digoxin or Lanoxin for atrial fibrillation. (4) Lugol's iodine orally or rectally. (5) Oxygen tent may be needed.

3. **Tetany (hypoparathyroidism).** Parathyroid glands situated behind thyroid gland (often buried within thyroid tissue in goitre). May be damaged, bruised or accidentally removed during surgery.

Signs and symptoms. 2–7 days post-operatively. Often vague. Muscle weakness, irritability, numbness (pins and needles) or cramps in extremities. Muscle spasm — carpopedal spasm of hands and feet.

Diagnosis. Trousseau's sign positive: sphygmomanometer cuff placed round arm and if blood calcium level is low, muscles go into spasm. Tapping facial nerve as it emerges from skull behind ear causes twitching of facial muscles (Chvostek's sign). Serum calcium level determined.

Treatment. Emergency — intravenous injection of calcium gluconate 10%, 10–30 ml. Must be given slowly as rapid infusion to patient receiving digitalis may result in cardiac arrest. If spasms difficult to control — parathyroid extract 100–200 units until critical period has passed.

4. **Infection.** Of wound: may cause cellulitis of neck in severe case. Stitch abscess or granuloma. Tracheitis: treated with moist inhalations.

5. **Respiratory obstruction.** Causes: haemorrhage as above; laryngeal oedema; tracheal collapse; bilateral laryngeal nerve

damage — may be bruised or stretched. If unilateral, hoarseness results which gradually decreases as nerve recovers or as laryngeal function compensates for paralysed cord. Bilateral obliteration of nerves will necessitate permanent tracheostomy (p. 191).

6. **Myxoedema (hypothyroidism).** Occurs if too much gland removed.

Signs and symptoms. Weakness, fatigue, intolerance to cold, dry skin, falling hair (especially eyebrows), non-pitting oedema.

Diagnosis. Confirmed by lowered basal metabolic rate, reduced uptake of radioactive iodine, raised blood cholesterol.

7. **Malignant exophthalmos.** Following surgery there is a greater secretion of T.S.H. which aggravates exophthalmos. May endanger eye, e.g. corneal ulceration, limited ocular movements, blindness.

Treatment. Protect the eyes — dark glasses, eye shields, tarsorrhaphy (rare). Thyroid extract may be given in an attempt to reduce secretion of T.S.H. but must be carefully regulated by estimations of B.M.R. and is rarely successful. Orbital decompression occasionally necessary if eye continues to enlarge despite conservative treatment.

8. **Keloid scar.** Occasionally hypertrophied scar forms necessitating plastic surgery.

9. **Recurrence.** May occur if insufficient gland removed.

PARATHYROID GLANDS

HYPOPARATHYROIDISM (TETANY)
Occurs after accidental removal of parathyroid glands during thyroidectomy (p. 186). Rare otherwise.

HYPERPARATHYROIDISM
Oversecretion of parathormone.

Causes. (1) Adenoma (most common). (2) Hyperplasia. (3) Carcinoma of gland.

Signs and symptoms. (1) Excessive blood calcium and reduced blood phosphate, causing weakness, anorexia, nausea, vomiting, weight loss, generalized pain in joints and muscles, thirst, polyuria. (2) Excess calcium in urine. Predisposes to renal calculi. (3) Decrease in skeletal calcium. Soft spongy bones liable to spontaneous fracture, deformities and cyst formation.

Investigations. *Radiological.* Straight abdominal X-ray; intravenous pyelography; retrograde pyelography for renal outline and calculi. Skeletal survey for decalcification, pathological fractures and osteitis fibrosa cystica. Subperiosteal reabsorption of bone especially of hands and skull.

Blood tests. Raised serum calcium. Low serum phosphates. (Findings may be indefinite as levels constantly change.) Several specimens may be required. Serum alkaline phosphatase may be raised as a result of depleted blood phosphates.

Urine tests. Several 24-hour specimens to determine calcium and phosphate levels. Increased output expected.

Treatment. Surgical exploration if investigations are suggestive. Parathyroids located. Adenoma excised. In hyperplasia 3 glands removed and fourth subtotally resected.

Post-operative care. Transient tetany may occur 2—4 days after operation. Treatment, p. 189.

TRACHEOSTOMY

Artificial opening into trachea which may be temporary or permanent.

Reasons

1. To provide an airway in cases of (a) laryngeal obstruction — carcinoma; trauma, e.g. gunshot wounds, cut throat; impacted foreign objects; oedema of glottis following trauma, allergy, burns, e.g. from corrosive poisons; diphtheria (rare today). (b) Prior to surgery of tongue, larynx, jaw, when gross swelling anticipated. (c) Haemorrhage into subcutaneous tissues, e.g. trauma to throat, occasionally in reactionary haemorrhage after thyroidectomy. (d) Following laryngectomy or accidental damage to both recurrent laryngeal nerves, e.g. during thyroidectomy.

2. To improve ventilation and protect tracheobronchial tree from aspiration of secretions. Eliminates 'dead space' between trachea and nose in cases of hypoxia due to prolonged unconsciousness especially in head injuries; chest infections — chronic bronchitis, bronchopneumonia, emphysema; chest injuries especially where lungs bruised: cor pulmonale and patient too weak to cough up through dead space.

3. To provide effective positive pressure ventilation in chest paralysis due to head and spinal injuries; poliomyelitis; tetanus; myasthenia gravis.

Preparation. May be performed under local or general anaesthesia. May be emergency or elective. If elective, skin shaved from chin to midsternum.

Procedure. Position: recumbent with small pillow under shoulders to hyperextend neck. Head immobilized between sandbags or held by assistant. Skin prepared. Local anaesthetic injected. Incision usually vertical for emergencies, transverse in elective cases for cosmetic reasons. Bleeding controlled. Trachea opened. Skin and muscle retracted. Isthmus of thyroid gland moved or divided. Trachea drawn upward with sharp hooks and immobilized. Opening made between second and third or between third and fourth tracheal rings. Opening kept patent while secretions aspirated. Anterior section of one ring excised. Tube inserted and secured with tapes round neck. Incision closed round tube with sutures. Keyhole dressing applied.

Aftercare. Nurse in constant attendance to prevent asphyxiation. Physiology altered: air not warmed and moistened by nasal passages. Mucosa tends to become dry inhibiting cilial action and causing secretions to become viscid and tenacious. This may cause blockage of passages and atelectasis: cough reflex altered due to proximity to larynx and inability to close glottis; speech impossible unless tracheal opening closed.

ROOM AND EQUIPMENT. Air should be warm and relative humidity about 50%. Oxygen, suction apparatus, positive pressure respirator should be in room. Nebulizer or humidifier may be attached to tracheostomy or patient may be nursed in humid oxygen tent. By bedside should be bundles of sterile catheters (preferably with open ends and approximately half the size of the tracheostomy tube lumen); spare sterile tracheostomy tubes same size as one in situ; pair of tracheal dilators; bowl of 2% sodium bicarbonate solution to rinse used catheters and inner tracheostomy tube; forceps, swabs, scissors.

POSITION. Depends on conscious state. Lateral, well supported with pillows if unconscious, semi-upright to prevent chest complications if conscious.

Suction. Initially ¼–½ hourly or more often if there is

192

copious mucus. Later — as required and always before turning and after physiotherapy.

METHOD. Strict aseptic precautions. Nurse's hands washed and dried. Nebulizer removed. Mouth and pharynx aspirated and catheter discarded into sodium bicarbonate solution. Second dry sterilized catheter inserted into trachea with suction pinched off. Catheter passed gently until resistance felt (about 15 cm). If resistance felt before this, blockage has occurred and should be reported at once.

Suction performed by unclipping and gently withdrawing catheter with rotary movement. Irregular jabbing movements must not be used. Catheter discarded. If further suction required, fresh catheter must be used. Patient turned, if possible, and procedure repeated.

If mucus thick and sticky and difficult to remove a few drops of sterile water can be instilled into tube beforehand. (Sodium bicarbonate should not be used. It paralyses cilia and reduces effectiveness of natural defence system of upper respiratory tract.)

TUBES. Many varieties. Two main categories.

Metal inner and outer tubes. Outer tube secured by tapes around neck. Nurse must never remove outer tube. If it becomes dislodged accidentally, tracheal dilator inserted and doctor summoned at once. Nurses must never try to re-insert outer tube. Inner tube — removed for cleaning, hourly at first, and fresh sterile one inserted at once. Later interval increased 2—4 hourly and whenever necessary. If secretions thick, inner tube may be removed prior to suction and fresh one inserted immediately after.

Cuffed plastic tubes. Single tube with inflatable cuff — 2—15 ml — creates air-tight circuit. Ischaemia of tracheal wall must be prevented by deflating cuff 10—15 minutes each hour after aspirating pharynx and trachea.

TAPES. Knot placed where patient does not lie on it. Tied firmly enough to keep tube in situ but constriction avoided. Tapes may need to be renewed daily. New tapes secured before removing old ones.

DRESSING. Single layer petroleum jelly gauze applied around tube to prevent excoriation and flat split dressing round tube.

Opening must never be covered. Dressing changed when necessary.

SKIN SUTURES. Removed 5—7 days.

FLUID INTAKE. Orally if possible. Intragastric tube if unconscious. Care taken to ensure tube in stomach. Aspirated before each feed and pH tested. Rare complication — tracheo-oesophageal fistula. Any leakage from trachea during feeding reported immediately. Light diet may be started if patient conscious and tolerating oral fluids.

PHYSIOTHERAPY. If conscious, deep breathing exercises started at once and continued regularly. If unconscious, postural drainage and percussion to chest.

COMMUNICATION. Patient may learn to talk while cuffed tube deflated by occluding opening. Otherwise — pencil and paper supplied or slate and chalk, or signal system established, e.g. blinking eyes. Bell left with conscious patient with assurance that nurses will answer call immediately.

Removal. Patency of airway tested by placing spigot in metal tube. (Must never be done with cuffed tube while inflated.) Doctor removes tube. Small dressing applied until opening heals.

Complications. Chest: atelectasis, pneumonia. Surgical emphysema if tube does not fit adequately or if tube becomes blocked. Necrosis of trachea from cuffed tube or tube which is too long. Stenosis of larynx or trachea, aftermath of infection. Tracheo-oesophageal fistula.

Chapter 7

THE CHEST AND BREAST

SUPERNUMERARY NIPPLES
May have considerable amount of breast tissue beneath.

LOCATION. Below normal breast — line extending from middle of clavicle to middle of inguinal ligament.

TREATMENT. Excision if sore or unsightly.

INFECTION
Acute mastitis
Inflammation of breast tissue. Also used to describe other conditions (often hormonal) in which breast function impaired.

Causes. (1) Hormonal. (a) Increased maternal hormones can cause mastitis neonatorum. (b) Puberty. Usually resolves spontaneously in few days. (2) Infective. During lactation organisms enter from cracked or fissured nipples or occasionally along lactiferous ducts. Milk in breast favours microbial growth.

Signs and symptoms. Of inflammation (p. 38).

Treatment. (Specific.) Use breast pump rather than manual expression. Latter more likely to damage breast tissue. Breast feeding inadvisable during acute phase of infection — danger to babe. Treat cracked nipples with local application, e.g. tincture of benzoin compound. Support breast: suitable brassiere with sterile pad of cotton wool or many-tailed binder. Apply heat to area: soothes but may stimulate engorgement of breast. Cold local applications may relieve pain and congestion. Short-wave therapy may be beneficial in some cases not responding to other measures. Systemic antibiotics.

Prognosis. May resolve; suppurate and form breast abscess; become chronic.

195

Breast abscess

Cause. Result of mastitis during lactation. Common organisms: *Staphylococcus aureus,* occasionally *Streptococcus pyogenes.*

Signs and symptoms. Inflammation followed by swinging temperature and localized swelling which becomes fluctuant. General malaise.

Treatment. Conservative measures as above. Usually resolves with vigorous antibiotic therapy. Surgery necessary if pus forms.

(1) Aspiration with wide bore needle, instillation of local antibiotic. (2) Incision and drainage. If lesion slow to heal — irrigation and instillation of antibiotics.

Chronic mastitis

Causes. Result of acute mastitis or inadequately treated breast abscess. Specific infections: tuberculosis (often bovine type), syphilis, actinomycosis. Chronic cystic mastitis due to oestrogen activity. Premenstrual engorgement leads to hyperplasia both within and outside ducts. This may lead to blockage of ducts which in turn leads to cyst formation.

Signs and symptoms. May be exacerbations and recessions of inflammation or breast engorgement. Characteristic 'lumpiness' in breast on palpation; may be painful.

Treatment. Must be differentiated from carcinoma. If doubtful — surgical exploration, biopsy, removal of lump or affected section of breast.

Conservative measures. Reassurance that carcinoma is not present, wearing of tight brassieres day and night, avoidance of trauma.

NEOPLASMS
Benign

Fat necrosis. Hard lump of degenerated fat following injury.

PATHOLOGY. Injury breaks down some fat capsules and causes haematoma. Released chemical substances partly digest fat, producing irritant substances that cause inflammation which leads to development of fibrous tissue.

SIGNS AND SYMPTOMS. Hard painless lump appearing to be

attached to skin. Edges not well defined. If untreated — gradually disappears.

TREATMENT. Biopsy usually necessary to differentiate from cancer. Excision of lump.

Duct papilloma. SITE. In any ducts of breast. Most commonly near areola.

SIGNS AND SYMPTOMS. Vary. Blood, either fresh, or old and dark from nipple. Cystic swelling due to blockage of duct by growth.

TREATMENT. Surgical removal because papilloma nearly always undergoes malignant change. Usually whole segment of breast removed with tumour.

Fibroadenoma. INCIDENCE. Occurs usually between 16 and 30 years but may occur in later life.

SIGNS AND SYMPTOMS. Depending on proportion of gland to fibrous tissue. Lump may be either hard or soft. Size varies from pea to orange. Size tends to increase during menstrual period and pregnancy. Edges well defined. Freely movable. Painless.

TREATMENT. Usually removed because it tends to increase in size and cause pressure symptoms. Radical incision made over lump, capsule incised, tumour enucleated. Frozen section to determine absence of malignancy. Walls of cavity sutured, drainage tube left in situ, wound sutured. Drainage tube removed on cessation of drainage — usually after 48 hours.

Malignant

Carcinoma. INCIDENCE. One of most common malignant tumours in women between 30 and 50 years. Less common but more malignant in males.

SIGNS AND SYMPTOMS. 1. Lump: painless, freely movable with no clearly defined edge. Later, as growth infiltrates, may become fixed to overlying skin and underlying muscle.

2. Palpable axillary lymph nodes.

3. Nipple retraction or elevation (tumour attached to skin).

4. Skin reddened and oedematous (does not involve hair follicles). Looks like orange peel (peau d'orange) due to infiltration into subcutaneous lymphatics and skin itself.

5. Blood-stained discharge from nipple (cancer is intraductal).

6. Ulceration of skin.

Early diagnosis essential for complete cure. Any lump in breast assumed malignant until proved otherwise.

SPREAD. Accelerated during pregnancy and lactation. (1) Intraductal. (2) Infiltration to fascia, muscles and skin. (3) Lymphatic: axilla, neck, other breast, liver. (4) Blood stream: mainly from lymphatic involvement and close proximity of thoracic duct. Common areas for metastases: lungs, brain, liver, bones especially ribs, spine, pelvis, femur, humerus, skull.

TREATMENT. Depends on stage of disease.

Stage 1. Lump in breast only: mastectomy and either removal of, or radiotherapy to, axillary nodes.

Stage 2. Lump in breast and palpable axillary nodes: same treatment.

Stage 3. Lump involves skin and underlying muscle.

Stage 4. Distant metastases.

Stages 3 and 4: palliative treatment only – simple mastectomy, radiotherapy, cytotoxic drugs, hormone therapy or endocrine surgery.

Paget's disease of nipple. Carcinoma of nipple or areola and large mouths of lactiferous ducts.

INCIDENCE. 3% of all breast cancers. Age usually over 50 years. Males and females.

SIGNS AND SYMPTOMS. Nipple itchy and burning. May be accompanied by superficial erosion or ulcer (may be mistaken for eczema). Blood may be expressed from breast.

DIAGNOSIS. Confirmed by biopsy.

TREATMENT. As for ordinary carcinoma of breast.

Mastectomy

Radical. Skin incision 1 in round tumour. Nipple removed and incision extended into axilla and down towards midline. Skin flaps retracted over wide area. Pectoralis major reflected and pectoralis minor removed. Axillary lymph nodes, all axillary connective tissue and pectoralis major dissected out. Care taken not to damage nerve of Bell. Methods of drainage vary: large drainage tube with several holes cut into it placed down from axilla and brought out through lower stab wound, plus small corrugated tube at lower end of suture line. Wound may require skin graft to ensure adequate closure.

Extended simple. As radical but pectoralis major not removed.

Simple. Breast only removed.

Pre-operative preparations. (Specific only.) PSYCHOLOGI-CAL. Because operation is mutilating, patient assured that breast loss can be disguised by use of artificial breast made of either sponge rubber, birdseed or cotton wool.

INVESTIGATIONS. Include full blood examination, blood for grouping and crossmatching, chest X-ray to exclude metastases in lung, skeletal survey (to exclude metastases).

PHYSIOTHERAPY. Essential to prepare patient for post-operative period. Pain, or fear of pain, may limit breathing, arm movements and movement in bed.

SKIN PREPARATION. Extensive area. All front of chest from axilla to umbilicus and down affected side to elbow including axilla, and to midline of back. Area of thigh may need prepara-tion for skin graft.

Post-operative care. Specific.

Shock. Usually profound therefore all preventive measures important.

Arm. Supported, either sling, firm binder or pillow.

Position. On recovery from anaesthesia gradually elevated to semi-upright position and leaning toward affected side to facilitate drainage by gravity and to help prevent pulmonary complications.

Physiotherapy. (1) Chest and legs. Must be commenced im-mediately consciousness returns and continued regularly until danger of pulmonary and vascular complications has passed. Ensure adequate analgesia in early stages before starting exercises. (2) Arm. Usually wrist movements only for first 48 hours to prevent wound breakdown and reactionary haemorrhage. Arm and shoulder movements gradually introduced to prevent stiffen-ing and contracture, until by tenth day patient should be able to touch back of head with ease. Full range of movement may not be recovered for several months depending on amount of muscle tissue removed.

Wound care. Main complication − collection of blood and/or serum which may cause tension and breaking down of suture line. Two drain tubes, smaller drain into dressing, larger axillary drain connected to gentle suction to ensure adequate removal of blood and/or serum. Underwater drainage to prevent ascending infection. First dressing. In 24–48 hours when small drainage tube removed. May be necessary to float dressing off with normal saline if serous ooze has dried. Wound inspected carefully for tension or haematoma. When redressing, axillary drainage tube dressed separately so that main dressing may remain undisturbed until sutures ready to be removed in 8–10 days. If skin graft employed, dressing of donor area left undisturbed for 10 days. Axillary drainage tube, shortened daily and removed when drainage has diminished, from third to fourth day onwards.

Nursing care. Patient will need assistance in cutting meat, dressing, sponging, etc. until arm movements are satisfactory.

Prosthesis. At first brassiere is filled with cotton wool. Later, carefully made prosthesis containing either birdseed (similar weight to normal breast) or sponge rubber may be fitted.

Radiotherapy. (p. 80.) Will not be commenced until wound completely healed. Course usually lasts 6–8 weeks.

Medical checks. Essential for early detection of recurrence or metastases. Patients are advised to return to doctor every 2 months for 2 years, then every 6 months for 5 years and then every 12 months for 10 years.

Complications. (Post-operatively.) *General.* Shock. Haemorrhage. Pulmonary complications. Vascular complications.

Specific. Necrosis of suture line from tension delays healing and postpones radiotherapy. Damage (usually temporary) to nerve of Bell – results in winging of scapula. Lymphoedema from obstruction to veins draining arm and removal of lymph nodes. If arm becomes grossly enlarged and useless plastic operation may be needed to restore utility. Limited shoulder movements from scar tissue and contracture – prevented by vigorous physiotherapy as above. Recurrence.

PNEUMOTHORAX

Air in pleural cavity as a result of disease or injury. May be intrapleural, i.e. between the 2 layers of pleura (most common form), or extrapleural: between parietal pleura and chest wall.

Causes. TRAUMATIC. Due to open 'sucking' wound of chest wall or an air leak in injured lung. (1) Penetrating injuries – knife or bullet. (2) Fractured ribs following crush injuries or severe blows puncturing lung. (3) Surgical: thoractomy (p. 208). Accidental damage during abdominal or thoracic surgery or during injection of local anaesthetic into brachial plexus.

SPONTANEOUS. Due to tearing of visceral pleura. (1) Alveoli enlarge due to emphysema stretching pleura until it tears. (2) Cysts. Emphysematous blebs or bullae behave similarly. (3) Infections. Inflammatory process weakens and destroys small area of pleura: tuberculosis, pneumonia.

INDUCED. (Artificial.) Air blown into pleural space via a needle. Formerly used as treatment in tuberculosis to rest lung. Almost completely superseded by modern chemotherapy.

Types. CLOSED. (Simple.) Chest wall remains intact but air enters and leaves pleural cavity during breathing through hole in either the lung or the tracheobronchial tree.

TENSION. (Valvular.) With each inspiration air enters pleural cavity from lung through hole in visceral pleura, or from exterior through hole in chest wall and parietal pleura. During expiration soft tissues close hole and air cannot leave (valvular action). Affected lung gradually compressed against mediastinum. In severe cases, mediastinum pushed against opposite lung.

OPEN. (Sucking.) Air enters and leaves pleural cavity through hole in chest wall. As air is drawn in through wound, less air is drawn in through tracheobronchial tree. Vicious circle soon established − diminished air through normal passageway causes deeper inspirations, these suck more air through chest wound and less still through nose into lungs.

Signs and symptoms. Vary with amount of air entering pleural space. Pain in chest radiating to diaphragm and referred to shoulder or occasionally to abdomen. Diminution or absence of breath sounds on affected side. Diminished chest movements. Mediastinal flutter in open pneumothorax, with each inspiration mediastinum shifts to opposite side. Increasing dyspnoea, cyanosis and anxiety. Increasing percussion note becoming tympanic. Audible 'sucking' in open pneumothorax.

Diagnosis. Confirmed by X-ray.

Treatment. (1) Ensure chest wall intact − occlusive dressing placed over wound as a first-aid measure then wound closed surgically. (2) Aspiration of air. Small needle or trocar inserted through chest wall (usually second intercostal space) and small plastic tube or fine catheter may be inserted. Suction applied and continued until lung re-expands. Underwater seal drainage (p. 211) usually applied for 24 hours after lung re-expands and only when X-ray shows complete re-expansion, tube or catheter removed. May take 3–5 days.

Complications. Unless pleura thickened by inflammation or covered with blood clot, air in pleural cavity gradually absorbed.

1. Mediastinal displacement and compression of other lung. Indicated by tracheal displacement as palpated in neck, increasing dyspnoea, cyanosis, tachycardia, apical heart beat heard in abnormal position – in sixth or seventh intercostal space when right lung collapsed, on opposite side when left lung collapsed.

2. Infection. Causes – open wound, lung tissue damage, stagnation of fluid in pleural space.

3. Paradoxical respirations. Difficult to detect. Increasing dyspnoea and cyanosis. Air is drawn into unaffected lung during inspiration both from exterior in normal manner and from affected lung. During expiration air passes from unaffected lung to the outside and some into the affected lung. Thus respiration is occurring from one lung to the other and oxygenation is inadequate.

HAEMOTHORAX

Collection of blood in pleural cavity. (Haemopneumothorax: bleeding associated with air in the pleural cavity.)

Causes. From lung itself, from chest wall, from diaphragm or mediastinal vessels, e.g. aneurysm.

Pathology. Blood in pleural cavity slow to clot (movement of lung thought to remove fibrin thus keeping blood fluid). Blood also acts as irritant thus adding effusion fluid to blood in pleural cavity. As amount increases lung movements restricted. In time fibrin becomes organized to form a dense, inelastic skin of adhesions over lung surface preventing re-expansion.

Signs and symptoms. Depends on extent and any associated injuries. Shock may be present and severe. Dyspnoea and cyanosis usual.

Treatment. 1. Haemorrhage: rest, blood transfusion, oxygen and general measures to overcome shock (p. 15).

2. Re-expansion of lung. Immediate removal of blood (within

24 hours) by aspiration. Aspirations may need to be continued daily to prevent clot formation and thickened pleura. Pneumothorax apparatus may be needed during aspiration to adjust intrapleural pressure if it is desirable to maintain pneumothorax to keep lung partly collapsed.

3. Removal of blood clot. (a) Enzymatic debridement: injection into pleural space of fibrinolytic enzyme, e.g. Varidase, followed in 12–18 hours by complete aspiration. (b) Decortication: surgical removal of thick fibrinous skin formed over lung. Indicated if conservative measures fail (after 3–5 weeks' trial) or if infection present.

SURGICAL EMPHYSEMA

Air in subcutaneous tissues.

Causes. 1. *Thoracic injuries* – puncture wound in chest wall, air drawn in but unable to escape; pneumothorax, usually associated with fractured rib; tracheostomy, leakage of air round wound.

2. *Fractures* – where a puncture wound is involved, other than in chest wall, e.g. tibia, small amounts of air may be trapped in tissues.

3. *Gas-forming organisms,* e.g. *Clostridium welchii* forming gas gangrene.

Signs and symptoms. 'Crackling' sensation of skin on palpation (may cause pain). May spread rapidly especially from chest where continuous pumping action of respiratory muscles hastens process.

Treatment. Usually none required, as air absorbed, but underlying cause should be treated promptly.

PLEURAL EFFUSION

Accumulation of fluid in pleural space.

Causes. Infections: tuberculosis of pleura or underlying lung; pneumonia; lung abscess; small emboli; injuries to chest wall; subphrenic abscess; neoplasm of pleura or lung; heart or kidney failure with generalized oedema.

Signs and symptoms. Increasing shortness of breath. Dullness of chest to percussion. Pyrexia may be present depending on cause.

Diagnosis. Confirmed by X-ray and aspiration of fluid.

Treatment. Treat underlying cause if possible. Aspirate via Martin's syringe and needle (p. 215).

EMPYEMA

Collection of pus in pleural cavity.

Causes. *Acute.* (1) Spread of infection from lungs — pneumococci, staphylococci, streptococci, tubercle bacilli. (2) Blood-borne infections (rare). (3) Contamination as result of surgery or trauma.

Chronic. (1) Following acute. (2) Retained foreign body. (3) Osteomyelitis of rib. (4) Underlying disease of lung which prevents re-expansion.

Signs and symptoms. Vary with amount of pus, degree of lung compression and underlying disease. Chest pain, cough, dyspnoea, malaise, swinging temperature, general toxaemia, leucocytosis.

Diagnosis. Confirmed by percussion and X-ray.

Treatment. General measures to overcome toxaemia (p. 45).

Antibiotic therapy. Systemically and occasionally locally, i.e. injected into pleural space after withdrawal of pus. Culture and sensitivity determine appropriate antibiotic.

Removal of pus. An empyema cavity will become sealed off by adhesions between the layers of pleura. Hence pneumothorax will not occur from treatment. Chest aspiration via Martin's syringe (p. 215) daily until only 50 ml can be removed on successive days. If pus too thick to remove via needle, self-retaining catheter introduced into cavity either by trocar or via small incision. Drainage via underwater seal apparatus. Open drainage — rib resection, large bore tube inserted into cavity, shortened gradually according to rate of healing and lung re-expansion. Decortication indicated — when infection uncontrolled by above measures; expansion of lung prevented by thick exudate. Combined with pulmonary resection when severe underlying lung disease present, e.g. bronchiectasis, lung abscess, fibrosis.

LUNG ABSCESS

Localized collection of pus within lung.

Causes. 1. Infection from pneumonia, bronchiectasis,

penetrating chest injuries, spread from perinephric or subphrenic abscess.

2. Obstruction by neoplasm in bronchus or lung, inhaled foreign object, embolus (from infection of clot or from resulting infarct).

Signs and symptoms. Mild pyrexia and malaise. Cough and pleurisy may be present. Slight haemoptysis indicating communication between abscess cavity and a bronchus. Contents of abscess may be expectorated — copious quantities of foul purulent sputum. Rapid development of clubbing of fingers.

Investigations. Full blood count reveals leucocytosis and lowered haemoglobin. Sputum examination for causative organism or cancer cells. Chest X-ray, tomography, bronchography. Bronchoscopy.

Treatment. CONSERVATIVE. Treat cause if possible. Antibiotics. Postural drainage. Physiotherapy to help patient cough up all purulent material. High protein diet with supplementary vitamins. Copious fluid intake. Correct anaemia. Bronchoscopy — to promote drainage in selected cases.

SURGICAL. Indicated if no improvement from medical measures within 10—21 days. (1) Drainage of cavity through large catheter inserted via bed of resected rib. (2) Segmental resection or lobectomy. (3) Pneumonectomy for carcinoma.

Complications. Rupture of abscess into pleural space. (Tension pneumothorax.) Massive haemoptysis. Blood-borne spread of infection to other parts including brain abscess.

BRONCHIECTASIS

Infection of lung characterized by distension and loss of elasticity of bronchi.

Pathology. If bronchus obstructed mucus will dam up distal to blockage and cause distension. Infection of stagnant fluid causes inflammation and erosion of bronchial walls. Fibrous tissue forms, and walls are permanently weakened. Increased pressure inside the bronchi, e.g. from coughing, or decreased pressure in tissues surrounding bronchi, e.g. from fibrosis, causes dilatations to occur in weakened sections.

Causes. Congenital defect of bronchial walls. Following childhood infections — whooping cough, measles, scarlet fever, primary tuberculosis, pneumonia. Inhaled foreign objects. Plugs of mucus. Neoplasm.

Signs and symptoms. Chronic cough with purulent sputum, more profuse on morning rising. Occasionally haemoptysis which may be severe. Repeated attacks of sinusitis and chest infections. Moist râles heard over affected areas. Clubbing of fingers in severe cases. General signs and symptoms of toxaemia.

Treatment. CONSERVATIVE. Postural drainage. Physiotherapy. Avoidance of respiratory infections and prompt treatment if they occur. Correction of associated conditions, e.g. sinusitis. Aerosol inhalations to aid free expectoration of sputum.

SURGICAL. Removal of affected segments in one or both lungs. Indications. Younger patient with disease confined to one or two lobes. (Operation may be performed up to 60 years but best results obtained in children.)

PULMONARY TUBERCULOSIS

Infection of lung tissue by *Mycobacterium tuberculosae.*

Cause. Primary infection by inhalation of organisms. Commonly affects apices of upper and lower lobes.

Signs and symptoms. None in early stages. Often detected during routine chest X-ray. Later cough increasing in severity and worse on rising. Sputum increasing in quantity and becoming purulent. Haemoptysis which may be severe. Anorexia, weight loss. Malaise. Night sweats. Moderate evening pyrexia in early disease. Swinging pyrexia in advanced disease.

Diagnosis. Confirmed by: (1) Positive Mantoux test. (2) Chest X-ray and tomograph. (3) Idientification of tubercle bacilli in sputum, collected during bronchoscopy, laryngeal swabbing, gastric lavage on waking. (4) Raised E.S.R.

Treatment. CONSERVATIVE. (Largely eliminates need for surgery.) Rest until temperature steady, appetite improved, weight increasing, E.S.R. falling. Chemotherapy – combinations of streptomycin, isonicotinic acid hydrazide (Isoniazid, I.N.A.H.), para-amino salicyclic acid (P.A.S.). (Sensitive pairs of drugs used to prevent emergence of drug resistant strains of tubercle bacilli.)

SURGERY. *Indications.* Failure of medical treatment after trial of 1–2 years. Persistence of positive sputum. Useless lung, e.g. severe fibrosis, persistent haemoptysis, secondarily infected.

Types. 1. Resection. (a) Wedge for small superficial lesion. (b) Segment, commonly for apical lesions. (c) Lobectomy for whole lobe. (d) Pneumonectomy for whole lung. (e) Pleuropneumonectomy – lung within the parietal pleura.

2. Collapse therapy – thoracoplasty. (Pneumothorax and phrenic nerve crush rarely performed now.)

Complications. Spread of disease occurs in 5–10%. Largely prevented by conversion of sputum from positive to negative pre-operatively.

NEOPLASM
Benign
   Rare. Differentiated from malignant by biopsy.

Malignant
   Primary carcinoma.

Incidence. More common in men than women (8:1). More common in 50–70 year age group but not uncommon after 30 years. Susceptibility greater in cigarette smokers and those resident in industrial areas where air polluted with fumes and smoke.

Signs and symptoms. *Early.* May be asymptomatic and remain 'silent' for years. Often detected on routine X-ray.

Later. Depends on size and site. May include cough with slight sputum often blood stained; clubbing of fingers may be an early manifestation; wheeze followed by atelectasis due to blockage of a bronchus; pleural effusion with blood-stained fluid if tumour close to visceral pleura; spread of tumour to nearby organs, e.g. to chest wall causing pain, phrenic nerves causing paralysis of diaphragm, recurrent laryngeal nerves causing hoarseness. General signs: malaise, loss of weight, cachexia.

Spread. Lymphatic – mediastinal, paratracheal and supra-clavicular nodes. Blood-borne metastases to brain, liver, adrenal glands, bones.

Investigations. X-ray – straight chest, tomogram, bronchogram, pulmonary angiogram. Sputum for malignant cells (not always reliable). Bronchoscopy with biopsy. Aspiration of pleural fluid for cells.

Treatment. CURATIVE. Resection – thoracotomy and pneumonectomy.

207

Contra-indications. Inadequate remaining healthy lung tissue, e.g. if emphysema present, or widespread involvement of both lungs. Poor general health. Evidence of metastatic spread. Inaccessibility, e.g. main bronchus or mediastinal organs involved.

PALLIATIVE. Radiotherapy, may relieve pain, cough or bronchial obstruction. Instillation of radioactive gold into pleural space for pleural effusion. Intravenous nitrogen mustard (Thiotepa, 5-fluorouracil).

Types of thoracic surgery

Thoracotomy. Incision into thorax for exploration.

METHOD. Posterolateral incision, rib resected, and thorax opened through bed of rib, or via intercostal space (fifth, sixth or seventh usually). Intercostal approach preferred because chest more stable post-operatively and pain less. Opening widened with rib retractors. Ribs above and below may be resected if very wide approach needed.

Decortication. Removal of thick fibrous pleura from lung.

INDICATIONS. Haemothorax. Empyema. Inexpandable lung.

CONTRA-INDICATIONS. Bronchiectasis. Active tuberculosis. Carcinoma. (May be done in these conditions if combined with other procedures, e.g. thoracoplasty, resection.)

METHOD. Thoracotomy as above. If empyema present, sac may be opened and contents removed by suction. 'Pell' appears pearly grey. Margins incised and stripped from lung surface by blunt dissection. Parietal pleura may be stripped from chest wall. Extent of stripping may be small, e.g. around an area of atelectatic lung, or extensive, e.g. around a whole lobe. Haemostasis achieved, one or more drain tubes inserted via stab wounds. Lung inflated by anaesthetist and thorax closed. Drain tubes connected to underwater seal drainage bottles.

Lung resection. INDICATIONS. Bronchiectasis. Lung abscess. Tuberculosis. Neoplasm. Severe crush injuries.

AMOUNT REMOVED. Wedge, segment, lobe, whole lung.

AIM. To conserve as much healthy lung tissue as possible while removing diseased section without cutting into it. Parietal pleura may be removed if disease active and patient's general condition satisfactory.

METHOD. Thoracotomy as above.

1. *Wedge.* Small diseased section excised between clamps. Cut edges oversewn.

2. *Segment.* Segments separated by avascular plane of cleavage. Each segment supplied individually by bronchus and artery (venous drainage usually shared between segments). Clamping of appropriate bronchus results in deflation of segment when rest of lung inflated. Segment removed. Small bronchus divided and ligated, large bronchus carefully sutured. Healthy lung tissue drawn up by sutures to cover raw area.

3. *Lobectomy.* Pleural adhesions especially on diaphragm and between lobes. Interlobular fissure opened down to hilum. Lobular vessels identified and dissected individually. Artery and veins ligated between clamps and severed. Bronchus clamped and divided as close to main trunk as possible. Stump sutured with interrupted, non-absorbable sutures and buried in flap of mediastinal pleura. Some surgeons prefer to seal stump of bronchus with muscle graft.

4. *Pneumonectomy.* Pleural adhesions divided. Hilar structures dissected free. Pulmonary vein ligated first to prevent circulation of emboli mobilized from tumour. Artery ligated and severed. Bronchus divided close to its bifurcation from the trachea and closed as above. Phrenic nerve divided on affected side causing elevation of that half of diaphragm with reduction of space after pneumonectomy. Space further reduced by thoracoplasty either during operation or at a later date. In some cases of carcinoma the pericardium may be opened so that a more radical excision may be done. Also, lymph nodes of mediastinum may be removed.

COMPLICATIONS. Spread of infection into adjacent areas or opposite lung. Infection of residual space. Bronchopleural fistula from leaking stump of bronchus.

Thoracoplasty. Permanent collapse of part or whole of lung by removal of 2 or more ribs so that chest wall falls inwards and compresses lung against mediastinum.

INDICATIONS. (1) Tuberculosis — active lesion, usually causing cavitation, and not responding to medical measures. (2) Emphysema — rarely indicated, may be combined with decortication. (3) Following pneumonectomy to obliterate dead space. (4) Hyperexpansion of opposite lung following pneumonectomy.

(5) Grossly fibrosed lung when pneumonectomy cannot be performed.

METHOD. (1) 'De-roofing'. For small area. Overlying ribs removed. Saucerized cavity remains. Packed with gauze and allowed to heal by granulation. (2) Periscapular incision. Scapula mobilized and retracted. Periosteum elevated and ribs removed from sternum to transverse processes. First to ninth ribs removed usually in 2 or 3 stages with 2 or 3 weeks between stages. Periosteum preserved and new ribs grow in collapsed position.

Complications. Spinal deformity. Uncertain effect on lung.

PRE-OPERATIVE PREPARATION FOR
THORACIC SURGERY

Aims. 1. Patient in best possible physical condition and free from infection.

2. Respiratory efficiency at maximum level. Existing infections treated with conservative measures, e.g. lung abscess, active tuberculosis, bronchiectasis, bronchitis, sinusitis, oral sepsis.

Diet. High calorie, high protein, supplementary vitamin C. Copious fluids to reduce toxaemia and keep lung secretion fluid.

Blood tests. White cell count to check on activity of infection. Haemoglobin level to detect anaemia (treated if present, to improve respirations). Grouping and crossmatching if blood loss anticipated.

Physiotherapy. (1) Breathing exercises to improve respiratory efficiency, to give patient confidence for post-operative stage, aid relaxation, expel secretions from lungs. Exercises should include controlled diaphragmatic breathing, localized unilateral chest movements (various areas inflated by pressure against hands on chest), deep breathing (inflating balloons may be useful), postural drainage, discouragement of ineffective coughing. (2) Shoulder, limb and abdominal exercises to improve circulation, prevent deep vein thrombosis, shorten convalescence by reducing muscle wastage, prevent spinal deformities. Good posture encouraged. Warned of danger of scoliosis. Prevented by keeping shoulders level and avoiding bending sideways (mirror placed at end of bed so that patient can observe and correct faulty posture).

Careful thorough explanations given of patient's role in

post-operative period. Practise administration of oxygen may lessen post-operative fear and increase cooperation.

During surgery. Anaesthesia light as possible. Muscle relaxants used and respirations controlled by anaesthetist. Thoracotomy causes lung to collapse. Pulmonary and circulatory insufficiency with hypoxia must be avoided. Suction tube passed into affected bronchus prevents 'spillover' of infected material into opposite lung.

POST-OPERATIVE CARE (SPECIFIC)

Preparation. Adequate pillows as patient will be nursed in semi-upright position. Equipment: underwater seal drainage with or without suction pump. Oxygen and suction apparatus. Sputum mug. Position: anaesthetist will not allow return to ward until patient conscious because of danger of respiratory or cardiac arrest. Elevated to semi-upright position as soon as condition permits. (Armchair arrangement of pillows forbidden because of danger of scoliosis.) Observations: routine for shock and haemorrhage. Asphyxia — careful observations of colour and general condition ¼–½ hourly. Oxygen not always required but at first sign of hypoxia oxygen must be given. Drainage — colour, amount (over 300 ml in first 6 hours must be reported), consistency observed and recorded.

Physiotherapy. Commenced on recovery from anaesthesia to achieve full aeration of lungs. Complete mobility of chest wall to prevent atelectasis. Two-hourly deep breathing when awake. Coughing and expectoration (analgesics may be needed beforehand and wound supported during effort). Postural drainage — physiotherapist instructs nurse and patient in this procedure so that it may be carried out regularly. Ambulation as soon as condition permits after removal of sutures and drainage tubes. Leg, arm, shoulder and abdominal exercises encouraged while remaining in bed. Caution needed in shoulder exercises for first few days (tension on suture line), but encouraged to clasp hands behind head and to comb own hair.

Drainage. CLOSED. Into underwater seal drainage bottle. Wide topped 2–3 litre bottle containing exact quantity (so that subsequent measurement of drainage accurate) of fluid which may be sterile saline or water, sodium citrate, Dettol 5%,

Formalin 40%. Fluid level marked with strapping. Bottle may be emptied daily or not until fluid near air outlet, but each day's level marked on bottle. (Amount, colour and consistency of drainage observed.) Bottle has tightly fitting stopper pierced by 2 holes. Through 1 hole passes long glass tube, its distal end 2 cm below fluid level in bottle, its medial end connected by tubing to patient's drain tube. Through other hole passes short glass tube to act as air outlet while bottle fills with draining fluid. Suction may be applied to this air outlet to aid drainage and help lung re-expansion. Level of fluid in long tube rises on inspiration and falls on expiration. If fluid fails to 'swing' tube blocked; possible causes: (a) clots or fibrinous exudate in tubing or glass connection (tapered variety of connector worst offender); (b) kinking, twisting or collapse of soft tubing (patient lying against tube, tube tucked in with bedclothes, compression from securing safety pin); (c) fully expanded lung pressing against intrathoracic end of drainage tube; (d) long glass tube pressing against bottom of bottle.

Dislodgement of tubing avoided by: (a) tubing sufficiently long to reach bottle and allow free movement of patient; (b) tubing attached firmly to patient's skin with strapping to prevent tension during movement; (c) tubing anchored to bedclothes with safety pin which encloses tubing but does not pass through it; (d) tubing not so long that it can trail on floor.

Tubing clamped close to chest and close to bottle with special tubing clamps (always at hand) before: (a) emptying bottle; (b) adjusting tubing; (c) raising bottle from floor (if this is necessary the bottle must be kept below patient's chest level to prevent siphoning of contents back into chest cavity). If tubing accidentally dislodged or disconnected, tubing must be clamped with fingers at once until tubing clamps can be applied. Clamping is a necessary emergency procedure that should be discontinued at earliest possible moment to prevent lung collapse.

Drain tube removed 24–48 hours. When X-ray shows re-expanded lung. Dressing prepared, e.g. petroleum jelly gauze and dressing pad. The moment drain tube withdrawn, dressing applied and held firmly in position with strapping or elastoplast. Some surgeons place a suture in position during operation and this is tied by second person while the drain tube is removed. Dressing

212

may be removed in 1–2 days when hole has healed. Sutures removed 6–8 days.

'OPEN' DRAINAGE. i.e. into a dressing. Occasionally used if space being drained is sealed off from rest of pleural space.

Drugs. Analgesics – sufficient to make coughing painless but not enough to depress respirations. Antibiotics – to prevent or treat infections.

Dressings. Removed when sutures due for removal 7–10 days. Drainage tube dressed separately.

Diet. Nourishing. Copious fluids.

Occupational and diversional therapy. If hospitalization to be prolonged, e.g. with tuberculosis, every effort made to prevent boredom.

Observations for complications. (1) Atelectasis. (2) Spread of original infection. (3) Pneumonia. (4) Empyema. (5) Broncho-pleural fistula – patient will suddenly cough up fluid sputum. Should lie on affected side to prevent flooding of sound bronchus, until surgical repair can be effected. (6) Haemorrhage or effusion. Detected by drainage. If drain tube has been removed there will be a mediastinal shift, rapid pulse and respirations, apex beat moved to sixth or seventh intercostal space. Immediate aspiration is necessary. (7) Tension pneumothorax due to air leak from cut lung surface. (8) Paradoxical respirations may follow thoracoplasty – chest wall on affected side drawn inwards during inspiration and pressed outwards during expiration – controlled by firm pressure over affected side and encouragement of diaphragmatic breathing.

SPECIAL INVESTIGATIONS
X-rays

Plain. X-ray of thorax without use of any contrast medium.

Indications. (1) Lung diseases: tuberculosis, pneumonia, emphysema, etc. (2) Thoracic injuries: pneumothorax, haemo-thorax, fractured rib, etc. Heart enlargement.

Preparation. Non-specific. Upper clothing removed as buttons, pins, etc. show on X-ray. Gown that ties at front worn. No strapping applied before X-ray of ribs (strapping may simulate linear fracture on X-ray).

Tomograph. Serial views focused at intervals of 1 cm from back to front and from side to side through lung substance.

Indications. Details of size and position of neoplasm or cavity. Demonstrates lung disease not evident on plain X-ray.

Preparation. As for plain X-ray.

Bronchogram. Contrast medium, e.g. Neohydriol, introduced into bronchial tree which is outlined on X-ray.

Indications. Bronchiectasis. Neoplasm. Lung abscess.

Preparation. Nothing by mouth at least 3 hours before to avoid danger of vomiting. If necessary, period of postural drainage (pus and sputum prevent proper filling of bronchi and coughing less likely).

Method. Throat anaesthetized by sucking anaesthetic lozenge or spraying with local anaesthetic. Radio-opaque fluid trickled over back of tongue. Position patient to spread medium evenly throughout bronchi. X-rays taken in different projections. (Alternatively local anaesthetic injected into front of neck and contrast medium injected directly into trachea via cricothyroid ligament.)

Aftercare. Nothing to eat or drink for 3 hours until effect of local anaesthetic has completely worn off (danger of inhalation of food or drink). Postural drainage to help eliminate contrast medium.

Bronchoscopy

Direct examination of tubes from larynx to bronchi via bronchoscope.

Indications. (1) Diagnosis: haemoptysis; unexplained cough; suspected neoplasm; bronchiectasis; pulmonary abscess; tuberculosis. (2) Treatment: removal of foreign body; biopsy or samples of fluid; reinflation of lung in atelectasis; introduction of radio-opaque substances.

Contra-indications. Upper respiratory tract infection; recent meal; laryngeal abnormalities (should be examined indirectly first with mirror).

Preparation. Nothing to eat or drink for 4 hours. Pre-operative medication, Omnopon 10–20 mg or morphia 10–15 mg to allay anxiety and relax patient. Atropine 0.25–1 mg to limit secretions. Usually done under local anaesthetic.

Method. Similar to oesophagoscopy. Trachea and bronchi

214

examined systematically. Right bronchus easy to enter but patient must turn head to right to enter left bronchus. Foreign objects can be removed with special forceps or by suction. Biopsy or specimen taken as necessary.

Aftercare. No oral food or fluids for 3 hours (local anaesthetic). Careful observations for complications. Oedema of glottis (report dyspnoea at once). Pneumonia (unless otherwise ordered patient nursed in left lateral position or modified Sims' position until anaesthetic has worn off, to minimize risk of inhalation of infected material).

Chest aspiration (paracentesis thoracis)

Removal of fluid or air from pleural space by means of needle introduced through intercostal space.

Indications. Relieve respiratory embarrassment. To collect specimen. Introduce drugs, e.g. antibiotic, cytotoxic drugs.

Conditions. Pneumothorax. Haemothorax. Pleural effusion. Empyema.

Preparation. Procedure carefully explained. Patient asked to warn doctor if about to cough (linctus or 'cough sweet' may be given). Patients warned not to move. Area shaved if necessary. Bed protected with mackintosh and drawsheet.

Method. Position: usually sitting up leaning forward over pillow on bed table. Unaffected side kept warm with small blanket. If needle to be inserted into side of chest, arm supported above head. Local anaesthetic injected. Special needle inserted and connected to a 2-way tap. Martin's syringe used to aspirate fluid and specimen saved. Drugs instilled as necessary.

If large quantity of fluid to be aspirated or if pus thick, Potain's aspirator may be used instead of syringe. Aspirant bottle has special stopper with 2 taps. Pump attached to one tap and air pumped out of bottle. This tap then turned off and tubing from needle in patient's chest attached to other tap. When this tap is opened partial vacuum in bottle draws fluid from patient's chest.

Needle withdrawn and hole painted with antiseptic (strapping and collodion avoided as they tend to keep area moist and delay healing).

During procedure nurse observes patient closely for signs of collapse. Patient must be kept warm.

Aftercare. Patient lies with affected side uppermost (prevents pus leaking along needle track causing sinus or abscess). Observe for complications. Haemothorax. Surgical emphysema. Collapse — too rapid or excessive removal of fluid may result in failure of body's compensatory mechanisms.

Chapter 8

THE CARDIOVASCULAR SYSTEM

THE HEART

CONGENITAL ABNORMALITIES
PATENT DUCTUS ARTERIOSUS

Failure of ductus arteriosus to close after birth.

Pathology. High aortic pressure forces blood through ductus into pulmonary artery causing extra strain on right side of heart which may fail. More common in girls than boys.

Signs and symptoms. Murmur, usually systolic at first, later becoming diastolic as well. Heard at second-third intercostal space to left of sternum. High pulse pressure (difference between systolic and diastolic pressure). Water-hammer or collapsing pulse.

Investigations. X-rays: enlargement of left atrium and ventricle, increased pulmonary vascular markings, expansile pulsation of pulmonary artery.

E.C.G.: normal or hypertrophy of left ventricle.

Complications. Heart failure. Subacute bacterial endocarditis.

Treatment. Surgical division or ligation of ductus.

COARCTATION OF AORTA

Narrowing of aorta, commonly at site of ligament between aorta and pulmonary artery (remnant of ductus arteriosus).

Pathology. Thought to be due to defect in closing mechanism of ductus arteriosus. Blood pressure high in head and upper extremities and low in lower parts of body. More common in boys than girls.

Signs and symptoms. Minimal in early childhood. Heart failure may occur in infancy. Older children: hypotension in lower parts of body, numbness of legs, popliteal pulse diminished or absent, evidence of increased collateral vessels in abdominal wall. Hypertension in upper parts of body — headaches, epistaxis, giddiness especially on bending forward.

217

Investigations. X-ray may show enlarged heart. Arteriography shows site of stenosis. E.C.G. usually shows left ventricular hypertrophy.

Complications. Heart failure especially in early infancy. Cerebral haemorrhage. Intermittent claudication.

Treatment. Surgery. Ideal age: 10–15 years when aorta has reached adult size. Excision of stenosed portion and end-to-end anastomosis. Arterial graft may be necessary.

ATRIAL SEPTAL DEFECT

Persistent patency of foramen ovale so that blood passed from right to left atrium.

Pathology. Oxygenated blood shunted from right to left atrium. May be associated with atrioventricular valve defects. In time increased pulmonary vascular resistance develops. More common in girls than boys.

Signs and symptoms. Growth may be retarded. Heart enlargement may cause bulge of left side of chest. Systolic murmur.

Investigations. X-ray: heart enlargement especially on right side, enlarged pulmonary vessels, small aortic shadow. E.C.G.: right ventricular hypertrophy (may resemble heart block).

Treatment. Open heart surgery and closure of defect, early unless marked pulmonary vascular resistance.

FALLOT'S TETRALOGY

Four defects — pulmonary stenosis, intraventricular septal defect, dextroposition of aorta so that it communicates with both ventricles, hypertrophy of right ventricle.

Pathology. Limited quantity of blood enters pulmonary artery because of its stenosis. Hypertrophy of right ventricle improves this but also shunts more blood into left ventricle and aorta. Aorta carries mixture of oxygenated and deoxygenated blood.

Signs and symptoms. Cyanosis as soon as ductus arteriosus closes (so-called 'blue baby'). Dyspnoea especially after exercise but may be continuous. Child may adopt characteristic posture — squatting on heels to facilitate breathing (increases blood supply to head and restricts it to legs). Cyanotic and fainting spells due to cerebral hypoxia. Clubbing of digits usually present by 2 years of age. Physically, but not mentally, retarded. Loud harsh systolic murmur.

Investigations. Haemoglobin reveals polycythaemia. X-ray shows 'wooden shoe' contour of heart: apex rounded and elevated above diaphragm. Pulmonary artery concave. Right ventricle enlarged. E.C.G.: marked predominance of right ventricle.

Complications. Heart failure. Untreated only 10% of cases reach adult life. Subacute bacterial endocarditis.

Treatment. Ideal age: 6—8 years if possible. Open heart repair of intraventricular septal defect and relief of pulmonary stenosis. Palliative measures — anastomosis of subclavian to pulmonary artery.

INJURY
CARDIAC TAMPONADE

Accumulation of blood or fluid in pericardial sac. Prevents adequate filling of heart during diastole.

Cause. (1) Small wound in heart, e.g. result of crush injury. (Large wounds cause rapid death from exsanguination.) (2) Acute pericarditis with effusion.

Signs and symptoms. Acute: pallor, sweating, cyanosis, dyspnoea, hypotension, distant or inaudible heart sounds, pulse weak, irregular or paradoxical (becomes weaker on inspiration), distended neck veins, unconsciousness or disorientation.

Investigations. Venous pressure elevated. Chest X-ray may show normal heart shadow. Fluoroscopy: diminished or absent cardiac pulsations, E.C.G. may be normal or show arrhythmias, or pattern similar to pericarditis.

Treatment. Position: semi-upright (because of dyspnoea). Morphia and oxygen as indicated. Blood prepared for transfusion. Aspiration of pericardium. Long needle inserted and fluid aspirated via 20—30 ml syringe and 2-way tap. If bleeding continues, thoracotomy and suture of heart.

Complications. Recovery rapid if patient survives heart wound. Occasionally — constrictive pericarditis.

INFECTIONS
ACUTE PERICARDITIS

Acute infection of pericardium usually with effusion.

Causes. Many. Infections: pneumonia, empyema, tuberculosis. Generalized oedema: carcinoma, uraemia, congestive cardiac failure. Allergy. Anticoagulant therapy. Trauma.

Signs and symptoms. Cardiac tamponade if fluid develops rapidly. Chest pain. Friction rub before development of fluid. General signs of infection if that is the cause.

Investigations. E.S.R. raised. X-ray: 'water bottle'-shaped shadow of the heart. Pericardial fluid examined in laboratory.

Treatment. Cardiac tamponade as above. Purulent pericarditis: systemic antibiotics, intrapericardial antibiotics. Drainage via extrapleural pericardiostomy.

CHRONIC CONSTRICTIVE PERICARDITIS

Reduction of diastolic filling action caused by adherent pericardium.

Cause. Result of inflammation of pericardium especially in tuberculosis. May follow rheumatic pericarditis or haemopericardium.

Pathology. Heart gradually compressed by thickening pericardium. In tubercular pericarditis, fibrous tissue may become hardened with lime salts so that heart encased in stony wall. Severe interference with heart's action results in inadequate filling during diastole and increased venous pressure. Cardiac tamponade.

Signs and symptoms. Dyspnoea. Generalized weakness. Abdominal distension. Tachycardia and paradoxical pulse. Low systolic blood pressure. Low pulse pressure. Pleural effusion. Enlarged liver. Ascites. Scrotal swelling. Ankle oedema.

Investigations. X-ray — pleural effusion, enlarged heart. E.C.G. diminished amplitude.

Treatment. Pericardiectomy if diagnosis made early enough. Palliative: thoracic and abdominal paracentesis.

MITRAL VALVE STENOSIS

Narrowing and stiffening of mitral valve due to contraction of scar tissue.

Cause. Most commonly a sequel to endocarditis following rheumatic fever, chorea and acute nephritis. Congenital stenosis rare.

Pathology. Deposition of scar tissue gradually contracts. Progressive narrowing results from fibrous union of free edges of valve. Deposits of calcium occur gradually and chordae tendinae may become cross fused, further reducing mobility and allowing regurgitation. Effects — at first cardiac output reduced during exercise, later also at rest. Increased pressure exerted by left ventricle to maintain adequate output. This raises pulmonary pressure which eventually raises pressure in right ventricle.

Signs and symptoms. May be history of rheumatic fever. Dyspnoea, at first during exercise and only slight. Later becomes severe with attacks of paroxysmal nocturnal dyspnoea (cardiac asthma). Orthopnoea may occur. Poor peripheral circulation with cold hands and feet, peripheral cyanosis with typical malar flush (peripheral vasoconstriction occurs to compensate for reduced cardiac output). Cardiac arrhythmias, e.g. atrial fibrillation.

Complications. Chronic bronchitis and emphysema. Pulmonary oedema. Congestive cardiac failure with generalized oedema. Emboli from stagnating blood in left atrium may lodge in brain, viscera or periphery.

Investigations. X-ray shows enlargement of left atrium; later, enlargement of pulmonary artery and right ventricle. Cardiac catheterization and/or angiography may detect associated aortic valve stenosis and/or incompetence. E.C.G. indicates ventricular strain or right heart predominance. E.S.R. to exclude active rheumatic heart disease.

Treatment. *Conservative*. Treat heart failure: rest, restricted fluids and salt, diuretics, digitalis. Emboli: anticoagulant therapy to prevent further clotting.

Surgical. Contra-indications: active rheumatic process, bacterial endocarditis, severe mitral incompetence, severe heart failure. Valvotomy — open or closed heart surgery. Complications: embolism, atrial fibrillation, syndrome of chest pain, pyrexia, cough. Total replacement of valve with prosthetic ball-valve or plastic cusps.

AORTIC VALVE STENOSIS

Cause. Congenital. Rheumatic heart disease. Often associated with mitral stenosis. Atherosclerosis.

Pathology. Similar to mitral stenosis. Leads on to left

ventricular dilatation and hypertrophy with later pulmonary back pressure and congestion and eventual strain on right side of heart and congestive cardiac failure.

Signs and symptoms. Fatigue and palpitation. Later, angina, syncope, left ventricular failure. Harsh systolic murmur. Blood pressure normal or low. Diminished pulse pressure. Forceful apical beat.

Investigations. X-ray: left ventricular enlargement. E.C.G.: left ventricular hypertrophy. Cardiac catheterization shows extent of lesion.

Treatment. *Conservative.* As for mitral stenosis.

Surgical. In selected cases under 40 years of age who improve with conservative care but are not adequately controlled.

CARDIAC SURGERY

Pre-operative preparation (Specific). Dangers must be clearly explained to patient or parents. Cooperation gained by careful explanation of apparatus, e.g. oxygen tent, underwater drainage, cardiac monitor, intravenous transfusion. Physiotherapy — as far as possible, exercises needed in the post-operative phase are taught, e.g. breathing exercises. Co-existing conditions treated, e.g. heart failure, anaemia, polycythaemia, respiratory infections.

Investigations (in addition to those above). Full blood examination, E.S.R., grouping, crossmatching. Urinalysis. Weight (for estimation of fluid replacement post-operatively).

Closed heart surgery

Operations performed on heart or great vessels without opening chambers.

Patent ductus arteriosus. Thoracotomy. Mediastinal pleura opened, avoiding phrenic and vagus nerves. Recurrent laryngeal nerve identified and preserved. Ductus isolated (may be necessary to open pericardium), ligated and sutured. (May reopen if ligated only.)

Coarctation of aorta. Approach as above. Aorta clamped above and below stenosis. Narrowed section removed. End-to-end anastomosis established or synthetic graft inserted. If neither of these possible hypertension in upper parts of body may be relieved by short-circuit operations. Subclavian artery divided and inserted into wall of pulmonary artery thus diverting blood from aorta back into lungs. (Collateral vessels take care of blood supply to arm.)

Open heart surgery

Incision. As for thoracotomy (p. 208) or sternotomy.

Congenital repairs. ATRIAL SEPTAL REPAIR. (Surface or blood cooling.) Right atrium opened. Defect repaired by approximation with silk sutures.

VENTRICULAR SEPTAL REPAIR. (Extracorporeal cooling.) Right ventricle opened with vertical incision avoiding coronary vessels. Defect sutured directly.

FALLOT'S TETRALOGY. (Extracorporeal cooling.) 'Total' correction — repair of septal defect, relief of pulmonary stenosis, resection of right ventricular wall.

Valve repairs. MITRAL VALVE. Valvulotomy (valvotomy). May be done in 3 minutes therefore requires no hypothermia. Small incision in left auricular appendage guarded by purse-string suture. Minute knife and dilator (valvulotome) attached to index finger. Passed through incision. Slit made in valve and same dilated. Great care taken to ensure no division or rupture of cusps otherwise valvular incompetence occurs.

AORTIC VALVE. Usually requires open operation with extracorporeal cooling. Transaortic approach. Fused cusps incised with scalpel or scissors.

Prosthetic replacement. Considered when restoration of patient's own valves not possible. Hypothermia with extracorporeal cooling.

MITRAL VALVE. e.g. Starr-Edwards ball-valve. Three parts: silastic ball situated in knitted teflon cuff contained in vitallium cage and ring. Various sizes. Action: sealing effect during systole, open during diastole.

Method. Thoracotomy. Heart-lung bypass. Left atrium incised. Blood evacuated. Valve and chordae tendinae removed. Prosthesis inserted and attached with interrupted sutures in teflon ring (normal tissue will grow into this thus making a more effective seal). All air removed from heart. Circulation re-established. Atriotomy closed.

AORTIC VALVE. e.g. Hufnagel cusps: Teflon or Dacron cloth

leaflets impregnated with silicone rubber; or ball-valve similar to mitral valve prosthesis.

Method. Usual approach by sternotomy. Heart-lung bypass. Aorta clamped at origin of innominate artery. Incision made and valve exposed. Coronary arteries cannulated and infused with oxygenated blood. One, two or three cusps removed and replaced with prostheses. Air removed. Incision closed. Circulation reestablished.

Other procedures

This is a rapidly expanding field in which the following procedures are being tried: (1) grafts of veins on to coronary arteries to improve supply to myocardium; (2) electronic pacemakers sewn into myocardium to maintain regular heart beat; (3) transplantation of semilunar valves from animals to man.

Hypothermia

Deliberate lowering of body temperature.

Indications. Cardiac surgery, to allow heart to stop beating for short time. Cerebrovascular surgery. Treatment in head injuries and subarachnoid haemorrhage.

Aim. To reduce tissue metabolism by depressing enzyme activity; reduces need for oxygen and protects vital cells (e.g. brain cells) from damage due to anoxia during circulatory interference.

Effects. BRAIN CELLS. At normal body temperature irreversible changes occur from anoxia in 3–4 minutes. At $28°–30°C$ time extended to 10–15 minutes. At $15°C$ cells survive for up to 1 hour.

CARDIOVASCULAR. Below $30°C$ reaction of blood altered, potassium lost, heart muscle becomes irritable, ventricular fibrillation occurs.

PERIPHERAL VESSELS. Vasoconstriction occurs and further cooling may be difficult unless superficial vessels made to dilate, e.g. by massage or giving vasodilating anaesthetic, e.g. ether.

CENTRAL NERVOUS SYSTEM. Loss of consciousness after $30°C$. Respiratory centre depressed. Breathing ceases at $20°C$.

Pre-operative investigations. E.C.G. Blood grouping and crossmatching. Antibody tests for cold agglutinins. Clotting and

224

bleeding times. E.S.R. Serum transaminase. Liver and renal function tests. Blood urea.

Pre-requisites. Shivering must not occur. Controlled by muscle relaxants, e.g. curare included with anaesthetic. Heat regulating centre depressed by giving drugs such as Largactil, Phenergan. Vasodilation encouraged by massage or ether anaesthetic. Fibrillation controlled with digitalis or procaine amide or defibrillator.

Methods. DRUGS 'LYTIC COCKTAIL'. Intravenous or intramuscular injection of combinations of chlorpromazine (Largactil), promethazine hydrochloride (Phenergan) and meperidine hydrochloride (Demerol). Causes $2°-4°C$ fall in temperature.

SURFACE COOLING. (1) Immersion in cold bath to which ice is added. (2) Water blanket − patient enclosed in special blanket through which cold water is running. Temperature controlled by battery-operated thermostat (patient rewarmed by raising temperature of water flowing through). (3) Refrigerated wind tunnel.

Advantages. No expensive equipment needed, no damage to blood vessels. *Disadvantages*. Surface damage may result from cold or from heat during rewarming. Difficult to rewarm patient quickly.

BLOOD-STREAM COOLING. Blood shunted through a cooling coil.

Advantages. Cooling not started until chest is opened; heart visible during cooling and fibrillation more easily controlled; temperature controlled more delicately; patient can be rewarmed more quickly.

Disadvantages. Blood may be damaged in journey through tubes.

EXTRACORPOREAL CIRCULATION. Various methods, e.g.:

1. Blood conducted from right atrium, through a pump, to pulmonary artery. Respirations maintained by positive pressure respirator. Blood conducted from left atrium via a heat exchanger and pumped back into body via femoral artery. Temperature reduced to $15°C$, cooler switched off while surgeon operates on cold, bloodless, stationary heart.

Advantages. Surgery easier; profound hypothermia gives more time; blood less damaged than by blood-stream cooling.

Disadvantages. Occasionally cerebral disturbance noted for about 1 week afterwards.

2. Heart-lung bypass. Blood conducted from superior and inferior venae cavae to machine for cooling and oxygenation. Returned to femoral artery. Aorta clamped near its semilunar valve. (Machine primed with 4 or more litres of compatible blood, heparin added to prevent clotting. Bubble chamber necessary to prevent air entering circulatory system.)

Disadvantages. Haemolysis and damage to platelets may occur. Brain and kidneys may be damaged by prolonged bypass.

Observations during hypothermia.

1. Respirations. Automatic and rhythmic with pneumoflator.

2. Activity of heart. Cardiac monitor.

3. Activity of brain. Electro-encephalogram if necessary.

4. Blood pressure — arterial and venous, continuously recorded.

5. Blood specimens frequently tested for oxygen and carbon dioxide content.

6. Temperature. Electric thermometers. Oesophageal (heart temperature). Rectal (peripheral temperature).

Rewarming. Patient's own heat-regulating centre would eventually restore normal temperature but is too slow. Aided by: placing patient in warm bath or warm air chamber; running warm fluid through covering blanket; rewarming blood stream when extracorporeal method used. Rewarming must not proceed too fast otherwise cerebral oedema and brain damage may occur.

Nursing care. PROTECTION OF SKIN. Oil, e.g. lanoline, mineral oil or cold cream applied to minimize tissue damage during surface cooling. Gentle massage aids vasodilation. Change of position every 2 hours.

Observations for complications. Hypersensitivity to cold, allergic reaction — urticaria. Frostbite. Fat necrosis (rare). Burns during rewarming. Cerebral oedema, convulsions. Haemorrhage from damage to platelets and use of heparin. Cardiac arrest: injection of calcium chloride found useful, defibrillator usually starts heart's action.

POST-OPERATIVE NURSING CARE, SPECIFIC

Preparation. Equipment must be to hand to deal with

asphyxia and cardiac arrhythmia or arrest. Special surveillance in an intensive therapy unit necessary for above possibilities and for cerebral, renal or liver failure.

Observations. Airway must be maintained. Oxygen may be given by mask or tent. Tracheostomy may have been performed. Frequent suction may be needed.

Vital signs. Pulse and E.C.G. monitor usually used – connected by wires to patient's chest. Any change in rate or rhythm noted and reported immediately. Temperature also monitored or taken rectally every 2 hours. (Following hypothermia, skin temperature may be taken per axilla ½-hourly until normal.) If temperature rises above 38.5°C it should be reduced. Hypothermia blanket may be used in severe cases. With slight elevation of temperature patient may remain in oxygen tent an extra day.

Conscious state. Any deterioration may indicate cerebral oedema or embolism. Colour and warmth of skin carefully observed.

Drainage. Underwater seal drainage connected (p. 211).

Fluid balance. Weakened heart will not tolerate overhydration or dehydration. Careful assessment of amount and type of fluid required guided by thirst, urinary output (catheter may be necessary for accurate measurement of output at short intervals), serum electrolytes, blood loss, tissue turgor. Intravenous infusion for first 24–48 hours. Oral fluids introduced slowly.

Position. Usually semi-recumbent to semi-upright but state of shock and ease of respirations may change this. Ripple mattress or sheepskin rugs may add to comfort and prevent pressure sores.

Pain. May be severe. Omnopon, pethidine or morphia may be required but care taken not to depress respirations. Pressure on wounds and tubes avoided during lifting and turning.

Physiotherapy. Started when patient recovers from anaesthesia – as for thoracotomy.

Ambulation. Depends on heart condition.

Remaining care. As for thoracotomy (pp. 208 and 211).

Complications. (1) Haemorrhage – may cause haemothorax or cardiac tamponade. (2) Emboli – cerebral, aortic or peripheral. (3) Pleural effusion. (4) Fibrillation. (5) Pyrexia, angina and pericardial rub — cause unknown. (6) Atelectasis. (7) Pneumonia. (8) Circulatory overloading.

SPECIAL PROCEDURES
Cardiac catheterization
Long fine nylon tube passed into heart chambers.

Indications. Cardioangiography. Measurement of pressures. Measurement of oxygen saturation.

Contra-indications. Pyrexia. Congestive cardiac failure. Any acute illness.

Preparation. Prophylactic chemotherapy 48 hours before. No oral food or fluid 6 hours before. Pre-medication usually for children only. Careful explanation of reasons for and method of procedure and role of patient.

Areas of insertion. (1) Median basilic vein. (2) Suprasternal notch into left atrium. (3) Via bronchus (bronchoscopy) into left atrium. (4) Via chest wall into apex and left ventricle. (5) Brachial artery. (6) Femoral vein. (7) Long saphenous vein in children.

Method. Skin prepared. Local anaesthetic injected. Small incision made in skin and vessel isolated. Stay sutures passed under vessel to maintain position. Catheter inserted and threaded into vessel. Position checked under image intensifier fluoroscope screen.

Oxygen saturation tests performed to determine congenital shunt faults. Blood taken from such places as pulmonary artery, right atrium, right ventricle. Samples taken during rest and exercise.

Pressure measurements. Catheter connected to electromanometer and continuous record of pressure taken during passage of catheter.

Continuous E.C.G. recordings made by usual leads.

Clotting of lumen of catheter prevented by continuous slow infusion of saline with small quantity of heparin.

Ventricular puncture. Special needle inserted directly into ventricle through third to fourth intercostal space.

Complications. Arrhythmias: reversion to normal rhythm occurs on removal of catheter. Embolism: clots or air. Infection: rare, avoided by strict aseptic technique. Mechanical injury: shock, haemorrhage.

228

PERIPHERAL BLOOD VESSELS

VARICOSE VEINS

Abnormal dilatation, elongation and tortuous alteration of veins.

Sites. Term most commonly applied to varicosity of long and short saphenous veins of leg. Other sites: haemorrhoidal veins (p. 139); testicular veins (varicocele, p. 379); oesophageal veins (p. 99).

Cause. Incompetence of valves. (1) Congenital weakness in walls of veins or in valves themselves. Appears to be an hereditary factor. Contributory factors: prolonged standing, increased intra-abdominal pressure, e.g. pregnancy, obesity, pelvic tumour, chronic cough. (2) Acquired. Following deep vein thrombosis, valves often destroyed especially in 'perforators'.

Pathology. Back pressure is transmitted down veins. When valves are deficient, pressure directed against walls. Subcutaneous tissue offers no support for superficial veins hence the dilated, elongated and tortuous veins bulge through under the skin. As valves become more and more inefficient, condition becomes worse and movement of blood along affected veins becomes slower and slower. Long saphenous vein affected most commonly.

Surrounding tissues and skin develop secondary changes such as fibrosis, chronic oedema and pigmentation. Atrophic changes may occur in skin (varicose ulcer).

Signs and symptoms. Extensive varicosity may be free of symptoms and ugly appearance may be patient's main concern, but minor varicosity may produce many symptoms, e.g. aching, burning sensation, fatigue in lower limbs, pain after prolonged standing, cramps. (Intermittent claudication is not a feature.) Later effects and complications: Ankle oedema. Phlebitis may follow slight injury. Thrombophlebitis. Eczema and ulceration. Rupture with profuse haemorrhage following slight injury.

Tests. *Trendelenberg.* Determines competence of valves at saphenofemoral junction and· in perforating veins. Veins are emptied by gravity by laying patient flat and elevating limb. Tourniquet applied around thigh and patient asked to stand. If veins fill very slowly or remain empty the perforating veins are competent. If veins fill rapidly saphenofemoral valve and perforators are incompetent. Exact site of incompetent perforators can be determined by placing tourniquet at successively lower levels.

Test for perforators. Firm rubber bandage applied from toes to upper third of thigh. Tourniquet applied to occlude long saphenous vein. Bandage unwound downwards and 'blow outs' detected.

Various similar tests may be employed to test efficiency of deep veins, e.g. studying effects of rest and exercise on obliterated or obstructed saphenous veins.

Venography. May be employed to test patency of veins and perforators.

Treatment

Conservative. Massage while leg in elevated position. Reduces oedema and improves circulation. Exercises improve pumping action of calf muscles. Elastic stocking and/or bandages applied from toe to knee or thigh to support superficial vessels. Intermittent elevation of leg. (Elastic stocking may be used as preventive measure if patient has a family history of varicose veins and is subject to any of the contributory factors, e.g. pregnancy or occupation that requires prolonged standing.)

INJECTIONS. Much controversy over the effectiveness of this method.

Indications. Early cases. Poor anaesthetic risk patients. Those in whom short segments of varicosity persist after operation.

Aim. Sterile sclerosing agent injected into vein, damages tunica intima and causes sterile, firmly adherent clot which eventually fibroses and occludes vein completely. Substances used: Ethamolin, sodium morrhuate 5%, hypertonic saline, quinine and urethane.

Method. Fine needle (number 25) inserted into vein and leg elevated to drain blood. 1—2 ml of agent injected and vein occluded above and below injection site for 2—3 minutes. Two or three areas treated at one session. Some surgeons advocate application of bandage to be worn night and day after injection, to keep opposing walls of vein in contact with each other and make subsequent fibrosis more effective. Injections repeated at fortnightly intervals. Patient advised to exercise to assist upward passage of blood and to keep legs elevated while sitting.

Surgery. LIGATION. May be combined with injection of sclerosing agent. Incision made over saphenous opening. Saphenous vein identified, cleared from surrounding tissues, and 3 in removed. Ends securely ligated. Also main tributaries. Several ml of sclerosing agent may be injected. Same technique may be employed at knee level. Similar technique at back of knee for short saphenous vein. Complications: Incision may have to be enlarged if vein difficult to locate. Tributary may be mistaken for main vein and sclerosing agent injected. Fluid may be injected into tissues. Tearing of vein or slipping of ligature may cause alarming haemorrhage — controlled by packing with gauze for 5 minutes and then suturing tear.

EXCISION AND STRIPPING. Vein exposed at groin and tributaries ligated. Also exposed at medial malleolus and stripper passed through vein from below. (Stripper consists of 35-in coiled spring with wire core. Small olive-head tip at leading end to pass through vein and large acorn head at other end.) Olive-head passed through vein and out at groin incision. Vein securely tied to stripper above acorn head which is too large to enter vein. Ties securing vein are left long enough so that they can be used to pull back the stripper if need be. Stripper pulled out through groin incision in series of jerks which tear the main vein from its tributaries. Haemorrhage prevented by application of pressure bandage from toes upwards to level of acorn head with each jerk of the stripper which can be felt under the skin. When stripper emerges completely with vein telescoped on it, wound in groin sutured and bandage completed. Stripper sometimes arrested at knee level and incision may be needed to free it before stripping can continue.

Several incisions may be made prior to stripping to locate and tie off perforating veins.

Post-operative care. POSITION. Foot of bed elevated on blocks to aid venous return. Bedcradle over lower limbs to take weight of bedclothes.

OBSERVATIONS. Foot to ensure adequate circulation. Leg to detect deep vein thrombosis (p. 21). Bandage to ensure even pressure and freedom from wrinkles.

AMBULATION. After 24 hours encourage walking, avoid standing and sitting. Elevate legs when sitting. Encourage ankle exercises.

SUTURES. Groin, removed fifth day; ankle, seventh day.

DISCHARGE. 7—10 days. Taught to apply own bandage which should be worn for at least 2 weeks.

Complications. Deep vein thrombosis. Recurrence. Infection — wounds; phlebitis. Haemorrhage — reactionary; secondary.

VARICOSE AND VENOUS ULCERS

Ulceration of lower limb due to impairment of blood supply and subsequent development of oedema.

Causes. (1) Stasis due to varicose veins. (2) Venous ulcer associated with disease of deep veins of leg.

CONTRIBUTORY FACTORS. Injury, usually minor. Obesity. Poor standard of cleanliness which leads to infection. Gravity, increases oedema around ankle. Systemic disease, e.g. anaemia, kidney disease.

Pathology. VARICOSE ULCER. Normally blood supply to skin, especially near medial malleolus and inner side of ankle, is limited because perforating veins drain blood into deep veins. When perforators are incompetent stasis and oedema result. Varicose ulcers are therefore due to incompetent perforators and not to saphenous incompetence.

VENOUS ULCER. Blockage of deep veins, e.g. due to deep vein thrombosis, causes back pressure along perforators into superficial veins. Venous stasis around ankle results, causing oedema, clotting within small vessels and eventual death of superficial tissues.

Signs and symptoms. VARICOSE ULCER. Brownish discolouration and thickening of skin (varicose eczema). Usually small shallow ulcer.

VENOUS ULCER. Deep and wide. Often 3—4 in in diameter with necrotic sloughing base surrounded by hard oedematous tissue.

Treatment. CORRECTION OF ASSOCIATED FACTORS. e.g. reduction of obesity, scrupulous cleanliness, treatment of anaemia, heart failure and renal disease, well-balanced diet especially vitamins.

REDUCTION OF OEDEMA. Exercise, encourage walking;

avoid sitting especially with legs crossed which impedes free circulation; physiotherapy with rotatory and dorsiflexion exercises. Elevation of limb especially when sitting. Foot of bed raised at night. Massage to remove oedema and improve tone of calf muscles (by physiotherapist or by patient himself 2—3 times daily) from toes to heel, round ankle and up leg to groin. Olive oil may be used as lubricant. Compression bandage applied from below upwards with firm even pressure. Prevents accumulation of blood and oedema around ankle.

Types of bandage. (1) Elastic bandage applied over dressing. One or two-way stretch depending on stage of ulcer. Removed while at rest. (2) Adherent bandage, e.g. elastoplast; Viscopaste (commercially prepared cotton bandage impregnated with zinc oxide and gelatin paste); Icthiopaste (commercially prepared coal-tar paste bandage especially for varicose eczema). Latter two dry out to form semi-rigid stocking which may be left on for up to 1 month.

HEALING. Often difficult. (1) Removal of slough — Eusol 1 in 2, Trypure Nova (enzyme preparation). (2) Local applications — Viscopaste or Icthiopaste as above. Non-adherent dressing, e.g. tulle gras, petroleum jelly gauze, Sofratulle (impregnated with antibiotic) — allow free escape of serum and encourage granulation. (3) Skin grafts — may not 'take' because of poor blood supply. Valuable aid to healthy granulation if blood supply can be improved. (4) Surgery — after preliminary conservative measures. (a) Ligation and injection of saphenous vein. (b) Direct ligation of perforating veins. (c) Excision of ulcer and skin graft. (d) Ligation of femoral or popliteal vein.

Complications. Infection. Malignant change if long-standing cases. Biopsy taken if any suspicion. Thrombosis of deep and superficial vein (p. 21).

ARTERIES

Any disease or injury to arterial wall may result in reduction of blood flow (ischaemia) or oxygen supply (hypoxia) to the area. If this state persists death of tissue may result. Some parts, e.g. upper limb have good collateral blood supply (smaller arteries around main vessel) which can enlarge to take bulk of blood flow when main artery occluded and surgery rarely needed.

CONGENITAL CONDITIONS
COARCTATION OF AORTA
See p. 217.

AGENESIS
Failure of development, and aplasia (failure to grow normally). Rare condition. May result in ischaemia or gangrene in infancy. May not manifest until later life. Diagnosis confirmed by arteriography. Treated by arterial transplant or bypass with arterial graft.

INJURIES
CONTUSION WITHOUT PENETRATION
Causes. Pressure from bone fragment, crushing injuries, foreign object in nearby tissues, e.g. 'near miss' by bullet.

Pathology. Reflex spasm results from irritation causing sustained contraction of arterial wall and ischaemia of nearby parts. Stasis in artery may cause thrombosis further obstructing blood flow.

Signs and symptoms. (1) Colour change in skin. Pallor and cyanosis giving mottled appearance. (2) Numbness, loss of sensation and later paralysis. Starts in most distal part, e.g. fingers or toes. (3) Absence of distal pulse. (4) Coldness. Affected limb appreciably colder than other one. (5) Pain. Usually described as severe cramp. (Four 'P's' — pallor, paralysis, pulselessness and pain.)

Treatment. Avoid (1) vasoconstrictors; (2) local heat; (3) elevation of limb. Surgery without delay. Exposure of artery and freeing from damaged tissue may be sufficient to relieve spasm. Cover segment with warm solution of muscle relaxant, e.g. 2% papaverine sulphate, for 10–15 minutes. If this fails to dilate vessel, small polythene catheter inserted into artery, brought out through skin puncture and perfusion of solution given at intervals for 48 hours.

PENETRATING WOUND
Cause. Knife (especially among butchers), gunshot, complicated fracture, crush injuries.

Pathology. Small wound may be sealed with haematoma

which is gradually absorbed. Larger wound causes extravasation of blood into surrounding tissues. If severe, this may compress smaller vessels thus occluding collateral circulation. Clot which is not absorbed creates a traumatic arterial aneurysm.

Treatment. Control haemorrhage with pressure dressing. Avoid tourniquet if possible. Blood transfusion according to state of shock and amount of blood lost. Immediate surgery if circulation of limb threatened.

(1) Debridement of wound. (2) Suture of damaged area if laceration small and there is no further arterial damage. Vein graft may be needed. (3) If artery badly lacerated — excision of damaged segment. Continuity restored by (a) end-to-end anastomosis, or (b) graft to bridge gap. (4) Ligation of artery provided there is good collateral circulation.

ARTERIO-VENOUS FISTULA

Abnormal communication between artery and vein.

Cause. Congenital. Penetrating injury where vein and artery lie close together.

Common sites. Femoral, popliteal, tibial, axillary, brachial and carotid vessels.

Pathology. Veins dilate because of pressure of arterial blood which enters. Coldness in area distal to fistula. Varicosity of affected vein. Ulceration of part in which circulation deficient. Tachycardia if fistula large (slows if fistula occluded). Total blood volume increases, heart dilates and hypertrophies to compensate for blood flow through fistula. May result in congestive cardiac failure.

Signs and symptoms. Pulsation in veins. Fluid thrill in veins. Bruit (continuous buzzing sound) heard on auscultation.

Treatment. Surgery delayed for following reasons: (1) danger of ischaemia slight as some blood still passing through artery; (2) risk of infection until original wound healed; (3) anatomy altered, especially in presence of haematoma, making surgery technically difficult; (4) collateral circulation usually develops within few weeks; (5) spontaneous closure of fistula may occur.

Repair. Fistula excised. Primary anastomosis between ends of artery. Prosthesis inserted if there is any tension on artery. Vein repaired if possible, otherwise ligated below fistula.

ANEURYSM

Disease or trauma weakens arterial wall, which dilates and presents a pulsating bulge.

Causes. (1) Congenital. (2) True aneurysm — atheroma, infection (arteritis), syphilis, polyarteritis nodosa. (3) 'False' aneurysm: injury weakening arterial wall or partial division of wall.

Types. (1) Fusiform: general all-round bulging due to generalized weakening of wall. (2) Saccular — sac-like bulging of one area due to localized weakening of wall. (3) Dissecting — endothelial lining ruptured due to injury or atherosclerosis, blood passes between endothelium and muscle wall. (4) Traumatic — clot fails to absorb and organizes so that its outer portion forms a wall while blood still circulates through its inner parts.

Pathology. Atherosclerosis most common cause of aneurysm in aorta. Wall of artery unable to withstand high blood pressure. Fibrous tissue replaces elastic tissue. Wall balloons out.

Results. Severe pain due to stretching of artery wall. Sudden rupture may occur with torrential haemorrhage. Thrombosis from turbulent eddies in aneurysm. Embolism — pieces of thrombus break off and lodge in smaller arteries.

Signs and symptoms. May be asymptomatic unless pressure occurs against neighbouring organs or aneurysm bursts. Pressure symptoms. (1) Thoracic. Trachea — dyspnoea; oesophagus — dysphagia; recurrent laryngeal nerve — hoarseness; superior vena cava — distended neck veins. (2) Abdominal. (More common below origin of renal arteries.) Pain — intermittent, due to enlargement or intramural dissection. Peripheral emboli and thrombosis. Rupture — sudden severe pain, shock, signs and symptoms of internal haemorrhage. Femoral or popliteal aneurysm. Firm pulsating mass associated with bruit. Distal circulation may be occluded by thrombi or emboli causing signs and symptoms of ischaemia (p. 237).

Treatment. Ruptured aortic aneurysm — surgical emergency. Minimum preparation. Abdomen cleared of clot and free blood. Aneurysm excised and prosthetic graft inserted. Occasionally, on opening abdomen aneurysm found to be intact. Sudden bulging responsible for severe pain and shock.

ACUTE OBLITERATIVE CONDITIONS
ARTERIAL EMBOLI

Embolus, usually portion of thrombus, lodged in vessel obstructing onward flow of blood.

Causes. Origin in heart: rheumatic heart disease, myocardial infarction, bacterial endocarditis, congestive cardiac failure, atrial fibrillation. From blood vessels: atheromatous plaques.

Common sites. At bifurcation of vessels: aorta into common iliac arteries, femoral artery into superficial and deep, popliteal into anterior and posterior tibial arteries, brachial into radial and ulnar arteries.

Pathology. Causes obstruction to onward flow of blood. Initiates widespread vasoconstriction in vessels which could have established collateral circulation. Damaged intima, and stasis in distal vessels causes further thrombosis. Ischaemia and hypoxia occur in distal parts. Most common area affected — lower limb. Other areas possible, notably brain and kidneys.

Signs and symptoms. Sudden pain at site of lodgement. Later pain in distal parts, described as severe cramp. Numbness and tingling. Coldness. Pallor, cyanosis and mottling. Absence of distal pulse. Hyperaesthesia, anaesthesia, weakness or paralysis.

Treatment. Immediate embolectomy, preferably within 12 hours.

EMERGENCY TREATMENT OF ISCHAEMIC LIMB. Keep limb at room temperature. Apply bedcradle and leave open at ends. Oxygen to part reduced, metabolism at a minimum. Do not apply heat or cold. Heat increases oxygen demand and hastens gangrene. Cold reduces ability of existing haemoglobin to release oxygen with similar result. Do not elevate limb. Pressure in distal parts is already reduced. It may help to elevate *head* of bed so that part is more dependent. Prevent damage to part. (Tissues are more susceptible to infection and paralysis may render patient incapable of feeling injury.) Constant and careful observation needed and report immediately any sign of injury. Avoid pressure — sheepskin rugs under heels, pillow or rubber block under ankle to lift heel from bed, no constricting clothing. Maintain cleanliness — gentle washing, no vigorous massage. Do not cut nails unless specifically asked and then exercise great caution. Encourage collateral circulation. While keeping part exposed apply gentle heat to rest of body by extra blanket or electric blanket. This encourages reflex vasodilation in affected part. Observe carefully that hypotension does not occur as a result.

Alcohol in small amounts may be given as it encourages vasodilation. Smoking forbidden as it encourages vasoconstriction. Pain relieved with morphia, omnopon, pethidine. Sedation with barbiturates encourages relaxation and vasodilation. Injection of local anaesthetic around sympathetic ganglia inhibits sympathetic impulses and results in vasodilation.

GENERAL MEASURES. Correction of anaemia and heart failure. Relief of pain. Injection of heparin to prevent extension of clot, usually given intravenously so that effect diminished by time patient ready for surgery, thus risk of haemorrhage lessened.

SURGICAL TREATMENT. *Embolectomy.* May be performed under local anaesthetic unless abdominal incision necessary for embolus at aortic bifurcation. Amputation if limb is obviously gangrenous.

CHRONIC OBLITERATIVE CONDITIONS
ATHEROSCLEROSIS

General thickening of arterial wall with consequent narrowing of lumen. Partial or complete blockage may occur.

Incidence. Commonly males over 40 years.

Cause. Related to ageing process, diabetes, excessive cigarette smoking, excessive cholesterol intake.

Site. Can affect any artery including coronary and cerebral vessels. More common in vessels supplying leg: aorta, iliacs, femoral, popliteal and tibial arteries.

Pathology. As lumen narrows, blood supply to specific areas reduced. Collateral circulation improves and provides sufficient oxygen and nutriment to tissues while at rest. If part is exercised hypoxia occurs and severe pain results. Patient forced to rest and pain gradually diminishes (intermittent claudication). Collateral supply may be sufficient to prevent gangrene but great care must be taken and part observed for early signs of gangrene. Thrombosis in affected vessels may occur at any time and result in acute obliterative condition as above.

Signs and symptoms. Intermittent claudication. Occurs in calf muscles if femoral or popliteal vessels affected. In thigh or gluteal

238

muscles if aorta or iliac vessels affected. Walking distance varies from few yards to indefinitely according to adequacy of collateral supply. Ischaemic pain described as gnawing ache with occasional spasms of sharp pain. Coldness of feet. Rest pain: may be due to simple ischaemia, sepsis or extensive arterial involvement. Throbbing pain worse when limb is warm as in bed. Relieved by cooling limb to room temperature or hanging over side of bed in dependent position.

Colour (dependent rubor) indicates ischaemic paralysis of skin capillaries. Pallor on elevation. Prolonged 'flushing time' (after elevation of normal limb, colour returns to foot in seconds when it is lowered. Anything over 20 seconds is considered evidence of arterial disease).

Absence or weakness of pulse in vessels distal to blockage.

Atrophic changes in skin, subcutaneous tissues and muscles, e.g. thinning of limb, loss of hair, shiny smooth skin, thickened or deformed nails. Sweating, or absence of sweating, guide to degree of sympathetic activity.

Diagnosis. Confirmed by arteriography.

Treatment. CONSERVATIVE. In addition to emergency measures on p. 237. Advise patient regarding prevention of injury. Avoid extremes of heat and cold. Keep skin soft and pliant with twice-daily applications of lanoline. Two pairs of socks worn for warmth. Well-fitting shoes and hose: no pressure areas. Avoid constrictive clothing and garters. Great care with cutting nails; soak feet 10–15 minutes before cutting. See chiropodist regarding difficult nails, corns, bunions, etc. Report minor foot injuries to doctor. Never walk barefooted.

Improve collateral circulation by (1) walking until onset of pain, then resting for 3–4 minutes. Repeated 7–8 times daily. (2) Breathing exercises which improve circulation generally. (3) Buerger's exercises – not to be used if infection or wound present – patient lies horizontal and elevates leg at 45° for 2 minutes, then dangles leg for 2 minutes while exercising ankles and toes, then rests leg horizontally for 2 minutes. Repeated 5 times each session 3–5 times daily. (4) Sleep with head of bed raised on 4-in blocks.

Diet. Normal well-balanced diet advocated by some. Reduced cholesterol intake by others.

If diabetes present — stabilize and control.

Vasodilator drugs, e.g. Priscol — little or no value.

SURGICAL. (1) Thrombo-endarterectomy. (2) Arterial graft. (3) Sympathectomy. (4) Amputation.

Complications. Infections; ulceration; gangrene; muscle contractures.

THROMBOANGIITIS OBLITERANS (BUERGER'S DISEASE)

Episodes of segmental inflammation and thrombosis occurring in blood vessels.

Cause. Unknown. May be associated with smoking.

Incidence. Males between 25 and 40 years. More common in Jews.

Pathology. Occlusion of arteries following inflammation. Ischaemia. Infection and/or gangrene. Quiescent periods lasting months or years. Arteries of leg most commonly affected. Superficial thrombophlebitis usually present.

Signs and symptoms. Similar to atherosclerotic ischaemia. Differences: Younger age group. Rest pain more pronounced. Colour changes — may not blanch on elevation. Usually bilateral. Intermittent course (atherosclerosis usually less dramatic and more persistent).

Treatment. As for atherosclerosis. Patient must stop smoking.

RAYNAUD'S PHENOMENON

Intermittent attacks of vasoconstriction in extremities, usually fingers. Precipitated by exposure to cold.

Causes. PRIMARY (RAYNAUD'S DISEASE). Abnormal response to cold by peripheral arteries. Hereditary factor.

SECONDARY (RAYNAUD'S PHENOMENON). Result of systemic disease, e.g. hypertension; atherosclerosis; scleroderma; some drugs, e.g. ergot; beta blockers; local obstruction, e.g. abnormality of cervical rib, intravascular thrombosis.

Signs and symptoms. Precipitated by cold or emotional stress. Following phases may last from seconds to hours depending on severity. (1) Pallor due to ischaemia. (2) Cyanosis due to hypoxia. Fingers feel numb and may ache. (3) Erythema. Metabolites produced in above stages and cause excess vasodilation. Sensation of burning and tingling. (4) Return to normal when metabolites washed out. (5) If attack prolonged, gangrene at tips of fingers.

Treatment. CONSERVATIVE. (1) Warmth — warm clothing and gloves and heating of environment. (2) Avoidance of emotional stress. (3) Vasodilator drugs, e.g. Priscol 25—50 mg, 3 times daily.

SURGICAL — only in severe cases. Recurrence common. Sympathectomy.

SURGERY OF BLOOD VESSELS
REPAIR
Indications. Damage due to injury or disease, e.g. aneurysm from atherosclerosis.

Methods. Artery exposed. Haemostasis achieved. Devitalized tissue removed. Continuity restored by end-to-end anastomosis or graft. Anastomosis — fine silk (0000) on atraumatic needles (16—20 mm). (Larger for aorta, 00 silk and 40 mm needles.) Continuous or intermittent sutures (mattress type most effective as edges are everted). Patency tested by releasing distal haemostat first (slower, more gentle flow). Persistent ooze arrested with muscle graft. Drainage of wound avoided — tends to promote infection.

GRAFTING
Indications. Congenital defect; injuries; arteriovenous fistula; aneurysm; obliterated artery.

Types. (1) Replacement — whole segment. (2) Patch — small hole repaired. (3) Bypass — short circuit of blood flow around obstruction, end-to-side anastomosis of prepared graft.

Materials. ARTERIAL. Homologous (i.e. taken from another body usually during autopsy. Sterilized in antibiotics or chemicals and then stored in frozen state, or freeze dried and stored at room temperature). Disadvantages: Sterilization uncertain. Supplies and facilities for storage not always available. Liable to development of aneurysm.

VENOUS. Homologous, as above. Autogenous, i.e. from same patient. Saphenous vein used because of its structure. Because of its valves must be reversed when inserted in place of an artery. Results variable. Some appear to take on characteristics of artery. Others result in dilatation and tortuosity because of relative inelasticity. Thrombosis and aneurysm may result. Bypass vein grafts have proved very successful. Vein patches also successful. Used for repairing incisions or injuries in arteries. Occasionally aneurysm results.

SYNTHETIC. Regarded as superior to above methods. More easily available in any shape or size. Knitted or woven tubes of Dacron, Terylene, Teflon or other synthetic material. Flexible and crimped to prevent kinking. Inert in tissues and water repellent (prevents thrombosis). More successful in aorto-iliac replacements than femoropoliteal (latter tends to obstruct more easily and become infected). Some material grafts are 'preclotted' by being dipped in blood before insertion; minimal ooze of blood when clamps released.

INCORPORATION. All grafts develop fibrous tissue around them (penetrates into interstices of synthetic grafts) and develop a lining of smooth, flattened, pavement cells thought to be derived from monocytes of blood.

EMBOLECTOMY

Method. Artery exposed. Site of clot sometimes recognizable by bulging area with pulsation above and immobile constriction below. Artery ligated above and below clot. Longitudinal incision made and artery gently 'milked' to express clot through incision. Forceps and suction may be used but with risk of breaking clot. Fogarty's catheter may be used. Threaded into artery beyond clot, bag inflated and catheter and clot removed. Proximal ligature removed and blood should flow through and remove any residual clots. If blood does not flow, lumen of vessel gently explored with blunt probe. Artery may need to be opened at higher level. Proximal ligation reapplied and artery repaired as above.

ENDARTERECTOMY

(Disobliteration. Rebore.) Removal of central obliterative core while leaving outer layers of vessel untouched.

Pathology. Atheromatous changes in vessel wall create plane of cleavage so that diseased portion can be removed without damage to healthy layers.

Method. (1) Small areas. Longitudinal incision through outer layer, identification of plane of cleavage. Diseased core and any clot in vicinity dissected out. (2) Larger area. Incisions made to divide core at each end of blocked segment and stripping loop threaded over core and pushed along artery. Core may then be pulled free. Any loose pieces of atheroma trimmed until satisfactory flow established. Vessel closed as above.

In any of above operations, hypothermia prevents interference with blood supply to vital areas which may cause irreversible damage.

CARE OF PATIENT

Pre-operative preparation

Dangers of operation explained to patient. Investigations: chest X-ray, E.C.G., haemoglobin estimation, arteriogram. Blood grouped and crossmatched. Physiotherapy for chest. Care of ischaemic limb if necessary (p. 237). Blood transfusion started immediately prior to operation because of expected blood loss.

During surgery

Accurate estimation of blood loss so that replacement can be accurate to prevent prolonged hypotension with thrombosis of graft and renal failure.

Post-operative care

Position. Flat while unconscious then gradually elevated to semi-upright position as condition improves. Bedcradle over legs and affected leg exposed to room temperature.

Observations. Routine for shock, haemorrhage, asphyxia. Half-hourly observation of limb — peripheral pulse, colour, temperature, sensation, swelling. Oedema common, due to increased distal blood flow. After aorto-iliac surgery observe urinary drainage (catheter in situ). Danger of renal hypotension and haematuria from anticoagulant drugs. Gastric suction and intravenous infusion (danger of paralytic ileus from handling of gut to expose aorta). Position changed 2-hourly.

Exercises. Legs, to prevent further thrombosis. Commenced slowly. Chest — deep breathing and coughing. Limb protected against injury and infection.

Ambulation. Gradual to ensure sound healing.

Drugs. Analgesics used only when really necessary as most tend to cause some hypotension. Anticoagulants – commenced on fifth day and continued indefinitely. Dose according to prothrombin level.

Discharge. Tenth–eleventh day in uncomplicated cases.

Complications. Shock. Haemorrhage: leakage round graft, failure of graft to take, secondary infection. Thrombosis: may need further embolectomy. Minor nerve damage especially following popliteal operation. Paralytic ileus. Dangers associated with long-term use of anticoagulants.

SYMPATHECTOMY

Removal of certain sympathetic ganglia resulting in vasodilation of peripheral vessels served by those sympathetic nerves.

Indications. (Very limited success.) Raynaud's phenomenon, thromboangiitis obliterans, poliomyelitis (circulation of limb improves). Need largely superseded by vasodilator drugs and 'chemical sympathectomy', i.e. injection of local anaesthetic or alcohol into ganglia.

Method. CERVICOTHORACIC – UPPER LIMB. Incision made above clavicle and second and third thoracic ganglia removed. Care taken to avoid injury to numerous blood vessels in area – subclavian, thyrocervical, vertebral and internal mammary arteries.

LUMBAR – LOWER LIMB. Incision made below tip of twelfth rib extending towards umbilicus. Sympathetic chain located between vertebral bodies and psoas muscle. First and second lumbar ganglia removed. Care taken to avoid damage to aorta, inferior vena cava, peritoneum and ureter.

Post-operative care. Observation of limb for signs of obstructed blood flow. Care as for ischaemic limb and arterial graft (p. 237, 241).

GANGRENE

Macroscopic death of tissue accompanied by putrefaction.

Causes. *Arterial obstruction.* (1) Intra-arterial: embolus, thrombus, atherosclerosis, injury or infection of arterial wall, degenerative changes due to ageing diabetes. (2) Vasospastic states: Buerger's disease, Raynaud's phenomenon, ergot poisoning. (3) Extra-arterial compression: injudicious use of tourniquet, pressure from splints, plasters, bed, patient's weight, strangulation of blood supply to viscera.

Injury. Local damage to tissue, e.g. crush, burn, blow. May actually destroy tissues or obstruct blood flow by oedema or coagulation of blood vessels in burns. Direct violence may sever arterial supply.

Infection. Gas gangrene (p. 47); carbuncle, boil (p. 41). Cells may die from direct assault by organisms and their toxins which may spread to small blood vessels, destroying them also, or because of oedema obstructing blood flow.

PREDISPOSING CAUSES. Diabetic patients more prone because of: (1) Disease of artery walls — calcification tends to occur at earlier age. Sclerosis narrows lumen and thrombosis more likely. (2) Peripheral neuritis. Results in loss of sensation and loss of awareness of injury. (3) Excess sugar in tissues favours rapid development of micro-organisms.

Pathology (1) Sudden development in previously healthy limb indicates embolism. Obstruction of arteries and veins occurs — so-called 'wet' gangrene. Oedema causes tense skin on which blisters may develop. Colour changes from white (arterial obstruction) to grey-blue, to mottled bluish-purple. Infection and putrefaction follow quickly. (2) So-called 'dry gangrene. Occurs gradually as collateral circulation fails. Tissues wither, becoming dry, wrinkled and dark brown-black (mainly from disintegration of haemoglobin). Greasy to touch. Not as easily infected.

Small areas of gangrene can be absorbed. Larger areas, if uninfected, slough away. If infection occurs tissues separate as inflammation spreads into surrounding previously healthy tissues. Suppuration may occur very rapidly. Patient may become acutely ill from toxic absorption. Zone of demarcation between healthy viable part and gangrenous area. Zone coloured pink due to hyperaemia and is extremely sensitive to touch (hyperaesthesia). Line of separation exists immediately between demarcation zone and gangrenous portion. Layer of granulation tissue extends into gangrene and becomes fibrosed when it is unable to receive adequate nutrition. Severe and progressive ischaemia evidenced by rapid spread of gangrene and sudden appearance of patches of gangrene in previously healthy areas.

Signs and symptoms. Ischaemia. Colour changes. Line of separation. Hyperaemia and hyperaesthesia of zone of demarcation. Pain at first, later — anaesthesia as nerve endings destroyed. Skin either wrinkled and dry or swollen, tense and blistered.

Treatment. CONSERVATIVE. Aims — rest and protect ischaemic limb while waiting for development of collateral supply; prevent infection of 'dry' gangrene by protecting from trauma and pressure, keeping dry; prompt and vigorous treatment of infected gangrene to prevent spread — systemic antibiotics, local powder antibiotics, removal of slough (p. 59), stimulation of granulation (p. 59).

SURGICAL. Sympathectomy may delay gangrenous process in some conditions, e.g. vasospastic states. Embolectomy. Arterial replacement. Amputation may be necessary to prevent further spread, remove useless and unsightly area, save patient's life by removing source of toxaemia.

SPECIAL INVESTIGATIONS
ANGIOGRAPHY

Introduction of opaque contrast medium into some part of cardiovascular system to demonstrate radiologically the course, walls or lumen of heart or vessels.

Preparation. Routine pre-anaesthetic preparation if general anaesthetic to be used, e.g. for children under 14 years, nervous patient, mentally confused or restless patients. Local anaesthetic usual. Explanations by radiologist reinforced by nurse. Test dose of medium given previous day to exclude allergy. No oral food for 3–6 hours beforehand. Skin prepared, shaved if necessary, antiseptic applied, e.g. alcoholic chlorhexidine 0.5%. Bowel cleared of gas if aortogram. Bladder emptied before leaving ward. Sedation, e.g. barbiturate (Nembutal 100–200 mg).

Methods. Vary with site. Two main types.

DIRECT SUBCUTANEOUS PUNCTURE. Preliminary nick made in skin with scalpel (keeps needle sharp; decreases likelihood of blockage). Needle inserted into vessel. Length of flexible polythene tubing connects needle to syringe to prevent dislodgement of needle. Contrast medium injected, e.g. diodine, Hypaque 75%, Pyelosil (all water-soluble iodine compounds). Radiographs taken.

SELDINGER CATHETERIZATION. Large bore needle inserted into vessel. Guide wire inserted some way along vessel and needle withdrawn. Fine catheter inserted into vessel over guide wire. Guide wire removed. Catheter threaded into chosen area under fluoroscopic screening.

Types

Arteriography. AORTOGRAM. Visualization of contrast medium in aorta and its branches. Usually under general anaesthetic. Approach: abdominal aorta. Most common areas (1) 9 cm left of spine and 2 cm above iliac crest; (2) just below angle of twelfth rib. Needle length varies from 6–18 cm.

Aftercare. Observations ¼–½ hourly for signs of internal haemorrhage. Dressing removed in 24 hours.

RENAL ARTERIOGRAPHY. Renal artery visualized. Similar to aortography.

PERIPHERAL ARTERIOGRAPHY. e.g. femoral artery, brachial artery.

Aftercare. Check of distal pulse ½-hourly for 4–6 hours, to ensure no obliteration of vessel by haematoma. Half-hourly observation of dressing for visible subcutaneous haematoma. Remove dressing in 24 hours.

CEREBRAL ANGIOGRAPHY. (p. 328.)

Venography (phlebography). INDICATIONS. Condition of deep veins of lower leg in varices (p. 230). Portal hypertension (p. 158).

METHOD AND AFTERCARE. As for arteriography.

Cardiac angiography. Visualization of medium in heart chambers through retrograde passage of catheter via brachial artery or inferior vena cava. Injection of medium directly into heart chamber.

INDICATIONS. Assess – heart size accurately; condition of valves; intracardiac communication.

Coronary angiography. Injection of bolus of contrast medium into aorta just above aortic valve or directly into each selected coronary branch.

DANGERS OF CARDIAC AND CORONARY ANGIOGRAPHY.

1. Hypersensitivity reaction to contrast media.

2. Mechanical injury to heart chamber or large vessel: haemorrhage and shock.

3. Accidental injection of medium into myocardium: myocardial infarct.

4. Cardiac failure due to elevation of pulmonary artery pressure.

5. Arrhythmias: cardiac arrest following ventricular fibrillation.

248

Chapter 9

BONES AND JOINTS

FRACTURES

Complete or incomplete break in the continuity of a bone.

Cause

Direct violence. Occurs at point of impact.

Indirect violence. Break occurs at a point remote from area of impact, e.g. fall on knee produces fractured neck of femur.

Muscular violence. Muscle contracts with such force as to break bone where it is inserted, e.g. violent contracture of quadriceps (as in attempt to prevent falling) may fracture patella.

Pathological. Bone weakened by disease, e.g. cyst, osteoporosis, rickets or congenital bone fragility (fragilitas ossium), or neoplasm (especially metastases) may break spontaneously or as result of trivial injury.

Classification

Extent. *Simple* (closed). Break in bone which does not communicate with atmosphere through wound in skin or mucous membrane.

Compound (open). Break in bone communicates either directly or indirectly with atmosphere through wound in skin or mucous membrane.

Greenstick. Incomplete break in bone. Broken on one side and bent on the other as piece of green wood. Occurs in children in whom calcification is incomplete.

Comminuted. Shattered bone. Bone broken into more than two pieces.

Complicated. Break in bone invloving serious injury to important neighbouring structures, e.g. nerve, blood vessel or adjacent organ, e.g. lung from fractured rib.

Pattern. *Transverse.* Break approximately at right angles to axis of bone. Usually due to direct violence.

249

Oblique. Break at an oblique or sloping angle to the axis of the bone. Usually due to indirect violence or to rotational force.

Spiral. Bone has been twisted apart and break 'spirals' along axis of bone.

T-shaped. Bone broken across and also fissured longitudinally, e.g. lower end of humerus extending into elbow joint.

Linear (fissure or crack). Break in bone without any displacement, e.g. skull or patella.

Depressed. Edges of fractures driven below level of surrounding bone, e.g. skull (p. 298).

Impacted. One segment firmly driven or jammed into the other. Usually a result of indirect violence. Force needed to separate parts.

Crush. Form of impaction in which bone is compressed, e.g. body of vertebra.

Associated structures. Separated epiphyses. Fracture involves growing cartilage and end of bone which may result in subsequent restriction of growth. Can only occur in children before ossification of epiphyses.

Articular. Fracture of joint surface of bone.

Avulsion. Piece of bone has been torn loose with accompanying attachment of tendon or ligament.

Signs and symptoms

Any of the following may be present. (1) Pain at site of injury. (2) Local tenderness. (3) Deformity due to change in contour or alignment, soft tissue swelling. (4) Loss of function due to pain, muscle spasm, instability of bone. (5) Bruising. Subcutaneous haemorrhage. May appear below site of fracture as blood may travel by gravity. (6) Abnormal mobility. (7) Crepitus. Grating sound or sensation heard or felt when broken ends rubbed on each other. Do not test for 6 or 7. Merely note their presence. History may be obtained of patient actually feeling or hearing bone breaking. In compound fracture bone may be visible protruding through skin.

Diagnosis and subsequent treatment

Determined by X-ray. Shock usually present to some degree. Signs and symptoms of haemorrhage may also be present.

Healing of fractures

Bone consists of organic framework (osteoid) filled with inorganic substances (calcium phosphate and carbonate). Healing fairly rapid process. Three stages:

1. Clot forms around broken ends as result of accompanying haemorrhage. Serum, white blood cells and fibrin form an exudate; organizing clot filled with granulating tissue.

2. Soft callus formed to provide temporary stop gap. Exudate replaced by new blood vessels and connective tissue in which cartilage is deposited.

3. New bone tissue forms. Bone cells — osteoblasts — invade callus laying down new bone in thin bars. Excess bone removed by other cells — osteoclasts — until eventually bone regains normal contour.

Factors necessary for healing. (1) Haematoma formation. (2) Contact of bone ends and no interposition of other tissues. (3) Continued immobilization until callus able to withstand stress. (4) Good blood supply.

Union of bones

Clinical union. Callus firm enough to hold bone ends together with weight bearing.

Minimal times in healthy adults. Fingers and toes: 2 weeks. Radius, ulna, clavicle: 4—6 weeks. Humerus: 6—8 weeks. Tibia and fibula: 8—10 weeks. Femur: 12—14 weeks.

Signs of union. No pain on manipulation. No mobility at site. X-ray shows healing.

Normal union. Depends on patient's general health, age, site of fracture and efficiency of treatment in relation to sepsis, haematoma formation, contact of bone ends.

Abnormalities of union. NON-UNION. Failure of bone to unite caused by (a) impaired blood supply; (b) interposition of muscle or other substance between bone ends; (c) infection; (d) incorrect immobilization.

Treatment. Bone graft after foreign material removed.

DELAYED UNION. Bone fails to unite firmly after time considered to be normal for that bone. Caused by (1) impaired blood supply; (2) age; (3) incorrect immobilization; (4) associated disease.

Treatment. Prolonged immobilization.

MALUNION. Bone ends unite but with poor apposition. Weakness and/or deformity results. Causes as above.

Treatment. None may be necessary. Fracture may need to be reset in correct anatomical position.

Complications of fracture

Specific. (1) Simple converted to compound. (2) Local damage: nerves, blood vessels, muscle maceration, joints, viscera, e.g. lung, spinal cord, bladder damage. (3) Infections: wound and/or bone; specific infections: tetanus, gas gangrene. (4) Non-, delayed or malunion. (5) Local pressure sores: plaster or traction. (6) Fat embolism: rare complication; thought to be due to fat globules liberated from bone marrow. May lodge (a) under skin causing petechial haemorrhage; (b) in lungs, signs and symptoms simulate pneumonia; (c) in brain, causing drowsiness, mental confusion, pyrexia, unconsciousness. Diagnosis confirmed by finding fat globules in sputum and urine. No specific treatment. Careful nursing.

General. (1) Shock. (2) Haemorrhage. (3) Chest complications: pneumonia, pulmonary embolism. (4) Pressure sores. (5) Bladder infection. (6) Renal calculi. (7) Delirium tremens: usually included in complications because of high proportion of patients who suffer fracture because of inebriation and are used to a high alcohol intake but denied same while in hospital.

Treatment

First aid. *Simple fracture.* Avoid unnecessary movement which could cause pain, shock, damage to other structures or disrupt haematoma. Method: Reassure patient by one's presence, calm efficient manner. Keep patient warm and comfortable. Do not move unless in danger. Arrange transport, preferably ambulance. Immobilization of fracture by immobilization of joints above and below fracture with slings or splints. (If ambulance is within easy reach, best left for qualified first-aider or doctor.) Doctor will give analgesia on arrival.

Compound. Prevent infection. Stop haemorrhage. Treat fracture as above. Method: Arrest haemorrhage preferably with digital pressure. Do not apply direct pressure over bone ends.

252

Avoid use of tourniquet unless absolutely necessary (because of danger of gas gangrene in devitalized tissue). Cover with sterile dressing if possible, otherwise surgically clean, e.g. freshly laundered handkerchief.

Definitive principles of treatment. Restore normal continuity and function of part. Reduce, retain, re-educate.

Reduction. Anatomical realignment of bone ends under local or general anaesthesia. Methods: (i) Closed — manipulation only. (ii) Open — under direct vision — all compound, unstable and complicated fractures.

Immobilization. Retention of bone ends in position after reduction until clinical union achieved.

Methods: (1) Splinting: External — plaster of Paris, Thomas' splint. Internal — screws and plates, wires, pins (e.g. Smith-Petersen) and plates; intramedullary nails (e.g. Kuntscher's), bone grafts either homogenous or synthetic (denatured, sterilized bone), e.g. Kiel. (2) Traction. Pull exerted manually or by mechanical devices to overcome muscle spasm which would cause over-riding of bone ends. Methods: (a) Skin traction (non-operative). Adhesive strapping arranged to exert pull on skin and therefore indirectly to skeleton. (b) Skeletal (operative). Traction applied directly to bone by means of pins or wires passed through long bone, or tongs anchored in skull.

Rehabilitation. Restoration of normal function if possible. Otherwise, educate other functions to compensate so that patient may be returned to useful place in community. Commences from time of admission. (1) Explanations of injury, treatment, time factor and possible results. (2) Socio-economic factors referred where necessary to medico-social worker. (3) Diversional or occupational therapy to relieve boredom, re-educate muscle function and provide remuneration. (4) Physiotherapy. Stimulates circulation thus encourages healing. Prevents stiffness of joints not immobilized, wasting of muscles. Develops muscles needed for crutch walking, lifting, etc. Restores injured limb to full capacity.

Compound fracture. First aid (see p. 252). Definitive treatment. Aim to prevent infection. Treat as surgical emergency.

PRE-OPERATIVE PREPARATION. *Treat shock and haemorrhage.* Admit to resuscitation unit. Look for and report presence of tourniquet. Bed warm but not over-heated. Foot of bed on blocks. Analgesics to relieve pain. Blood grouped and crossmatched. Transfusion if needed. Rest. Oxygen.

Observations. Assess degree of shock and detect haemorrhage. Pulse, blood pressure, colour and general condition ¼-hourly. Local dressing left undisturbed to minimize infection. Report any bleeding. Distal pulse and sensation to detect damage to nerve or artery.

Prophylactic drugs. Antibiotics: usually crystalline penicillin 2 million units immediately and 1 million units 6-hourly. Tetanus prophylaxis. If previously immunized: booster dose of tetanus toxoid. If not, tetanus antitoxin serum 1,500 units after test dose of 150 units. Anti-gas gangrene serum 10,000 to 20,000 units may be given (effectiveness in doubt).

Preparation for theatre. As soon as general condition permits. Formal admission, permission for anaesthesia, urine test, visit from minister of religon, pre-operative medication. (Clothing removed, but if unable to do so without disturbing fracture, may be cut along seams or left in place until patient anaesthetized.) If possible X-ray should be taken.

OPERATION. First preparation. Dressing removed. Wound covered with sterile gauze. Limb washed with soap and water, shaved and dried. Antiseptic lotion applied. Second preparation. Surgical team regowns and gloves. Area is again painted with antiseptic lotion and draped. Debridement (surgical toilet). Removal of all foreign material and dead and devitalized tissues from wound. Exploration of wound and removal of clot and foreign objects. Radical removal of fat and devitalized muscle (minimal amounts of skin removed). Minimal amounts of bone and periosteum removed. (All sequestra must be removed.) Repair to damaged structures – nerves, tendons, organs, muscle, skin. Open reduction. Internal fixation contra-indicated because of danger of infection. If unavoidable because of instability, non-irritating substances will be used and massive doses of antibiotics given. Closure of wound. Complete if wound less than 12 hours old, clean, and sutures not under tension, i.e. enough skin left to effect adequate closure. Partial closure if wound contaminated or older than 12 hours, sutured later when infection subsides and healthy granulation tissue present. Skin graft – when insufficient

254

skin left for closure. Relieving incision — instead of skin graft. Incision made lateral to original wound thus allowing skin across wound to be sutured without tension over fracture site. Relieving incision heals by granulation.

IMMOBILIZATION. Plaster of Paris with or without a window to allow dressing of wound. Traction.

POST-OPERATIVE CARE. Routine, with specific observations of damaged limb in plaster or traction (p. 260).

SPECIFIC COMPLICATIONS. (1) Wound infection: careful observation for temperature, especially swinging type, together with rapid pulse and pain. (2) Secondary haemorrhage — observe for general signs and symptoms and extent of blood stain on cast. (3) Gas gangrene (p. 47). (4) Tetanus (p. 45).

Management of traction

Indications. To overcome muscle spasm and prevent over-riding of bone ends following fracture. To reduce dislocation of joints. To correct or prevent muscle shortening and deformity. To relieve pain from muscle spasm, e.g. from infective arthritis, or displaced intervertebral discs.

Methods. SKIN. Used successfully in children, elderly patients, poor-risk surgical patients when only slight traction needed. Traction force diffused over wide total area therefore damage to any specific tissues unlikely.

Disadvantages. Moderate amount of traction only can be applied because of relative elasticity of soft tissues. Cannot be used successfully on patients with well-developed muscles.

SKELETAL. Fine wire (Kirschner) or thicker pin (Steinmann) passed through bone and horseshoe-shaped stirrup applied to both ends of wire or pin. Action of Kirschner wire improved by placing it under tension. Where traction is needed to cervical vertebrae curved calipers may be inserted into burr holes on each side of skull.

Bones used for traction: skull, olecranon process, femoral condyle, tibial head, malleolus, calcaneum (os calcis).

Advantages. Greater amount of traction applied. Less discomfort for patient.

Disadvantages. Introduction of organisms along course of pin. Bone necrosis from pressure (in children pin may pull through

255

bone). Tearing of skin from excessive traction. Operative procedure usually requiring anaesthetic. Looks cruel.

PULP TRACTION. Suture or wire passed through pulp of digit and attached to splint which encircles it. Rarely used because of inconvenience but does keep digit immobilized satisfactorily.

Dangers of traction. Excessive pull causing delayed or non-union of fracture, tearing of bone and skin. Damage to arteries and nerves. Prolonged immobilization — osteoporosis, muscle wasting, joint stiffness. Skin sores from pressure.

Forms of traction. FIXED. Pull exerted between two fixed points, e.g. Thomas' splint — padded ring which fits over thigh and lateral bar which is continuous on both sides. Flannel slings are applied between lateral bars and leg rests on these. Lateral bars extend several inches beyond patient's leg. Applied to leg with ring in contact with skin over ischial tuberosity. Skin or skeletal traction applied and tied directly to distal end of splint. Thus traction is being applied at end of splint and countertraction by ring of splint.

BALANCED, SLIDING OR WEIGHT TRACTION. Pull exerted by two mobile opposing forces separated by raised structure to balance each other. e.g. for fractured femur weights attached to skin or skeleton extensions while countertraction applied by patient's own weight. Balance attained by elevating foot of bed. Tendency for patient to slide to head of bed counteracted by pull of weights. In cervical traction weights applied to skull via caliper and countertraction by patient's own weight when head of bed is elevated.

Application. SKIN TRACTION. *Equipment required.* Varies according to different surgeons' preferences, e.g. elastoplast or perforated zinc oxide plaster or Ventfoam (ventilated cotton-backed foam rubber which adheres to skin when bandaged firmly in place). Crepe, flannelette or domett bandages, adhesive felt or latex foam to protect bony prominences. Tincture of benzoin compound. Shave tray. Depending on form of traction — spreader (thin wooden block with holes for passage of traction cords so that cords or strapping do not press on malleoli). Pulley cords. Weights. Bedblocks. Safety pins. Pillows. Slings. Splints.

Preparation of patient. Relevant explanation to ensure cooperation. Explanations also given to relatives who may consider that apparatus appears cruel. Ensure firm base on bed (fracture boards if necessary) and comfortable mattress. Ensure privacy. Wash and dry leg thoroughly observing any abrasions which should be reported immediately. Shave leg if necessary taking particular care not to cause any skin damage. Paint limb with tincture of benzoin compound which eliminates allergic reaction to strapping and assists adhesive properties. Protect bony prominences with adhesive felt or latex foam or orthopaedic wool.

Applying extensions. Measure length of required adhesive strapping. Apply to lateral aspect of limb using trochanter and malleolus as guide for central line. Commencing at malleolus, work upwards stretching material sideways, thus preventing wrinkles and accommodating limb contours. Incorporate spreader and proceed in similar manner on medial side. On no account must material become wrinkled or adherent to crest of tibia or patella, causes pressure sores, immobility of patella and tearing of skin.

Bandage then applied evenly and firmly avoiding reverse spirals as double thickness causes pressure. Patella must remain uncovered to check knee is slightly bent.

Splint or sling applied as necessary.

Traction applied, e.g. (1) extension tapes tied to splint or foot of bed (fixed traction). (2) Pugh's traction — spreader incorporated into adhesive leaving 6-in space to heel to permit ankle movements. Cord attached to spreader and passed over pulley at bed end. Weights attached to cord. (3) Gallows (Bryant or vertical) traction used for children whose overall weight is insufficient to provide adequate countertraction and would necessitate constant readjustment. Both legs are flexed at hips and suspended by traction to overhead beam. Buttocks must not rest on bed. Pugh's traction is used and cords are either attached directly to beam, or indirectly via pulleys to the cot ends where weights are then attached. Traction controlled and hip rotation prevented by applying traction to both legs. Occasionally one leg left out of traction to provide additional countertraction or after bony union is reasonably solid. Hamilton Russell traction (can be modified and used with skeletal traction as well). Leg rests on sling which passes under slightly flexed knee, and on pillow which extends from knee to ankle. Heel free from bed to prevent pressure sores. Traction exerted through a 4-pulley system. Actual pull appears to be in direction other than that required — (a) vertical pull at knee, (b) 2 parallel ropes exerting horizontal pull on lower limb. Resultant of these 2 forces is maximum traction corresponding to line bisecting angle between (a) and (b), thus pull is on femur not on knee or lower limb. As a result of the 2 parallel horizontal pulls, actual amount of weight required is halved, i.e. a 4-lb weight will exert an 8-lb pull.

Patient able to move freely in bed and can be nursed in semi-upright position, helping to prevent pulmonary complications. Pressure sore on heel prevented. Patient encouraged to move freely in bed ('monkey chain' provided) thus other pressure sores prevented.

SKELETAL TRACTION. *Equipment.* For skin preparation. Instruments — Johanson's drill or Kirschner wire introducer, Kirschner wires or Steinmann pin, selection of stirrups, spanner, pliers, wire cutter, strainer.

Depending on form of traction may require Balkan frame, Thomas' splint, footpiece, Pearson's knee attachment, cords, weights, slings, pins, adhesive plaster, Braun's frame, bedblocks.

Preparation of patient. Routine pre-operative preparation.

Method. After preliminary skin cleansing, small incision made in lateral aspect of leg. Wire or pin bored through bone by drill or introducer and small incision made in medial aspect when elevation of skin seen — to prevent tearing. Pin or wire attached to arms of stirrup. Wire strained taut with strainer and made secure by having nuts tightened. Corks may be attached to ends of wire to prevent scratching from same. Wire or pin should be firmly embedded and unable to move. Cords attached to stirrup. Traction applied with aid of various devices, e.g. Thomas' splint, Braun's frame.

Nursing management. AIMS. Comfort patient, physical and psychological. Maintain constant traction until clinical union achieved. Prevent complications of prolonged bed rest.

BED. Firm base. Fracture boards if necessary. Soft mattress. Bedclothes arranged in separate packs for trunk and limb not in traction. Patient must be kept warm and bed tidy at all times (important for patients' morale). Bedcradle may be used if both legs in traction to ensure that bedclothes do not hamper efficiency of traction. If overhead frame, 'monkey bar' used to enable patient to lift himself and thus help to prevent pressure sores and hypostatic pneumonia. Bedclothes necessary when patients' own weight is countertraction.

WEIGHT. Determined by surgeon. Nurse ensures that blocks remain in position especially during ward cleaning. If blocks removed, even for short time, effectiveness of traction lost. Frequent inspection of pulleys to ensure running smoothly and freely, not squeaking (may not be noticed by busy nurse but will be source of intense irritation to patient), in correct position. This will be determined by surgeon but must be understood and maintained by nurse.

Cords. Must pass over pulleys in straight line (height of pulley adjusted to keep line level with long axis of limb); not frayed or knotted and passing freely over pulley (changing bedclothes accomplished while manual traction maintained).

Weights. Ensure securely attached to cords, hanging freely at all times (i.e. not resting on floor or bedframe or bed); constant traction applied (may be necessary for another nurse to steady weights, lifting them carefully when patient raised, then lowering them carefully); avoidance of accidental movement of weight (e.g. knock with chair or mop — very painful for patient).

POSITION OF PATIENT. Varies from recumbent to semi-upright, the more upright the patient the less effective the countertraction.

CARE OF LIMB IN TRACTION. *Position.* Hip slightly abducted, thigh slightly flexed (latter should not exceed 20° between bed and thigh). Patella pointing to ceiling — quick guide to position of limb. Knee slightly flexed (5°). Foot supported and at right angles to leg; various forms of support used, e.g. footpiece on Thomas' splint or Braun's frame, piece of adhesive plaster applied to sole of foot and attached to weights. May be internal or external rotation or in neutral position according to form of treatment. Heel must be free from pressure from bed or splints.

Warmth. May be covered with small blanket. Foot covered with sock.

Physiotherapy. Encourage movement where possible to prevent muscle wasting and improve circulation, e.g. quadriceps and foot exercises.

Thomas' splint. Must be accurate fit. Measure thigh prior to application and use correct size ring. If ring too large it causes pressure sores on surrounding areas; projects over external genitalia and creates difficulties with micturition and defaecation. If ring too small causes pressure sores by pressing on inappropriate places. Must be maintained in correct position: in contact with skin over ischial tuberosity to provide countertraction. Leather should be kept soft by frequent washing with saddle soap or application of olive oil. Skin under ring washed and dried thoroughly several times a day and area of weight redistributed, i.e. skin pushed and/or pulled by fingers above or below ring. Patient taught to do this himself. Supporting slings adjusted to normal contour of leg to keep ⅓ of leg above lateral bars and ⅔ below. Must not be pulled so tight as to cause necrosis around pin. Deep vein thrombosis may result. Constant observation to prevent sagging of slings — unsupported tissue becomes oedematous.

OBSERVATIONS. *Extremities.* Temperature change, especially coldness; colour — report pallor indicating pressure on arteries; cyanosis (venous congestion due to pressure); swelling due to oedema from pressure or lack of exercise or deep vein thrombosis (may also cause pressure on blood vessels and nerves); numbness, tingling, loss of sensation (nerve damage); pain (pressure and infection).

Bandage. Check that it is not too tight and causing pressure on limb.

Itch. May be due to allergy to skin traction equipment.

Pressure. Under ring of Thomas' splint; around ankle; under heel.

Position of: Sling under knee extension in Hamilton Russell traction; pillow, soft, extending from knee to ankle — heel must be free of bed.

Dressings. Daily or more often if necessary to points of entry and exit of pin, e.g. petroleum jelly gauze or gauze soaked in antiseptic. Some surgeons prefer use of plastic skin sprayed around area — Nobecutane.

DIET. Protein and vitamin C may be increased to aid healing. Adequate roughage to prevent constipation. Copious fluids also prevent constipation — and renal stasis, calculi formation. In recumbent position patient needs help with cutting food. Small meals at frequent intervals, aid digestion.

DAILY HYGIENE. Daily sponge. Patient needs assistance for inaccessible parts: toes, back, nails. Hair washed weekly. Pressure area care — diligent examination of all pressure areas for redness. 2—4 hourly position change. Use of bed-aids to prevent pressure, e.g. pillows, air-ring, sheepskin, bedcradle. Massage of pressure areas to stimulate circulation. Bladder: position may present difficulties with micturition. If patient's condition permits may be elevated with pillows to achieve more normal position. Bowels controlled by diets and fluids. If constipation occurs, mild aperient or suppositories may be employed. In obstinate constipation: enema. Patient encouraged to be as independent as possible in regard to personal hygiene.

PHYSIOTHERAPY. Chest: deep breathing to prevent pulmonary complications. Upper limbs: prepare for crutch walking. Joints not immobilized, especially limb not in traction; full range of movement 3—4 times daily. Limb in traction, as above (p. 259).

PSYCHOLOGICAL PROBLEMS. Relevant explanations at time of treatment. Encourage independence as much as possible. Financial: arrange visit from medico-social worker. Boredom: establish satisfactory nurse-patient relationships so that patient feels warmly accepted, encourage visits from relatives and friends, encourage rapport between other patients, diversional and occupational therapy according to patient's interests and abilities (may provide some financial remuneration as well).

Removal of skin extension. Do not 'rip off' quickly — may cause raw area which is painful and may become infected. Soak off adhesive plaster with some form of adhesive remover, e.g. methylated ether or Zoff. Remove gently and beware of tearing skin especially in the elderly. Wash skin, dry and apply oil to restore normal nutrition as soon as possible.

Plaster of Paris

Bandages impregnated with gypsum — fine white mineral (hydrated sulphate of calcium). Heated to $250°C$ to remove water of crystallization.

Action. When water added crystallization occurs and plaster sets giving off heat during process.

Factors affecting setting. Accelerated by adding salt, alum, hot water, hard water. Retarded by adding alcohol, borax, citrates, cold water, soft water or when applied over padding, or if atmosphere humid. Weakened by atmospheric moisture being absorbed, very hot water, stirred or moulded beyond its setting point. Hardened by blood soaking into plaster, french chalk (talc).

Indications. Immobilization: fractures, joint disease, e.g. tuberculosis, severe sprains, pedicle skin graft, e.g. from arm to ear when arm and head need immobilization; prevention and correction of deformities, e.g. prevention of foot drop by maintaining limb in position of function, correction of congenital dislocation of hip with frog plaster. Permit active weight bearing to stimulate circulation and speed recovery and prevent complications of long bedrest.

Advantages. 'Tailor made' for each patient so should fit exactly. Can be applied to any deformity and maintain required position. Allows early ambulation. Easy to apply, requires minimal equipment and is relatively inexpensive. Is light in weight and can be worn for months without discomfort.

Disadvantages. Immobilized joints become stiff and muscles weaken. May press on skin leading to sores and infection. Pressure on blood vessels and/or nerves causing ischaemia, gangrene, paralysis and contractures. Itching due to dead skin which normally flakes off and is washed away. Some patients are allergic to plaster – dermatitis results.

Types of applications. CAST. Entirely encases an area: *cylinder* encases extremity; *body* encases entire trunk; *hip spica* encases all of one leg and either all or to knee of other leg and extending upwards to waist.

SPLINTS OR MOULDS. Supports but does not completely encase an area.

Equipment for application. Plaster bandages of suitable size to area. Bowl of water (43°C) sufficiently full to allow complete immersion of bandages without spilling. (Thin smear of petroleum jelly in bowl facilities cleaning after use.) Padding – felt sponge, orthopaedic wool, stockinette, unsterile gloves, plaster apron and boots, plastic or canvas covering for table and floor, plastic or mackintosh sheet to protect patient's clothing, plaster knife, scissors, shears, bandages and slings.

Padding of plasters. PADDED. Firmly fitting cotton wool bandages applied over part and under plaster. (Stockinette may be applied first.) Or two or more layers of felt may be applied, holes being made in this for bony prominences.

Indications. Recent injury, operation, forcible manipulation where there is danger of oedema. Thin patient with well-defined bony prominences.

Advantages. Allows for oedema. Allows more muscular movement thus encouraging circulation to fracture area.

UNPADDED. Plaster applied directly to skin; is uncomfortable to hirsute patients on removal and electric cutter must never be used. Application over *stockinette* is just as good a fit therefore no advantage gained in applying direct to skin.

Indications. (For unpadded or stockinette only.) Where there is no risk of swelling and no exaggerated bony prominences.

Method. May be done under general anaesthetic. If not, patient's cooperation must be gained by relevant explanations. If splint or mould being made — dry plaster measured and cut as necessary. Plaster *bandage* immersed in water and bubbling ensues. Remove from water as soon as bubbling ceases, to minimize loss of plaster. When removing excess water squeeze gently from both ends simultaneously and not from centre. When *slab* is immersed it is folded and index finger inserted into open ends. When bubbling has ceased it is opened out quickly, smoothed and then applied. Limb held in desired position, bandage rolled firmly around, frequently pressed with thumb and heel of hand to ensure contact with limb and even spread of plaster. Each turn conforms to shape of limb (small pleats at edge of bandage aid shaping and change of direction), and covers two-thirds of previous turn. Both hands used to smooth plaster during application. Careful moulding important over bony prominences during setting. This is done with thumb and heel of hand. Plaster polished with french chalk — does not get as dirty as rough plaster and is more durable.

HANDLING WET PLASTER. Avoid finger imprints and flattening from hard surfaces. Support plaster with cupped hands never with fingers. Keep moving hands up and down plaster while holding. Support on soft surface, e.g. mackintosh-covered pillow, and never allow to rest on hard surface, e.g. edge of bed, table or trolley, hard mattress. Heel must be kept free of pressure even from soft pillow.

DRYING OF PLASTER. Left exposed to atmosphere at room temperature for 24 hours. Avoid use of artificial heat to dry because (1) plaster dries unevenly and tends to crack and may become soft in patches, (2) extra heat in addition to heat given off by plaster may be sufficient to burn patient (this is not felt by patient and may become infected). Check for complete drying — plaster white, odourless and shining. Cast firm, hard and resonant when tapped.

Aftercare of plaster. Elevate lower limb on pillow, foot of bed may also be elevated; upper limb, pillow or support in sling at right angles to body, e.g. sling supported by intravenous stand. Wash plaster from fingers or toes while wet. Expose to room temperature (although plaster is warm at first, later, when chemical reaction has ceased, it becomes cold so patient must be kept in warm atmosphere). Ensure fingers or toes are on view, e.g. bedclothes folded back over bedcradle.

OBSERVATIONS. Half-hourly plaster checks. Mainly for pressure. Oedema. Plaster shrinks as it dries. Pressure on nerves, blood vessels and skin.

1. *Colour.* Normally pink. Blanching test: when gentle pressure applied on nail it blanches but quickly returns to normal. Slow return of colour indicates early pressure on blood vessels. (Check with other limb for control time.) Cyanosis — venous congestion — should disappear on further elevation of limb. Pallor — suggests arterial obstruction.

2. *Temperature of digits.* Normally warm. Cold — arterial obstruction. Hot — venous congestion.

3. *Swelling.* Causes — venous congestion; result of original trauma; position change of limb during or after application of plaster.

4. *Pain.* Localized and intense — may be due to pressure or infection (intense local pain — early indication of gas gangrene).

5. *Numbness or tingling.* Nerve pressure.

6. *Loss of sensation or movement.* Nerve pressure. Should any of the above occur, action must be taken immediately and not deferred for any reason whatsoever. Continued pressure quickly results in gangrene or paralysis.

264

Elevate limb and encourage patient to exercise toes.

Report to doctor. Ensure plaster cutters are to hand.

If doctor not available and symptoms do not abate plaster must be split (see later).

After examination of limb tape the two sections of the cast securely together.

Other observations. Area of blood on plaster, e.g. following compound fracture. Area should be marked in ink and time and date written on plaster. If spreading, another coloured ink can be used to differentiate. Edges of plaster for chafing (see plaster sores, below). Temperature — onset of infection. Unusual odours — plaster sores, gas gangrene (mouse-like odour). Difficulty with micturition or defaecation.

Plaster sores. Sores occurring under plaster due to pressure.

CAUSES. *Badly fitting plasters.* Unevenly applied; too tight (especially unpadded plasters when swelling occurs); too loose (especially padded plasters when swelling has subsided); unprotected bony prominences.

Indentations. Finger prints; flattened surfaces.

Damaged plaster. Cracked; rough edges; indiscriminate trimming of plaster edges; softened area.

Foreign objects between skin and plaster. Most common cause — patient tries to relieve an itch wih knitting needle, ruler, etc., loses same and cannot retrieve it.

SIGNS AND SYMPTOMS. Local: burning sensation under plaster; local heat, may be felt through plaster; swelling of extremities; offensive odour; purulent discharge evident on plaster. General: irritability; restlessness especially at night; rise in temperature; general malaise.

TREATMENT. (1) Do not ignore patient's complaints of local pain and burning under plaster. (2) Window may be made over painful area. (3) Remove cause if possible, e.g. thin layer of padding; splitting of plaster at extremities; reinforcing area of plaster; bivalve plaster and strap together with adhesive tape; change plaster. (4) Eusol dressings to wound to remove slough. (5) Granulations encouraged by exposure to sunlight, infra-red rays, specific lotions or creams, e.g. scarlet red, lotio rubra. (6) Skin grafting may sometimes be necessary.

Ambulation. For limb — commenced after 48 hours. Special heel may be incorporated into plaster or patient may be permitted no weight bearing but must walk with crutches.

Discharge. Instructions: when to return to doctor; keep limb elevated when possible to prevent swelling; continue frequent movement of digits — report any disability at once; report immediately blueness, whiteness, pins and needles; burning, swelling, pain, discharge, odour; keep plaster dry.

Removal of plaster cast. Bivalving: cutting plaster in two equal parts.

REASONS. To relieve pressure or inspect limb if patient complains of pain. Change dressing or remove sutures. Remove foreign objects. When clinical union is achieved.

EQUIPMENT. Cast saw, plaster knife, plaster shears, spreaders, canvas or plastic sheet to place under cast.

METHOD. Electric cutter may be used but on padded casts only, as blade gets hot from friction. Many patients also object to noise. Pencil lines are drawn down sides of limb ensuring that bony prominences are avoided. Limb supported on firm base. Patient given assurance that the procedure will not hurt (if patient has been hurt in the past by incorrectly used shears he may be terrified and have no confidence in the cutter). Limb held steady by assistant. Blade of shears inserted between padding and plaster with whole length of blade in contact with padding. If only point used, patient may be cut. Small amount nibbled at a time. Patient's complaints of pain or discomfort must not be disregarded. When both sides have been cut, upper portion may be removed.

REMOVAL OF LIMB FROM PLASTER. Sudden loss of support is painful and alarming. Therefore support whole limb and do not lift leg by foot alone. Do not allow sudden changes of position of limb.

Aftercare of limb. Gently wash and thoroughly dry. PHisoHex or alcohol may be needed to remove thick yellow or brown crusts (consists of sebaceous material and dead skin). Oil or lubricating cream applied. Swelling often occurs after plaster removed. Prevented by elevating limb at intervals during day, avoiding long periods when limb is appended and bandaging to support limb during day time.

SPECIAL FRACTURES

Jaw

Cause. Direct violence, e.g. sporting accidents, fights, traffic accidents.

Areas. For descriptive purposes fractures of face divided into thirds. Upper: frontal bone and skull; middle: zygoma, malar and nasal bones, maxilla; lower: mandible.

Type. Almost always compound through mouth, nose or maxillary antrum.

Signs and symptoms. Pain on movement of jaw. Irregularity in tooth alignment. Difficulty in speech and closure of jaw. Crepitus on movement of jaw.

Treatment. FIRST AID. Barrel bandage to provide firm upward pull and immobilization.

PRE-OPERATIVE PREPARATION (Specific). Maintenance of clear airway. May be necessary to nurse patient in prone position with forehead supported on pillow so that tongue may not occlude airway and secretions and blood may drain out of mouth. Management of associated injuries, e.g. cerebral damage, eye injuries, facial lacerations, shock. Emergency pre-operative preparation (p. 2). Shave off stubbly beard in males. Some surgeons advocate lubrication of angles of mouth with lanoline base ointment.

SURGERY. Removal of any teeth where fracture goes through socket. Reduction – essential to re-establish alignment of teeth, normal bite. Manipulation alone may suffice, or wires, elevators or disimpaction forceps may be required. Open reduction may be necessary.

IMMOBILIZATION. Lower jaw wired to firm unyielding support which may be: (1) Upper jaw: upper and lower teeth wired together; when teeth missing, special splint made (Gunning's) to fit over gum; mandible wired to this. (2) Pin: inserted through cheek into maxilla; protruding ends wired to mandible. (3) Plaster head cap: Gunning's splint fitted to teeth or gums of fractured mandible and wired to cap.

POST-OPERATIVE CARE (Specific). Pair of wire cutters must be on hand in case of asphyxiation which may necessitate opening mouth. Observations while unconscious – colour and respirations to detect early onset of asphyxiation. Amount of bleeding – should be minimal – evidenced by obvious discharge from mouth, swallowing action by patient. Infection easily acquired from stagnant saliva and decomposing food particles. Mouth irrigations (with Higginson's syringe to provide some pressure, with fine metal or rubber catheter). Antiseptic mouthwash, e.g. glycerine thymol compound 1 in 8 or hydrogen peroxide 1 in 4 or sodium bicarbonate 1 in 160, 2-hourly. Patient should be taught to manage procedure himself as soon as possible.

Diet. Fluids only during immobilization. As much variety as possible. Taken through straw or rubber tube. As oedema subsides semi-solid material taken through spaces between teeth. Avoid hot foods and presence of pips and skins. (Intragastric feeding indicated only rarely when fluid cannot be taken into mouth.) Foods that dissolve in mouth may be given but anything requiring chewing not given until union complete. Talking prohibited. Pencil and paper provided.

Ribs

Cause. Usually direct violence. Occasionally spontaneous fracture from severe coughing; sixth–ninth ribs.

Pathology. Break usually occurs near angle of rib. Severe displacement rarely occurs as muscles hold parts in position. If displacement occurs, organs may be damaged – pleura, lungs (pneumothorax and/or haemothorax), liver, spleen, kidneys, colon.

Signs and symptoms. Localized pain at fracture site, aggravated by breathing and coughing. Limitation of movement on injured side. Tenderness and crepitus at fracture site.

Treatment. Union is spontaneous and treatment aimed at alleviation of discomfort and prevention of complications.

IMMOBILIZATION. Skin over area shaved if necessary. Tinct. benzoin co. applied. Chest strapped with zinc oxide adhesive plaster. Application – patient breathes out as far as he can then holds breath while prepared strips are applied. Extend from beyond midline anteriorly to beyond midline posteriorly. Vertical strips applied over ends for neatness and to prevent curling up.

Disadvantages. Affords relief but restricts respiratory movement and breathing capacity.

INTERCOSTAL NERVE BLOCK. Long-acting local anaesthetic, e.g. 2% procaine, injected around fracture site (just below margin of injured rib and several normal ribs above and below). Repeated as often as necessary.

Contra-indication. Depression of breathing and cough with excessive doses of narcotics. Breathing exercises encouraged.

Complications. Haemothorax. Pneumothorax. Surgical emphysema. Atelectasis. Pneumonia.

Sternum

Cause. Severe direct trauma. Vertical compression of thoracic cage and simultaneous fracture of thoracic spine.

Pathology. In direct trauma, sternum driven in from front reduces anteroposterior diameter of thorax reducing breathing capacity. Displacement seldom severe in compression type, though sternum angled backwards near junction of manubrium and body. Contusion of heart not uncommon.

Signs and symptoms. Severe precordial pain. Dyspnoea. Crepitus and deformity may be present.

Treatment. No special treatment. Sit patient in upright position. Relieve pain. Strapping of associated ribs.

Major chest injury: 'stove-in' or flail chest

Fracture of ribs and sternum. Paradoxical breathing: injured side moves inwards during inspiration as uninjured side moves outwards and vice versa.

Causes. Crush injuries. Direct violence, e.g. being thrown against steering wheel.

Pathology. Airway may be obstructed. Pleural cavity may become filled with blood and air. Thoracic cage loses rigidity.

Signs and symptoms. Paradoxical respirations. Severe pain, dyspnoea. Obstructed airway.

Treatment. Keep airway clear: suction. Tracheostomy may be needed. Drainage of pleural space: underwater seal drainage (p. 211). Traction of sternum restores full respiratory capacity: large towel clips inserted round ribs or sternum and weights (about 3 lb) attached. Traction maintained for 2—3 weeks.

Surgery. Internal fixation by intramedullary wires. Pain relief — analgesia or long-acting local anaesthetic may be injected.

Clavicle

Cause. Indirect violence by falling on outstretched hand, or direct violence.

Site. Most common: junction of middle and outer third. Less common: outer end.

Displacement. Lateral fragment downwards and medially (due to relative fixation of medial fragment and weight of arm).

Treatment. Displacement reduced as far as possible (perfect positioning of fragment not essential), by holding braced shoulders back with figure-of-eight bandage. Arm rested in sling for first week and then active shoulder exercises commenced when pain subsides. Healing occurs in 2—4 weeks. Bandages discarded after 2 weeks.

Scapula

Unless complicated by dislocated shoulder, no treatment.

Humerus

Fractured neck of humerus. CAUSE. Fall on outstretched arm. More common in elderly.

SIGNS AND SYMPTOMS. Swelling of shoulder. Restriction of shoulder movements.

TREATMENT. Conservative. Majority of uncomplicated fractures in elderly. Sling to support arm. Passive and active shoulder work commenced immediately and continued daily until fracture healed in 8—12 weeks. Younger age group: reduce; immobilize: abduction in shoulder spica or adduction frame for 6 weeks.

Surgery. Seldom indicated (unstable fracture only) open reduction and fixation with wires.

COMPLICATIONS. Joint stiffness in elderly. Prevented by early shoulder exercises. Nerve injury (axillary nerve). Treatment: wait for signs of returning function. If not evidenced in desired time (calculated from site of injury assuming nerve fibre regeneration to be 1 in per month), surgical exploration and restoration if possible.

Shaft of humerus. CAUSE. Direct violence. Violent muscular activity may produce spiral fracture; more common in adults than in children.

270

PATHOLOGY. Damage may be done to radial nerve (causing wrist drop), or to brachial vessels (less common).

TREATMENT. Unnecessary to procure perfect alignment, contact over ¼–½ fractured area sufficient. Complete immobilization. Most unite readily with minimal external splintage.

Stable fracture. Reduction, manipulation, immobilization. (1) Plaster cast upper arm only from axilla to elbow. (2) Full cast from axilla to wrist with elbow flexed at right angles. Support provided by sling.

Unstable fracture. Plaster shoulder spica. Shoulder is semi-abducted, elbow flexed at right angles. Trunk and whole of upper limb, except fingers, enclosed in plaster. Alternatively, open reduction and internal fixation (p. 253). Less cumbersome and more comfortable than above. Intramedullary nail inserted from above through greater tuberosity, or from below from just above olecranon fossa to reduce infection risk.

Supracondylar fracture of humerus. Important and common fracture in children.

CAUSE. Fall on outstretched arm.

DISPLACEMENT. Lower fragment displaced and tilted backwards.

DIAGNOSIS. Confirmed by X-ray. Often difficult to diagnose. X-ray of other elbow taken for comparison.

TREATMENT. Undisplaced fracture: 3 weeks' protection in an above-elbow plaster. Displaced fracture: treated as surgical emergency because of danger to median nerve or brachial artery. Reduction, manipulation. Lower fragment corrected by longitudinal traction on limb and with elbow flexed 90° or more, direct pressure applied behind olecranon (perfect alignment is not necessary, provided that lateral tilting is corrected in lower fragment). Immobilization. Plaster cast with elbow flexed at 90°. Traction indicated if (1) unstable fracture, (2) 2–3 unsuccessful attempts at reduction, (3) absent radial pulse does not improve with reduction (traction prevents displacement and further pressure on blood vessel).

COMPLICATIONS. Damage to brachial artery.

Causes. Injury by displaced fragment. May be completely severed or severely bruised thus occluding arterial flow by spasm or thrombus. Swelling, expected to increase 24–72 hours. Special care after plaster applied and any change reported immediately.

Effects. Vary. Severe impairment may result in gangrene of digits. Ischaemia results when vessel partially occluded. Sufficient blood passes through collateral vessels to supply needs of hand but changes occur in flexor muscles of forearm and occasionally peripheral nerve trunks. Fibrous tissue replaces muscle, wrist and fingers are drawn into flexion as result (Volkmann's ischaemic contracture). Sensory and motor paralysis of forearm may result if peripheral nerve trunks are also damaged by ischaemia.

Treatment. Any signs of impaired circulation in digits and patient's inability to fully extend fingers require immediate treatment. (1) Loosen external splint and bandage. (2) Further manipulation if necessary to replace displaced fragment. (3) Vasodilation encouraged in rest of body by application of heat. (4) Failure of above – operation – exploration and repair of brachial nerve if necessary. Established case: improve whatever function remains; physiotherapy and stretching splints to overcome muscle shortening. Surgery: muscle slide and muscle transfer operation may enable patient to retain limited use of hand. Median nerve damage: treatment on page 270.

Radius and ulna

Olecranon process. CAUSE. Fall on olecranon (point of elbow).

TYPES. Break without displacement. Break with complete separation of fragment. Comminuted fracture.

TREATMENT. Depends on type. Plaster for 2–3 weeks, elbow slightly flexed. Open reduction and internal fixation. Excision of all fragments and aponeurosis of triceps secured to stump of ulna (sutures passed through small holes drilled in ulna). Immobilized in plaster 3 weeks. Active exercises commenced 3 weeks after treatment in all types.

COMPLICATIONS. Non-union. Wide separation between fragments becomes bridged with fibrous tissue thus weakening power of extension. Treatment – in younger age groups only – excise scar and screw fragments together. Osteoarthritis if articular surface uneven. Constant use of arm particularly for heavy work will result in painful osteoarthritis after several years.

Head of radius. CAUSE. Fall on outstretched hand.

DIAGNOSIS. Often difficult. Does not always show clearly in X-ray.

SIGNS AND SYMPTOMS. Local tenderness. Impaired elbow movement. Sharp pain at lateral joint on extremes of rotation.

TREATMENT. Minimal damage — conservative — plaster for 3 weeks with elbow at right angles and forearm midway between pronation and supination. Active movements commenced after 3 weeks. Severe damage. i.e. — if radial head distorted — complete excision of radial head (never advised in children).

COMPLICATIONS. Rare. Joint stiffness. Osteoarthritis.

Shaft of radius and ulna. May occur alone or together.

CAUSE. Direct violence. Fall on hand.

TREATMENT. Accurate alignment essential. Slight disturbance interferes with relationship between radius and ulna. Results in impaired rotation and subluxation of radio-ulnar joint.

Conservative. Manipulation and full-length arm plaster with forearm midway between pronation and supination.

Operative. Open reduction and fixation.

Colles' fracture. Originally described as impacted fracture of radius 1½ in above wrist joint. Now extended to cover variety of fractures in which there is dorsal displacement of fragment of radius.

CAUSE. Fall with hand outstretched, wrist in dorsiflexion and forearm in pronation.

INCIDENCE. Common in any age group but more prevalent in middle and later years.

TYPICAL DEFORMITY. Because of dorsal and lateral radius displacement, articular surface points downwards and backwards. Impaction occurs of lower fragment into upper fragment and characteristic 'dinner fork' displacement is seen. Dorsal depression above fracture, below fracture there is marked elevation also involving hand (fingers simulating prongs of fork).

TREATMENT. *Minimal displacement:* reduction unnecessary. Wrist immobilized with splint extending from hand to elbow. Removed for hand exercises 3–4 times daily after 3 days. Splint discarded after 3 weeks.

Marked displacement: early manipulation. Plaster applied and moulded snugly over bones as safeguard against re-displacement. Cast may be full or incomplete covering ⅔ circumference of arm.

Advantage of latter: can be removed should swelling occur and can be tightened with bandages as necessary. X-ray after 1 week to ensure that re-displacement has not occurred (cannot be reduced if displacement persists for more than 2 weeks). Plaster left for 6 weeks. Finger, hand, elbow and shoulder exercises encouraged. Union far from consolidated but firm enough to prevent re-displacement. Active physiotherapy commenced to strengthen wrist and finger muscles.

COMPLICATIONS. (1) Malunion if displacement persists without correction, wrist weakens and unsightly deformity results. Treatment: surgical, bone ends realigned and internal fixation employed. (2) Median nerve damage. Usually mild and recovers within 6 months. (3) Subluxation of inferior radio-ulnar joint. (4) Joint stiffness, wrist and shoulder. Prevented by exercise.

Smith's fracture. (Reversed Colles'.) Displaced fragment of radius rotated forward and articular surface rotated anteriorly.

CAUSE. Fall on flexed wrist.

TREATMENT. As above.

Scaphoid bone

Cause. Direct violence, e.g. due to 'kick back' from starting handle when cranking vehicle. Also fall on outstretched hand.

Signs and symptoms. Often minimal and treatment not sought as hand can still be used.

Diagnosis. Difficult even with X-ray. Any tenderness in scaphoid region (anatomical 'snuffbox'), or impairment of wrist movements must have thorough radiological examination repeated in 2 weeks if not conclusive.

Treatment. Plaster extending from thumb, moulded firmly around first metacarpal, to halfway up forearm. Palm from proximal skin crease left free for full range of finger movements. Thumb is free to move at interphalangeal joint.

Complications. Common.

DELAYED UNION AND NON-UNION. Treatment unsatisfactory for both.

AVASCULAR NECROSIS. Blood supply to scaphoid is very poor. Main vessel enters distal half of bone and may be damaged. Proximal half of bone may die before damage is repaired resulting in 'crumbling' of bone. Diagnosed 1—3 months after injury by X-ray if history of pain and impaired wrist movement given.

Treatment. Nothing will restore full wrist movement. Surgical intervention essential as irregular dead bone fragment will lead to osteoarthritis. When fragments are removed wrist movements are limited. If above unsuccessful arthrodesis may be necessary to alleviate pain.

OSTEOARTHRITIS. *Causes.* Non-union (often because patient did not seek medical advice); avascular necrosis; repeated movement on damaged bone wears down articular surface.

Treatment. Mild cases: wrist support and avoid stress on wrist. Severe cases: arthrodesis.

Pelvis

Cause. Direct or indirect violence transmitted through lower extremities.

Types. Isolated (not involving pelvic ring). Multiple (involving pelvic ring).

Treatment. ISOLATED. Bed rest 2—3 weeks. Pelvic binder may be applied. Physiotherapy to lower limb commenced immediately.

MULTIPLE. (There must be fracture or dislocation to involve pelvic ring at two opposite points.) (1) Slight displacement. Rest until solid union 6—8 weeks. Avoid any form of weight bearing even sitting. Pelvic sling may be used to facilitate nursing. Lower limb exercises to maintain mobile joints and active muscles. (2) Disruption of symphysis pubis. Union achieved by either pelvic sling crossed to provide maximum compression. Short hip spica from waist to groin on unaffected side and knee on affected side. Open reduction and internal fixation with wires or plate and screws. (3) Maximal displacement. Reduce by traction either through lower end of femur or proximal end of tibia.

In most fractures of pelvis weight bearing is commenced after 6—8 weeks.

Complications. RUPTURED BLADDER. *Cause.* May be punctured by bone spike or torn in disruption of symphysis pubis.

Pathology. Extravasation of urine into perivesical space.

Signs and symptoms. Desire to micturate but unable to pass urine. Catheterization may reveal blood but not urine. Shock may be present. Diagnosis confirmed by cystogram.

Treatment. Surgical repair of torn bladder. Drainage of bladder by urethral catheter. Intermittent irrigation may be necessary to remove blood clots. Drainage of perivesical space by small drain tube.

RUPTURED URETHRA. *Cause.* Wide disruption of pubic symphysis.

Pathology. If micturition attempted perineum may bulge with blood and urine (membranous urethra most commonly injured). Prostate gland may be avulsed and dislocated upwards.

Signs and symptoms. Urethral bleeding. Retention of urine. (If condition suspected, warn patient not to attempt micturition.) Shock. Pain in abdomen or perineum.

Diagnosis. Confirmed by urethrogram. Cystogram should also be done if possible, i.e. if catheter can be passed into bladder, to exclude bladder damage.

Treatment. If catheter can be passed, leave in position for 14–21 days. Surgical repair (suprapubic incision). Torn ends located and sutured over catheter if possible. Bladder may need suprapubic drain. Perineal laceration drained.

Complications. Urethral structure — periodic passage of urethral sounds for at least 1 year.

INJURY TO RECTUM. Rare. Blood found on rectal examination.

Treatment. Surgical repair. May need temporary colostomy (p. 130).

TEARING OF COMMON ILIAC ARTERY OR ONE OF ITS BRANCHES. Repaired by suturing or grafting (p. 241).

Femur

Neck. Common fracture in patient over 50 years.

CAUSE. Rotational force due to stumble or fall. Osteoporosis in elderly makes bone weak.

SIGNS AND SYMPTOMS. Lateral rotation of limb often up to 90°. Shortening of limb. Pain on movement of hip. If fracture impacted and adducted none of the above are present and patient may be able to walk (sometimes for several days before seeking medical advice).

DIAGNOSIS. Confirmed by X-ray. Anteroposterior and lateral views.

TREATMENT. *Unimpacted.* Essential that bone ends are in good alignment and strict immobilization enforced, e.g. open reduction and internal fixation with various modification of nails (Smith-Petersen, Thornton, Thatcher) and plates (Jewitt, McLaughlin).

Advantages: Active hip movements immediately. Early ambulation with crutches or sticks to avoid complications of prolonged bed rest but ideally weight bearing should be avoided for 3 months. Femoral head may be completely removed and metal prosthesis applied. (Arthroplasty) (Austin-Moore, Judet).

Impacted. Conservative treatment usually successful. Skin traction. Hamilton-Russell extension (p. 257), for 3 weeks after which ambulation on crutches encouraged. Weight bearing on affected leg contra-indicated 8—10 weeks. Some surgeons distrust conservative measures and treat as above.

COMPLICATIONS. More common in this area than in rest of femur. (1) Non-union. Causes — poor blood supply, haematoma removal with synovial fluid, inadequate immobilization. (2) Avascular necrosis. Blood supply to femoral head poor, 3 routes (a) vessel in ligamentum teres, (b) vessels in capsule reflected on to femoral neck, (c) nutrient vessel from femoral shaft. The higher the fracture the more complete the damage to vessels. If area avascular bone dies resulting in eventual collapse of femoral head or osteoarthritis in later years.

Treatment. Difficult. Varies with age of patient and area of non-union. (1) Nail removal. Does not improve function but relieves pain. Allows some movement — satisfactory for elderly patient. (2) Arthroplasty as above. Method of choice with best results. (3) Arthrodesis. Sometimes difficult to achieve satisfactory bony union and immobilization for long period is necessary. Pain relief and limited movement possible. (4) Various forms of osteotomy and internal fixation. Results uncertain. Only satisfactory if head of femur has satisfactory blood supply.

Trochanteric fracture. Any area between greater and lesser trochanters.

CAUSE. Fall. Mainly in elderly over 70 years.

PATHOLOGY. Union easier and with fewer complications than neck.

SIGNS AND SYMPTOMS. Similar to fractured neck of femur but pain concentrated over trochanter and bruising appears in 1—2 days. (Not seen when neck fractured because blood retained within joint capsule.)

DIAGNOSIS. Confirmation usually easy with X-ray.

TREATMENT. Unites readily. Conservative for poor-risk and young patients — Hamilton-Russell skin traction 8—10 weeks. (Plaster spica rarely used because of discomfort.) Operative — internal fixation with pin and plates (essential for aged patient when prolonged immobilization results in complications).

Shaft. CAUSE. (1) Direct violence. (2) Common site for pathological fracture from metastases.

INCIDENCE. Any age group.

PATHOLOGY. Shock and soft tissue injury common because violence is common and bleeding is usually severe. (0.5 litres can extravasate in simple fracture.)

SIGNS AND SYMPTOMS. Shock and internal haemorrhage. Severe pain in thigh. Deformity of limb. Uncommonly, injuries to sciatic nerve or femoral artery or vein.

TREATMENT. *Conservative.* Manipulation. Skeletal traction through tibial tuberosity or distal end of femur. If patient small with mild muscular development, skin traction may be sufficient. Adults — Hamilton-Russell. Children — Bryant's.

Operative. Internal fixation — long intramedullary nail — Kuntscher's.

INDICATIONS. (1) Elderly. Long period of recumbency contra-indicated. (2) When reduction and retention cannot be maintained satisfactorily. (3) To facilitate treatment of other injuries. (4) Facilitates nursing and allows early ambulation in fractures due to metastatic deposits. (5) Shorter hospitalization when economic needs are pressing.

AFTERCARE. No immobilization needed. Exercises of related muscles and knee joint. Early ambulation 2—3 weeks after operation. Weight bearing after evidence of bony union.

COMPLICATIONS. Delayed, mal- or non-union. Knee stiffness due to muscular adhesions, not due to knee damage. Treated by prolonged active exercises.

278

Patella

Cause. Direct violence or violent contracture of quadriceps muscle.

Treatment. Depends on type of fracture:

Transverse with no displacement. Aspirate any haemarthrosis, plaster from groin to ankle with knee slightly flexed. Commence active exercises after 3 weeks.

Separation. Achieve perfect alignment during operation and fix internally with screws and wires. Immobilize in plaster for 2 weeks, then commence intense exercises to mobilize knee joint and restore function of quadriceps muscle. Over 40 years, excise patella. In advanced years full range of movement of knee becomes difficult. Patella excised from surrounding aponeurosis of quadriceps muscle which is then reconstituted with sutures. Immobilize for 3 weeks with almost full extension. After 10 days active quadriceps and leg-raising exercises commenced. Function of knee only slightly impaired, full extension may be difficult but patient only aware of this when ascending and descending stairs.

Comminuted fracture. Excision of patella.

Tibia and fibula

Shaft. Direct violence common cause. Most common type of compound fracture.

TREATMENT. Fibula usually unites readily with no problems. Tibia. Careful alignment needed to prevent shortening. Reduction, open for compound fracture.

Immobilization. (1) Plaster. Full length from groin to toes with knee slightly flexed and foot at right angles. Ambulation. After 2–3 weeks if fracture stable. Walking heel or rocker incorporated into plaster. If unstable, walking deferred until sixth week but crutch walking allowed prior to this. Plaster removed 9–12 weeks when X-ray shows union. After this active physiotherapy for knee, ankle and foot. (2) Traction. For unstable fracture. Skeletal traction through calcaneum or lower end of tibia for 3–4 weeks. Then walking with closely applied plaster.

COMPLICATIONS. Damage to tibial artery or nerve.

Pott's fracture. Loosely applied term to describe any fracture of the ankle in which there is abduction and external rotation.

TREATMENT. Depends on type of injury.

Fracture without displacement. Below-knee walking plaster for 3—6 weeks.

Fracture with displacement. Reduction with careful replacement of fragments. Immobilization — either plaster 8—10 weeks or internal fixation with screws and then plaster 8—12 weeks.

COMPLICATIONS. (1) Stiffness of ankle. Gravity oedema results after removal of plaster. Controlled by application of crepe bandage — otherwise physiotherapy will not be effective. (2) Osteoarthritis. Due to poor alignment when ankle joint involved. May require arthrodesis if extremely painful.

DISEASE OF BONE

OSTEOMYELITIS

Acute or chronic inflammation of bone. (Originally term applied to infection of bone marrow.)

Acute

Cause. *Primary.* Direct implantation of organisms from penetrating wound, compound fracture, surgery of bone, intramedullary infusion or injections.

Secondary. Septicaemia or pyaemia from septic focus, e.g. boil or carbuncle.

COMMON ORGANISMS. Staphylococci, streptococci, pneumococci.

Pathology. Usually a history of previous injury, often minor. Organisms multiply in haematoma and initiate abscess formation. Abscess may spread (1) down bone marrow. Oedema and exudate cause pressure on shaft of bone and sequestrum (dead bone) forms; (2) on to surface of bone under periosteum or through periosteum to form abscess under skin which may rupture and form sinus; (3) into joints. In children under 3 years infection tracks to end of bone. After that age cartilage forms barrier through which pus cannot pass.

Signs and symptoms. Sudden, often dramatic onset of pyrexia (especially in infants) with accompanying severe toxaemia. In adults there may be no pyrexia. Local pain which may be so severe that child will not move part. Bone tenderness on palpation. Local redness, heat and swelling.

Investigations. Full blood examination: raised white cell count (leucocytosis). Erythrocyte sedimentation rate: commonly raised. Blood culture may isolate responsible organism from patient with pyrexia. X-ray shows no change until after 10–14 days. Early changes: thickening of tissues adjacent to infected area. Later changes: destruction of compact bone and changes in cancellous tissue.

Treatment. ANTIBIOTIC THERAPY. Commenced immediately – penicillin with another antibiotic, in case organism resistant to penicillin. (Broad spectrum antibiotics avoided because with prolonged treatment resistant strains may develop rapidly.) As soon as organisms identified, antibiotic of choice given.

PAIN RELIEF. Rest limb with splint (Thomas' or plaster). Also limits toxic liberation from area. Analgesics. Some surgeons advocate that as pain is a guide to improvement or otherwise, analgesics should be minimized.

GENERAL MEASURES TO OVERCOME TOXAEMIA (p. 45).

DRAINAGE. Abscesses in soft tissues, e.g. under skin, aspirated daily. After 24 hours if fever and pain persist, hole drilled in bone and pus expelled (with persistent pain pus is usually under pressure).

Complications. Bone necrosis leading to sequestrum formation – results in chronic osteomyelitis.

Chronic osteomyelitis

Cause. As for acute.

Types. REPEATED INFECTION. Area becomes red, swollen and painful but not as acute as original attack. May not manifest itself for weeks or months or even years after original attack.

Treatment. Rest and antibiotics.

SINUS FORMATION. Due to (1) sequestrum, (2) abscess.

Treatment. (1) Sequestrectomy. (2) Drainage; rest and antibiotics.

BRODIE'S ABSCESS. Chronic bone abscess (common site – cancellous extremity of bone).

Causes. (1) Sequestrum. (2) Infection with organisms of low virulence, i.e. do not cause an acute infection.

Treatment. General measures to overcome infection; sequestrectomy; drainage of abscess (healing often delayed because of depth of abscess. Repeated skin grafting or transference of adjacent muscle belly may be successful). Amputation no longer a favoured method but may be indicated if extremity no longer serving useful function, or is complicated such as by secondary sarcoma.

Tubercular osteomyelitis

Cause. *Mycobacterium tuberculosae* which reach bones and joints via blood stream from primary focus, e.g. lungs or kidneys.

Pathology. BONE. 'Cold abscess' (i.e. local collection of pus which does not invoke the usual hyperaemic reaction of inflammation and therefore does not feel as warm as other abscesses). Abscess forms as a result of coalescence of several small tubercles (small central area of caseation surrounded by body's defence cells). Results of cold abscess. May heal with formation of scar tissue. May form discharging sinus by tracking to skin. May spread inside fascial sheath of muscle and form sinus some distance from source of pus. May spread to other structures, e.g. joints.

JOINT. Tubercles form on synovial membrane which becomes thickened and secretion of synovial fluid increased. If untreated infection spread to hyaline cartilage and underlying bone.

Signs and symptoms. GENERAL. Malaise, weight loss, anorexia, night sweats, raised evening temperature.

LOCAL. Swelling due to effusion into joint space and oedema of soft tissues, resulting in restriction of movement, sensation of stiffness, limping. Pain — may be absent in acute stage but presents later due to muscle spasm guarding joint. Atrophy of muscles and deformity if untreated.

Investigations. X-ray. Of chest to locate primary lesion. Of affected area — may be no visible change for some days. Isolation of acid-fast bacilli-joint biopsy, affected lymph node, aspiration of joint fluid or pus from abscess. Evidence of general tuberculosis — positive Mantoux test, E.S.R. raised, may be some anaemia. Examination of sputum and urine for acid-fast bacilli.

Treatment. GENERAL. Of primary lesion. Rest, physical and mental; fresh air, i.e. adequately ventilated wards. High protein diet (reduced calories to prevent obesity), varied in type to encourage patient to eat. Copious fluids to prevent urinary infections and renal calculi. Drugs: combination of two of the following: streptomycin, para-amino salicylic acid (P.A.S.), isonicotinic acid hydrazide (I.N.A.H.).

SPECIFIC. Conservative in acute infections. Immobilization by splints and plasters. Aspiration. Surgery may be indicated in some chronic cases especially in weight bearing joints. (i) Synovectomy and debridement of as much infected material as possible. (ii) Arthrodesis when function cannot be salvaged.

Complications. Rarely seen with modern treatment where time of immobilization and severity of condition have been reduced. (1) Abscess formation (if presenting at skin is neither painful nor tender). (2) Sinus formation. (3) Tubercular meningitis from blood-borne spread. (4) Miliary tuberculosis — widespread dissemination of organisms via blood stream. (5) Amyloid disease — rare condition, amyloid material deposited in liver, kidney, spleen and intestines, due to protein loss from tissues without adequate intake for replacement, main cause — anorexia. (6) Deformity due to changes in bones and joints.

JOINTS

SPRAINS

Complete or incomplete rupture of ligaments or capsule as a result of a stretching force.

Cause. Sudden stress sufficient to break ligament or less severe force occurring while protective muscles are relaxed.

Signs and symptoms. History of injury. Local pain, aggravated by movements that cause tensing of injured ligaments. Local tenderness. Swelling due to fluid effusion and oedema. Abnormal position or movements.

Diagnosis. Confirmed by X-ray to exclude fracture.

Treatment. Encourage early ambulation, although if swelling marked — elevation of limb (e.g. ankle) and avoidance of weight bearing 2–3 days. Support joint with strapping (e.g. elastoplast, 2–3 weeks). Warm baths and supportive bandages (e.g. crepe), may assist reduction of swelling and pain. (First-aid treatment to prevent swelling — cold compress applied immediately after injury, usually effective.) Avoid external splinting though may be necessary to immobilize in plaster if painful or disabling but should never exceed 2–3 weeks.

DISLOCATIONS AND SUBLUXATIONS

Dislocation. Displacement of articular surfaces of joint in which there is complete disruption of apposition.

Subluxation. Displacement of articular surfaces but some contact is maintained between them.

Causes. CONGENITAL. e.g. knee, hip.

PATHOLOGICAL (spontaneous). No injury sustained. Usually secondary to some other disease in which either relaxation of the joint capsule (e.g. rheumatoid arthritis or subacute infections), or unequal pull of muscles (e.g. in poliomyelitis, cerebral palsy) occurs.

TRAUMATIC (commonest cause). Stress injury sufficient to pull articular surfaces apart, or may occur when muscles are relaxed. Common joints involved — shoulder, elbow, ankle, interphalangeal.

Intracapsular. Dislocated articular surfaces remain within an unbroken joint capsule.

Damage to capsule. More common. (i) Capsule and reinforcing ligaments torn at iniury. (ii) Capsule not torn but peeled away from bony attachments. (iii) Avulsion by bone fragment.

RECURRENT. Permanent damage of ligaments or articular surfaces results in repeated displacements. Usually an initial violent displacement. Joints commonly affected — shoulder, ankle, sternoclavicular, patellofemoral.

Treatment. (General principles.)

REDUCTION. By manipulation or, occasionally, open. Injury of soft tissues: allow to heal spontaneously. Occasionally sutured. Active movements commenced immediately or a few days after injury. Immobilization avoided unless (1) severe pain, (2) injury to main ligament responsible for joint stability, (3) danger of post-traumatic ossification, e.g. elbow, hip.

Complications. (1) Persistent instability leading to recurrent dislocations. (2) Joint stiffness due to (a) adhesions within and around joint; (b) post-traumatic ossification around joint (myositis ossificans); (c) post-traumatic painful osteoporosis (rare). (3) Osteoarthritis from uneven articular surfaces — damage to articular cartilage. (4) Infection — open reduction only.

Congenital dislocation of hip

Head of femur not in acetabulum.

Cause. Unknown. Thought to be due to abnormal posture in uterus.

Pathology. Acetabulum becomes filled with fibrous tissue and fat from rubbing action of displaced femoral head. Becomes flattened inward at rim from pressure of femoral head. Femoral head becomes flattened, conical and anteverted as it presses against ilium and rim of acetabulum to form new 'false acetabulum'. Soft tissues: capsule becomes thickened and stretched. Inserting muscles become shortened and contracted.

Signs and symptoms. Before weight bearing age: often other abnormalities present, e.g. talipes. Abnormality of buttock — unequal position of creases, elevation or depression of one buttock. Adductor tendon prominent as tight band when hip flexed. Abnormality of movement, e.g. limited adduction, constant external rotation. On palpation — absence of femoral head in correct anatomical position. Broadening of perineum.

After weight bearing. Slow to walk. Limp, unilateral, favouring of normal side, if bilateral, 'waddle' limp on each side alternately. Trendelenberg's sign — crease of buttock on unaffected side falls instead of rising when patient stands on affected leg with unaffected leg flexed at hip and knee. Shortening of limb and lumbar lordosis when patient stands. Telescoping, i.e. sliding of long axis of femur up and down in relation to stationary pelvis — can be demonstrated only when child completely relaxed.

Diagnosis. Confirmed after some months of life by X-ray (in first few months cartilaginous nature of bones does not permit accurate diagnosis because cartilage is not radio-opaque). Arthrogram — injection of radio-opaque dye into joint and X-ray taken. Useful as diagnostic aid and guide to effectiveness of treatment.

Treatment. Commenced as early in life as possible before other changes occur.

REDUCTION. (1) Abduction of limb only if in first 6 months of life. If this fails: (2) Manipulation under general anaesthesia, or (3) Longitudinal traction on frame followed by gradual horizontal abduction to coax head into acetabulum, or (4) Open reduction to remove any obstruction present, e.g. capsular folds, pads of fat or fibrous tissue in acetabulum, hypertrophy of ligamentum teres.

IMMOBILIZATION. (1) 'Frog' plaster — from waist to ankle with hip abducted and knee flexed. (2) Variety of 'mobile' splints which permit controlled movement while maintaining abduction of hip. Immobilization continued until X-ray shows acetabulum sufficiently developed to retain femoral head. Time varies from 6 to 18 months.

REHABILITATION. After prolonged immobilization physiotherapy must be carefully planned and instituted to restore and develop muscles so that gait is normal.

SURGERY – JOINTS
Arthrodesis

Fixation of a joint by removal of articular cartilages and restoration of continuity by apposition of bone ends.

Indications. (1) When muscles paralysed and fixation will permit some use of limbs. (2) Relieve pain in intractable osteoarthritis by limiting range of movement. (3) Joint destroyed by trauma and repair impossible.

Disadvantages. Added strain thrown on to other parts of body, e.g. arthrodesis of hip: strain on lumbar spine (may be overcome by strengthening muscles of area involved by exercise).

Method. Articular cartilage and any diseased or damaged tissue removed. Bony continuity achieved by (1) compression of bone ends, e.g. knee joint — Clovely's clamp; (2) internal fixation — wires, pins, plates, bone graft, bone chips.

Arthroplasty

Refashioning of joint to restore mobility by use of artificial replacements.

Indications. (1) Osteoarthritis resulting in marked deformity and crippling. (2) Some cases of fracture of head or neck of femur where blood supply impaired or when long immobilization contra-indicated.

286

Method. e.g. hip – most common joint affected. (1) Arthrotomy: incision into joint capsule. (2) Excision of joint capsule, any fibrous tissue in acetabulum, dead bone from femoral head, or complete femoral head removed. (3) Replacement: hole bored in neck of femur, pin inserted to which is attached vitallium, acrylic or stainless steel mould to replace head of femur.

Alternatively, if head of femur remains, a vitallium, acrylic or stainless steel cup is placed between head of femur and acetabulum (cup arthroplasty).

Post-operative care. Routine as for any extensive surgery. Limb immobilized either resting on Thomas' splint or between sandbags with degree of abduction or adduction as necessary, or skin traction. Physiotherapy to ensure stable mobile joint – first post-operative day, passive hip and knee movements. Patient encouraged to move freely in bed with help of 'monkey bar'.

Ambulation. On crutches, without weight bearing, movement of legs as in walking. Some surgeons advocate starting on first post-operative day if condition satisfactory or seventh–tenth day when sutures removed or fourth–sixth week if traction employed: Then graduation on to elbow crutches and stick with gradual weight bearing, then walking without support.

Menisectomy

Removal of meniscus (semilunar cartilage of knee).

Indications. Tearing due to sudden twisting movement of leg while weight is bearing on the knee (common among football players).

PATHOLOGY Medial meniscus more commonly injured than lateral.

Types of tear. (1) 'Bucket-handle': marginal longitudinal tear. Fragments remain attached at each end. Medial fragment displaced towards midline of joint. Condyle of femur passes through tear to 'lock' joint, i.e. full limit of extension impossible but some degree of flexion retained. (2) Incomplete longitudinal tear in either anterior or posterior horn in which torn fragments become pedunculated – remaining attached to body. The menisci are almost avascular hence spontaneous repair does not take place readily. Synovial fluid increased causing effusion. Haemarthrosis may also occur if injury extends to vascular tissues of joint, e.g. rupture of ligament.

SIGNS AND SYMPTOMS. History of twisting movement. 'Sickening' pain at anteromedial aspect of joint, increased with forcible rotation of leg with knee flexed at right angles. Locking of joint. Swelling of knee appears 12–24 hours after injury and subsides in about 3 weeks. Cartilage may slip back into proper position and knee resume normal function only to recur when similar injury sustained. Weakness and atrophy of quadriceps muscle may occur in injuries of more than 2–3 weeks' duration.

TREATMENT. *Conservative.* Rest; weight bearing prohibited, may be ambulatory on crutches, until healing complete and full range of movements possible. If pain severe, back splint applied with knee slightly flexed. Pressure bandage to reduce swelling. Occasionally aspiration may be necessary to remove gross effusion. Quadriceps exercises to prevent wasting. Commenced immediately and repeated several times a day.

Complications. Torn ligament forces joint into abnormal position. Osteoarthritis results from prolonged friction between surfaces not normally in contact.

Surgical. As described below.

Pre-operative care. Quadriceps exercises taught to patient so that they may be started immediately post-operatively. Some surgeons advocate 2-day skin preparation to minimize skin micro-organisms (risk of infection accentuated as operation performed in bloodless field).

Operation. Usually performed in bloodless field as blood tends to obscure view and makes operation technically more difficult. Esmarch rubber bandage applied in overlapping turns from toe to thigh with leg elevated. Considerable pressure applied. Second bandage applied to upper thigh and first bandage removed. Leg should be exsanguinated. Operation may continue for ½–1 hour before tourniquet is released. Danger of damage to peroneal (lateral popliteal) nerve if bandage applied too tightly around head of fibula. Oedema common post-operatively if bloodless field technique used.

Arthrotomy by oblique incision over medial side of knee joint. Meniscus removed and any associated damaged structures repaired (anterior cruciate ligament commonly).

Post-operative care. Limb elevated and protected with bed-cradle. Pressure bandage applied to control effusion. Remains in situ 4—5 days post-operatively. Quadriceps exercises started as soon as patient conscious and gradually increased in frequency. Careful observation of toes to ensure unimpaired circulation and to detect any nerve damage (p. 260). Weight bearing started when effusion subsides and when patient able to perform quadriceps exercises without pain. Ambulation without weight bearing necessary until this state achieved. Graduated exercises until patient can walk and continued until quadriceps tone equal in both legs.

HALLUX VALGUS

Lateral deviation of great toe at metatarsophalangeal joint so that great toe directed toward midline of foot and head of metatarsal prominent on inner side of foot. 'Bunion' — bursa over metatarsal head as protection from pressure. May become infected.

Cause. Badly fitting shoes. (Barefooted races do not suffer from this condition.) Aggravated by high heels. Predisposing factor: weak intrinsic foot muscles due to pressure from shoes or from infection.

Signs and symptoms. Pain. Metatarsalgia. Hammer toe deformity of second toe due to grossly deformed great toe lying under or over it. Osteoarthritic changes from persistent malalignment.

Treatment. *Conservative.* Relief of pressure over bunion by wearing roomy shoes and padding over area if necessary. Exercises to strengthen small muscles of foot.

Surgical. Keller's arthroplasty: wedge resection of proximal half of proximal phalanx. Or arthrodesis of metatarsophalangeal joint.

COMMON DEFORMITIES

Torticollis (wry neck)

Spasm or shortening of neck structures (commonly sternomastoid muscles) resulting in deviation of head towards shoulder and face turned to opposite side.

Cause. Congenital, very rare and associated with spinal abnormalities. Birth injury, common.

Pathology. Soft swelling (so-called sternomastoid tumour) arises in lower third of muscle during first week of life. Due to haematoma resulting from damage to sternomastoid muscle. Swelling resolves but resulting fibrosis causes ischaemia which produces an aseptic necrosis. This causes further fibrosis and gradual shortening of the muscle.

Signs. Head held to one side constantly. Sternomastoid muscle stands out like cord when head straightened. Asymmetry of face — smaller on affected side. Curvature of cervical spine. Elevation of shoulder on affected side.

Treatment. *Conservative.* Gentle manipulation daily, mother taught as soon as possible. Wearing of collar (deeper on affected side) may suffice if detected in early stages.

Surgical. Indicated when conservative measures fail or in cases which are not diagnosed early. Division of muscle, usually at lower end. Immobilization in over-corrected position, followed by exercises and wearing of collar. Nerves may be divided if spasmodic condition present.

SPINE
Scoliosis

Lateral curvature of spine accompanied by rotation of vertebrae.

Causes. Faulty posture in childhood due to congenital weakness and poor development of muscles. Diseases: spinal tuberculosis, poliomyelitis, occasionally rickets. Many cases are idiopathic.

Pathology. Whatever the cause, eventually the convex side of spine grows more rapidly than the concave side.

Treatment. Either control growth on convex side or increase compensatory curves.

Surgery. Removal of epiphyseal plates on convex side with resultant intervertebral fusion. Remedial exercises, removable braces, plaster jackets.

Palliative measures. Excision of portion of rib humps or scapula, to improve appearance only.

Kyphosis

Exaggerated thoracic curvature ('hump back') which is either rounded or angular.

Cause. Congenital; faulty posture; disease of vertebrae, e.g.

infection, malignancy, rickets, Paget's disease, osteochondritis (Scheuermann's disease); degeneration of intervertebral discs.

Treatment. Directed at cause where possible. Corrective exercises. Special spinal supports.

Lordosis

Exaggeration of concave lumbar curvature of spine.

Causes. Secondary to kyphosis; to balance abdominal protrusion in conditions such as rickets, obesity, pregnancy.

Treatment. Remedial physiotherapy to strengthen back muscles. Wearing of supportive belt.

Dupuytren's contracture

Thickening and induration of palmar fascia resulting in flexion deformity of third, fourth and occasionally middle fingers.

Cause. Unknown. Thought to be due to genetic influences. Contributory factors: occupations involving pressure on palms of hands.

Signs and symptoms. Nodules on medial side of hand and skin thickened and creased. Cord-like structures extend into fingers. Flexion deformities of fingers, often flexing completely against palms thus becoming useless and a nuisance in gripping movements.

Treatment. Conservative in early stages — splinting. Surgical — excision of affected palmar fascia.

Syndactylism

Webbing of fingers and toes. Congenital fusion of two or more fingers or toes, usually lower portion only joined by skin, occasionally bones may also fuse.

Treatment. Plastic surgery: provision of skin surfaces on affected side of digits and their bases.

LOWER LIMBS

TERMINOLOGY. *Varum (varus, vara).* Turning inwards towards midline.

Valgus (valgum). Turning outwards away from midline.

Coxa vara

Angle between shaft and neck of femur reduced (normal angle, 135°). Thigh appears to deviate towards midline of body.

Cause. Congenital. Acquired: slipping of femoral epiphysis, or injury to neck of femur.

Signs and symptoms. Limitation of abduction; obvious limp; positive Trendelenberg sign.

Treatment. Fixation in position of abduction and internal rotation or subtrochanteric osteotomy followed by fixation in abducted position and use of walking caliper later.

Genu valgum

'Knock knees'. Legs below knees deviated away from midline.

Causes. Poor muscle tone; trauma; rickets.

Treatment. *Conservative.* Splint at night; wedged inner side of soles and heels; knock knee brace: leather straps secure leg and thigh to light metal bar attached to outer side of boot or shoe.

Surgery. Severe cases only; osteotomy of lower end of femur.

Genu Varum

'Bow legs.' Curvature of lower limb so that wide space occurs between knees when standing.

Cause. Horse riding; trauma; rickets.

Treatment. Splinting; osteotomy.

Talipes

'Club foot.' Congenital deformity of foot so that it is twisted out of shape and cannot assume normal position.

Varieties. *Talipes equinus.* Plantar flexion — heel drawn up and toes extended downwards (similar to horse's hoof hence name). *Talipes calcaneus.* Dorsiflexion of foot so that toes drawn up and heel extended downwards. *Talipes valgus.* Heel turned out away from midline. *Talipes varus.* Heel turned inwards towards midline. Sole vertical towards other foot and patient walks on edge of foot.

Various combination of above: equino-varus, equino-valgus, calcaneo-valgus, calcaneo-varus.

Treatment. Various corrective splints. Tenotomy followed by immobilization in over-corrected position in plaster, followed by physiotherapy.

Pes cavus

'Claw foot.' Abnormal elevation of longitudinal arch of foot.

Cause. Congenital. Complication of some diseases of central nervous system.

Treatment. Mild cases: only difficulty is in obtaining comfortable shoes. Severe cases causing pain and difficulty in walking, corrective surgery to flatten arch.

Pes planus

'Flat foot.' Abnormal lowering of longitudinal arch of foot.

Causes. Congenital. Acquired — loss of muscle tone (overstrain, long period of immobilization; rickets).

Treatment. None necessary unless condition painful or foot useless. Pain: remedial exercises, pad in shoe to support arch. Rigidity: manipulation under general anaesthetic and remedial physiotherapy.

Ingrowing toenail

Free corner of toenail (usually great toe) embeds in soft tissue of nail fold.

Cause. Pressure from shoe forces carelessly trimmed nail edge into tissues. Ulceration occurs, becomes infected and granulation tissue gives appearance that nail is growing into toe.

Signs and symptoms. Discomfort. Pain when infection occurs plus signs and symptoms of inflammation.

Prevention. Careful trimming of toenails — cutting straight across and not trimming round curve of toe. 'V' cut out of centre of nail in persons subject to this condition.

Treatment. *Early case:* pledgets of cotton wool soaked in spirit placed under corner of nail daily and nail edges allowed to grow beyond skin fold.

Later case. Especially when infected: removal of small wedge of nail, i.e. the infected corner or removal of whole nail. Application of local antiseptics.

AMPUTATION

Surgical removal of limb or portion of limb. (Term also used for removal of other parts, e.g. breast, cervix of uterus.)

Indications. (1) Death of tissue — ischaemic gangrene, e.g. thrombosis, embolism, atherosclerosis, Buerger's disease. Gross uncontrollable infection, e.g. in osteomyelitis, gas gangrene. (2) Damage (irreparable): crush injury, gunshot wound. (3) Disease: osteosarcoma. (4) Disuse (complete): for persistent pain or if limb is nuisance, e.g. poliomyelitis, congenital deformity, paraplegia.

Pre-operative preparation. *Emergency surgery.* Very little time for any preparation of patient.

Elective surgery. Psychological adjustment. Careful explanation for necessity of so drastic a procedure by doctor, reinforced by nurse. (Occasionally the surgeon may withhold this explanation from the patient until after surgery, e.g. elderly ill patient with gangrene.) Further reassurance — explanation as to possible outcome and availability of wide range of prostheses.

Nurse must make sure that the patient or legal guardian has signed consent form to avoid any legal repercussions.

Physiotherapy to assist in crutch walking later and to prevent pulmonary complications.

Surgery. Level of amputation depends on site and type of surgery and ease with which prosthesis may be fitted to that area, e.g. amputation through joint results in bulky appliances and mechanical difficulties.

SITES. 1. Through ankle (Syme's operation). Satisfactory for those with good circulation, younger age group and those who do not object to having a bulky ankle. Disability is much less with this than any other amputation.

2. Tibial. Ideal site 5 in below knee. Cosmetic appearance of prosthesis satisfactory.

3. Through knee joint. Uncertain healing but recommended for bilateral amputee.

4. Mid-thigh. Ideal site 10–12 in below hip. This and (2) are most common types.

5. Greater trochanter level. High degree of disability results.

6. 'Hind-quarters.' For malignant disease of hip or thigh. Includes removal of half pelvis. (Abdominal incision necessary for exposure and tying of common iliac artery.) Similar patterns for upper limb.

EMERGENCY. Guillotine method. Skin, muscle and bone all divided at same level. Skin traction may be applied to skin of stump to prevent its contraction. Later when patient's condition improved and danger of skin infection passed, re-amputation performed with fashioning of stump to fit prosthesis.

ELECTIVE. Plans are made to ensure that stump is correct size and length to fit prosthesis. Bone end must be adequately covered with skin; muscle and fascia closed to prevent bone adhering to scar. Wound should heal by first intention with no infection and no haematoma (drain tube or tubes inserted).

Post-operative care. *Preparation of bed.* Divided bed or open cradle bed so that stump will be on view until danger of reactionary haemorrhage over. Tourniquet previously retained at foot of bed but may alarm patient. Digital pressure can be applied more quickly and effectively. Nurse should know where tourniquet is stored and how to use it if required.

Position of stump. Cloth placed over stump and anchored under sandbags — controls twitching of limb which is distressing for patient. Also prevents flexion-deformity of hip. Patient may sit on air-ring. Some surgeons advocate limb elevated on mackintosh-covered pillow to prevent oedema and aid venous return for first 24 hours. Leg must be removed from pillow after this time to prevent permanent flexion and contracture of anterior muscles.

Pain. May feel as if it originates in amputated limb — so-called 'phantom' pains — may be severe and require morphia for alleviation.

Drain tube. Simple rubber. Removed 36—48 hours. Additional holes cut in fine polythene tube may be left in wound and low pressure suction applied for 48 hours.

Wound. Minimal handling of stump for 8—10 days: reduces 'phantom' pains and aids healing of tissues. Dressing removed for extraction of drain tube. Observe for haematoma, infection and tension of sutures. When bandaging aim at even distribution of pressure over whole stump to aid absorption of oedema and shaping for future prosthesis. Avoid pressure which may impede blood supply and delay wound healing. Formerly, stress laid on production of conical shape but light pressure bandage (e.g. tubular cap of tubegauze type), plus exercises usually adequate to produce good shape of stump.

Sutures. Removed 7—10 days. May need to be done under general anaesthesia.

Physiotherapy. Routine for chest and sound limb. Stump: minimal until wound healed. Prevention of flexion deformity important; special exercises by physiotherapist but nurse should ensure that patient hyperextends stump at least 3 times daily. Development of muscles for fitting of prosthesis and effective walking later.

Ambulation. Because of upset in balance, patient must be taught balance when sitting up in bed, standing by bed, moving from bed to chair and back to bed. When this is satisfactory he is taught to walk on crutches. Final fitting of prosthesis delayed for 3–4 months because of changes in stump.

Emotional support. Patient often feels discouraged especially in relation to loss of independence. Nurse must take every opportunity to combat this. Diversional and occupational therapy necessary to prevent boredom and 'self-pity'.

Occupation. Patient may need to change from former occupation. Assistance should be sought from vocational guidance centre.

Complications. (1) Haemorrhage: reactionary. (2) Infection: may lead to secondary haemorrhage. (3) 'Phantom' pains: persistence depending on patient's emotional outlook; aided by development of outside interests and satisfaction of socio-emotional needs. (4) Skin adherent to bone: painful and requires further amputation. (5) Failure of healing, mainly due to poor shaping of skin flaps. (6) Crutch palsy: pressure on axillary nerves by improper use of crutches. May result in temporary paralysis of arms. (7) Flexion deformity: makes walking and fitting of prosthesis extremely difficult or impossible.

Chapter 10

HEAD, BRAIN AND SPINAL CORD

HEAD INJURIES

SCALP

Laceration

Bleeds freely. Less prone to infection than other areas but potentially more dangerous if infection occurs. Heals rapidly.

Treatment. FIRST AID: pad and firm bandage.

HOSPITAL. Clip and shave hair for 2 in around wound. Cleanse area thoroughly. Doctor may excise dead tissue and suture under local anaesthesia.

Haematoma

Collection of blood under skin. If under pericranium spread limited by suture lines of skull, but if in aponeurosis — extensive spread.

Treatment. Aspirate, strict asepsis essential. If in sutured wound — provide drainage tube.

FRACTURES OF THE SKULL

VAULT

Linear (fissured)

Single fracture line.

Simple. No involvement of skin or mucous membranes. May be damage to brain substance or blood vessels.

DIAGNOSIS. X-ray.

TREATMENT. Non-specific. Rest. Observations for brain damage (see later).

Compound. Communicates with atmosphere through scalp wound. Usually obvious but all scalp wounds should be explored thoroughly. X-ray conclusive.

TREATMENT. Surgical emergency. Strict asepsis essential.

Dead tissue, bone spicules, loose fragments and blood clot removed. Wound closed. If surgery delayed or if wound contaminated drainage tube provided. Antibiotics. Strict rest with observations for brain damage.

Depressed fractures

Edges of fracture line driven below level of surrounding bone. **Simple ('pond').** Buckling in of scalp without skin laceration. Appears as dint in skull. Confirmed by X-ray.

CAUSE. Blow from blunt object. Precipitate labour — sacral promontory. Instrumental delivery — blade of obstetric forceps.

TREATMENT. (1) None if area small, brain undamaged, not over important cerebral areas — motor, speech, etc. (2) Trephine (burr holes) made at edge of depressed area which is levered up through these holes. (3) Craniotomy. Burr holes made and bone between holes sawn through with Gigli saw. Flap of scalp and bone turned outward to expose brain and coverings. Devitalized bone removed, bleeding points arrested by diathermy or ligation or gelatin sponge. Dura mater repaired as necessary. Flaps replaced.

Compound comminuted fractures. Skull shatters like an egg shell, skin lacerated, dura mater and brain damaged, fragments or bone may be driven deep into brain.

CAUSE. Severe blow on head.

TREATMENT. Craniotomy as above with removal of foreign objects driven into brain. With depressed fracture symptoms of brain damage will not abate until pressure from bones relieved.

BASE

Bones much thicker at base hence severe trauma necessary to cause fracture.

Features. (1) Usually accompanied by brain damage. (2) Nearly always compound. Blood, cerebrospinal fluid may escape from (a) Anterior fossa: nasal sinuses and nose (epistaxis, rhinorrhoea); mouth; orbits (haematoma). (b) Middle fossa: nasal sinuses and nose; ears (otorrhoea). (c) Posterior fossa — nasal sinuses and nose; neck (suboccipital area haematoma). (3) Often damage to cranial nerves. Anterior fossa: anosmia; middle fossa: blindness, strabismus, fixed pupils, partial facial paralysis;

posterior fossa: deafness, facial paralysis, difficulty in talking and swallowing, extensive effects from vagus nerve damage.

Treatment. BRAIN DAMAGE. See p. 302.

FRACTURE. Of little importance except to prevent infection spreading to meninges. (Antibiotic cover.)

DISCHARGES. Cover ear with sterile dressing and leave to drain. Warn patient not to blow nose or to suppress sneezes (c.s.f. leaks will close spontaneously in 8–10 days in most cases).

BRAIN INJURIES

Local damage. May result from direct blow with resultant depressed fracture, or a penetrating injury, e.g. bullet wound.

Crush injury. When head compressed between two opposing forces brain may be damaged extensively.

Acceleration/deceleration injury. Cranium is a rigid, inexpandable box; brain has a consistency little more rigid than a jelly; attached only by blood vessels and nerves at base and by a few veins along midline superiorly.

Acceleration. If head made to move suddenly by a blow, brain remains momentarily still until hit by internal surface of bone at point of impact. It then wobbles like a jelly, striking the bones opposite to and at the point of impact. Number of movements depends on force of blow.

Deceleration. If head moving, then suddenly stopped, brain continues to move momentarily in original line of direction; strikes skull bones and then rebounds against opposite side of skull. These bounces may be repeated several times depending on original speed of movement and suddenness of stopping (e.g. head of motor cyclist thrown from machine).

Damage resulting from injuries

(1) Shaking of brain. (2) Bruising (contusion). Membranes not usually damaged but microscopic trauma resulting in small haemorrhages and oedema. (3) Laceration. Macroscopic evidence of brain damage. (4) Haemorrhage. Extradural, subdural and intracerebral. (5) Brainstem damage interfering with vital functions.

Signs and symptoms.

From this damage arise 4 definite groups of signs and symptoms:

299

Concussion. Loss of consciousness, may be transient or may last several days. May be accompanied by vomiting. Recovery usually complete but headache may be severe and persistent. Also amnesia of accident — retrograde amnesia.

CAUSE. Acceleration/deceleration injury. Shearing forces are set up by the shaking resulting in temporary paralysis of function. If base of brain involved there is interference with heart action, respiration and other vital functions.

FEATURES. Similar to shock: (1) loss of consciousness; (2) vital signs — rise in pulse rate, fall in blood pressure, shallow, sighing respirations, subnormal temperature which rises slightly later as blood and oedema absorbed; (3) pupils react equally, but often sluggishly to light; (4) muscle tone may be flaccid and sphincters relaxed.

Cerebral irritation. Period of irritability which may follow unconsciousness.

CAUSE. Thought to be due to irritation by blood on cerebral cortex. If persisting for longer than 48 hours may indicate increasing intracranial pressure.

FEATURES. (1) Conscious state. Usually follows unconsciousness from concussion; unaware of environment and confused in relation to time, place and personal details such as name, address, etc.; will not cooperate or answer questions rationally; may complain of headache and nausea; sensitive to noise and light (lies curled up on side with back to light). (2) Vital signs returning to normal. (3) Pupils react equally but sluggishly to light.(4) Exaggerated reflexes; restless; may become abusive if disturbed; (restlessness increases when patient desires to micturate or defaecate).

Cerebral compression. (Increased intracranial pressure.) Cranium is rigid and inexpandable hence any increase in pressure inside skull compresses soft brain substance.

CAUSES. (1) Oedema from injury or later from infection (meningitis). (2) Haemorrhage — extradural, subdural or intra-cerebral. (3) Foreign objects, e.g. bullet. (4) Piece of bone from depressed fracture. (5) Interference with free escape of c.s.f. from ventricles by haemorrhage or infection.

FEATURES. *Conscious state.* Increasing depth of uncon-sciousness shown by failure to respond to stimuli — firstly, failure

300

to respond to verbal commands, even shouting; next, failure to respond to mild skin stimulation, e.g. tickling; finally, failure to respond to painful stimuli, e.g. pressure on supra-orbital ridges. Reflexes are absent. May be a lucid interval with patient conscious and alert between the unconsciousness of concussion and that of compression; occurs in extradural haemorrhage when bleeding from middle menigeal artery must strip dura mater from skull before pressure can be exerted on brain. Also, during concussion, blood pressure is reduced and symptoms may not appear for several hours. If the haemorrhage is subarachnoid, blood may escape into ventricles and pressure may be days or weeks building up.

If concussion is prolonged, or if damage is severe, there may be no lucid interval.

Vital signs. Pulse: slowing rate and increasing volume. Blood pressure: rising systolic pressure and increasing pulse pressure. Respirations: slowing and becoming stertorous. Temperature: slight elevation but of no significance.

As pressure increases, circulation within brain impaired. A reflex compensatory action is initiated whereby heart action increases in strength but becomes slower, to force blood into cranial cavity. This further raises intracranial pressure and so a vicious circle is established which will lead to death unless steps are taken to relieve pressure.

Pupils. At first, slight pressure on oculomotor nerve on affected side causes stimulation and pupil on affected side constricts and does not respond to light. As pressure increases, nerve becomes fatigued. Pupil dilates and remains fixed. Further increase in pressure affects opposite oculomotor nerve and that pupil behaves similarly.

Muscle tone and activity. Slight pressure over motor area may cause localized twitching (uncoordinated movements which are spontaneous and repetitive) in specific muscles on opposite side to injury. Twitching becomes more generalized until fits occur. As the nerves fatigue there is flaccid paralysis.

Brainstem damage. May occur as result of direct blow in occipital region, or severe shearing stress from acceleration/deceleration injury, or from increasing intracranial pressure pushing down until it involves brainstem.

301

FEATURES. *Unconscious.* No response to any stimuli.

Vital signs. Pulse: weak and rate increasing. Blood pressure: falling. Respirations: become cyclic (Cheyne-Stokes type). Temperature: rapid rise to 41°–45°C, hyperpyrexia, sweat no longer produced but heat production by metabolism and muscle activity continues.

Pupils. Dilated and not reacting to light.

Muscle tone. Damage to midbrain or pons varolii results in sustained contraction of extensor muscle (decerebrate rigidity): head thrown back, back arched, limbs stiff and straight. Damage to medulla may cause flaccidity.

MANAGEMENT OF HEAD INJURIES

Aims. (1) Careful and intelligent observation to detect early onset of any significant change in condition. (2) Preservation of life and prevention of complications while patient unconscious. (3) Rehabilitation of conscious patient to maximum health for that patient.

Observations

Must be diligently and intelligently recorded. Nurse must be aware of which observations must be reported immediately to surgeon – those that are concerned with cerebral compression – as prompt surgical intervention may prevent permanent brain damage or loss of life.

Observations commenced as soon as possible to establish base lines from which any significant changes can be noted at earliest moment. The following should be charted clearly every half hour until consciousness returns.

Level of consciousness. (Degree of responsiveness.) Terms such as 'stupor', 'semiconscious', 'coma' are best avoided as they do not convey a clear-enough picture of patient's condition. (1) Whether alert or drowsy. (2) Whether answers to questions are rational or confused. (3) Response to stimuli (a) verbal commands, (b) cutaneous stimulation, (c) painful stimulation. Report immediately increasing drowsiness and increasing failure to respond to stimuli.

Pupils. Equality and reaction.

METHOD OF EXAMINATON. Often difficult if large

302

haematoma present. Use bright torch with narrow beam, open one eye and direct beam into it. Note whether pupil constricts then remove beam and note whether pupil dilates. Repeat with other eye. Next, open both eyes and while directing beam into one eye note the effect on the opposite eye. Repeat with other eye.

INTERPRETATION. Both eyes should constrict and dilate simultaneously when either eye is illuminated. With increasing pressure the oculomotor nerve is damaged. Affected eye fails to react to light whichever eye is illuminated but unaffected pupil continues to react normally to light in either eye. Damage to optic nerve at time of injury causes dilated pupil on affected side. Neither pupil reacts when the blind eye is illuminated but both pupils react when the unaffected eye is illuminated. Report immediately any change in pupil equality and failure of pupil to react in either eye.

Vital signs. PULSE AND BLOOD PRESSURE. Increasing pulse rate and falling blood pressure may indicate (1) concussion, (2) shock from other injuries, (3) continuing haemorrhage other than cerebral, (4) brainstem damage. In (1), (2) and (3) there should be a gradual return to normal. Continuing rise in pulse rate and fall in blood pressure should be reported immediately.

Falling pulse rate and rising blood pressure are most important indications of rising intracranial pressure and must be reported immediately. (Shock is unusual in head injuries uncomplicated with other damage.)

RESPIRATIONS. Shallow and rapid in concussion. Becoming slow and stertorous in increasing intracranial pressure and cyclic or Cheyne-Stokes type indicate deterioration and brainstem damage. Both should be reported at once.

TEMPERATURE. Rising temperature must be reported at once. May indicate infection or damage to heat regulating centre. If the latter, attempts must be made to maintain temperature at $35° - 36°C$ by external means (see p. 306).

Muscular tone and activity. WEAKNESS OF FACE, ARM OR LEG. Occurs on side opposite to head injury. Detected by (1) observing relative degree of movement on each side if patient restless; (2) observing, if unconscious, relative degree of grimacing in response to supra-orbital pressure; (3) arm or leg lifted and allowed to fall back. Flaccid paralysis denoted by lead-like fall.

TWITCHING OF MUSCLES. Site and time reported accurately and promptly. Helps surgeon to pinpoint area of increasing pressure.

GENERALIZED FITS. Report immediately.

REFLEXES. Doctor will test; any spasticity or flaccidity noted.

Blood and c.s.f. escape. May be differentiated from blood alone as fluid thinner and fails to clot. Blood may fill middle ear and if drum is not ruptured bulging causes severe pain (restlessness if patient unconscious).

Fluid balance chart.

Care of the unconscious patient

Maintenance of clear airway. POSITION. Assisting natural airway by gravity — lateral position to facilitate drainage of mucus and blood into cheek where it can be sucked out easily. If flat on back, elevate jaw to prevent tongue falling back and occluding airway.

SUCTION. Necessary to prevent inhalation of secretions. Perform whenever 'bubbly' and immediately before change of position to prevent 'spill-over' into other lung.

ARTIFICIAL AIRWAY. Laboured breathing contributes to cerebral congestion. (1) Endotracheal tube, cuffed, prevents inhalation of anything except air. Should not be in situ longer than 12–24 hours. Cuff deflated 5 minutes in each hour to relieve pressure against tracheal wall and prevent necrosis. (2) Tracheostomy may be performed for following reasons: if artificial airway still needed after 24 hours; if positive pressure ventilation required; if chest infection present and more efficient suction needed; to reduce 'dead space' of tract if laboured respirations continue. (Care of tracheostomy, see p. 192.)

OXYGEN. Given for cyanosis but ineffective if air passages obstructed. Must be given if any hypoxia because of danger of further cerebral damage.

PHYSIOTHERAPY. Percussion of chest may be performed by physiotherapist in conjunction with suction. With return of consciousness cough and swallow reflexes return and patient encouraged to expectorate.

Maintenance of general condition. FLUIDS. Previously thought that withholding fluids dehydrated the water-logged brain. Now believed it is better to provide adequate fluids but that there is no urgency to start until patient has been unconscious for 12 hours.

Intragastric feeding. Method of choice if patient unconscious, provided there is no vomiting, as calorie requirements sufficient for metabolism can be provided easily. First feeding should consist of 30 ml only followed by gastric aspiration 1 hour later to ensure that absorption is satisfactory. Increase to 60–75 ml hourly until normal fluid requirements are met – 2 to 2½ litres per day.

Intravenous infusion. Indicated if patient vomiting (tendency to vomit usually passes in 20 hours). Difficult to provide sufficient calories without overhydrating patient, e.g. 6 litres of 5% dextrose provides only 1,200 calories (1,800–2,000 calories needed for basal metabolism).

Fluid balance chart. All intake recorded – type, time and amount. All output recorded especially urine. Daily balance is guide to hydration, dehydration and overhydration.

DIET. No urgency to commence for 2–3 days. If then patient still unconscious and swallowing reflexes absent intragastric feeding commenced with evaporated skimmed milk with protein powders added, e.g. Casilan or Complan. Katabolism is often excessive and prolonged in some cases of head injury. Despite high protein intake the body fails to utilize it and progressive wasting results. In such cases anabolism stimulators may be tried: methandienone (Dianabol) 5 mg daily.

HYGIENE. *Skin care.* Daily sponge, attention to nails and hair. Pressure area care is an important nursing duty – regular turning, use of ripple mattress, sheepskin pads and bootees, bed dry at all times. (Turning also helps prevent pneumonia.)

Eyes. Often only partially closed and need special attention to prevent dryness and abrasion from bedclothes, towels, dust. Eye toilets or irrigation 2–4 hourly; instillation of castor oil drops 4-hourly; always close eyes after examination; antibiotic drops or ointment may be ordered. Occasionally the eyelids may be taped to prevent corneal ulcers from dryness or abrasion.

Ears and nose. When c.s.f. leaking warn patient not to blow nose and to suppress sneezes. Apply sterile pad lightly and change often. Do not pack or plug. Turn to affected side to encourage drainage.

Mouth. Frequent toilets especially when tracheostomy or Ryle's tube in position.

Elimination. Bladder. Retention of urine common and often cause of restlessness. Pass indwelling catheter with strict aseptic precautions and release 2–4 hourly. Retention with overflow: if continent and restless examine abdomen for distension and treat as above. Incontinence. Wet beds must be avoided. Condom drainage carries less risk of infection than catheterization but must be removed twice daily and penis, prepuce and glans cleaned and thoroughly dried. Alternatively, catheterize with strict aseptic precautions and change catheter once a week.

Bowels. Constipation best avoided by glycerine suppository or small enema. If given at same time on each occasion, convenient regular habit can be established. Be alert for impacted faeces — denoted by spurious diarrhoea (passage of mucus but not faeces). Diarrhoea — control by diet. Record size and nature of stool.

PREVENTION OF DEFORMITY. Spastic or flaccid paralysis may be present. Careful nursing needed to prevent permanent deformity, e.g. foot and wrist drop. Maintain functional position of limbs with pillows, footboard, splinting, bedcradle. Joints must never be hyperextended. Passive exercises — all limbs put through full range of movement several times daily.

TEMPERATURE CONTROL. With hyperpyrexia, unless metabolism is reduced, tissue wastage will result and this may constitute a threat to the brain in itself: body may 'burn itself out'. Temperature may be lowered by (1) reducing bedclothes and personal clothing, (2) tepid sponging, (3) wet sheet and fan, (4) drugs: chlorpromazine, phenergan, barbiturates, aspirin.

ANTIBIOTICS. Prophylactic cover to prevent (1) meningitis and encephalitis when compound fracture present, (2) pneumonia.

Increased intracranial pressure

Treatment depends on cause.

Oedema. Recumbent position. Gravity increases cerebral oedema. Foot of bed should not be raised unless other injuries

306

necessitate this. By osmosis, hypertonic solutions, e.g. magnesium sulphate 25–50%, glucose 50%, per rectum, dehydrate brain temporarily. Forced diuresis with Mannitol 15% intravenously may have same effect. Hypothermia (p. 224) occasionally used to prevent further oedema by lowering body metabolism.

Haemorrhage. EXTRADURAL. See p. 300.

SUBDURAL. Site in potential space between inner layer of dura mater and arachnoid mater. Causes: tearing of veins passing through space from cortex to superior sagittal sinus; intracerebral haematoma communicating with subdural space.

Acute. Accompanies severe head injuries with cerebral swelling. Rapid formation of haematoma of significant size causes rapid onset of signs and symptoms of cerebral compression.

Subacute. Minimal cerebral swelling. Some blood may escape into ventricles. Haematoma must reach significant size before signs and symptoms of gradually increasing intracranial pressure arise. Local and general signs and symptoms occur. Often appears 3–10 days after injury.

Chronic. Slow formation of haematoma. May become encased in fibrous membrane and enlarge slowly. History of head injury is often lacking as blow required is minimal. Can mimic any brain disorder but commonly simulates cerebral tumour.

INTRACEREBRAL. Bleeding within brain substance. Treatment usually ineffective as surgical intervention unable to arrest haemorrhage without damage to important brain structures.

Treatment. Surgical emergency. Pressure must be relieved before it affects brainstem causing permanent paralysis and disability. If haematoma is successfully removed later, disability remains.

PREPARATION. Routine for theatre as on p. 2. Shave entire scalp.

OPERATION Incision upper border of zygoma above external auditory meatus. Small hole made through skull using either trephine (circular saw with central pin) or burr.

Appearance through hole: extradural haemorrhage – blood clot presenting through hole; subdural haemorrhage – plum-coloured bulging dura; swelling of brain – dura bulging but of normal colour.

Extradural haemorrhage. Incision enlarged and hole in skull enlarged with rongeur forceps. Clot slowly evacuated by suction or broken up with blunt dissector and irrigated with normal saline. Middle meningeal artery identified and sealed by diathermy, ligation with suture or silver clip. If other vessels bleeding these must be located and dealt with similarly. If unable to identify, small graft from temporal muscle packed between dura and bone, dura sutured to pericranium to retain graft in position.

Subdural haemorrhage. Skull opening enlarged, dura incised while protecting underlying brain with director. Haematoma aspirated or flushed out. No attempt made to identify bleeding vessel. Usually seals itself spontaneously. Drain tube left in situ 48 hours. Exploratory hole may be made on other side as bleeding frequently bilateral.

Intracerebral haemorrhage. Skull hole enlarged to provide measure of decompression (must not extend beyond lateral fissure as cerebral cortex in danger of herniation).

Closure of wound. If drainage not necessary — bone disc replaced and muscle sewn without tension. Scalp closed in 2 layers to prevent infection and escape of cerebrospinal fluid.

Rehabilitation of conscious patient

Restlessness. Occurs during cerebral irritation. Patient must be protected from injuring himself. May become abusive and violent when disturbed, hence other patients must be protected. (1) Nurse in single room if possible. Room should be quiet, well ventilated and darkened. (2) Bed: padded head and cot sides. (3) Restraining straps tend to make patient more restless but must be advocated if patient in danger of injuring himself or if he continually removes Ryle's tube, intravenous tubes, catheters or dressing. (4) Sedation usually contra-indicated as drugs mask important vital signs especially pupil reactions. Phenobarbitone or paraldehyde may be given.

Position. Pillows are gradually introduced and unless patient complains of vertigo, headache, nausea or vomiting, upright position attained in 2–3 days.

Ambulation. Must be gradual — prone to headaches, vertigo, impaired memory and concentration; these tend to make patient anxious and nervous and may turn him into 'psychological' invalid. (1) Graduated exercises, especially when residual muscle

308

weakness exists. Rehabilitation programme and prognosis explained when paralysis persists. (2) Activities. Reading, talking, diversional therapy encouraged to stimulate an interest in life. (3) Sitting out of bed. Determined by (a) when patient can sit up without nausea, vomiting or headache, and (b) expresses a desire to sit out. Normal activities should be resumed gradually.

Discharge. Once patient ambulant, discharged to suitable environment; usually in about 3 weeks. May be ready to work 1 week later. When permanent damage remains, relatives may need explanations and encouragement in handling patient. Patient may need assistance in choice of new job.

Complications

Those requiring urgent surgery. (1) Depressed fracture. (2) Haemorrhage: extradural, subdural, intracerebral. (3) Intracranial abscess. (4) Jacksonian epilepsy.

Those not requiring surgery. (1) Epileptic fits. (2) Infection: meningitis, encephalitis. (3) Cerebral damage resulting in altered personality. (4) Persistent headaches. (5) Hyperpyrexia. (6) Diabetes insipidus. (7) Damage to cranial nerves.

VERTEBRAL COLUMN

FRACTURES AND DISLOCATIONS OF VERTEBRAE

Sites. Cervical (less common but potentially more dangerous); thoracic; lumbar.

Causes. (1) Direct violence, e.g. crushing injuries, gunshot wounds, severe blows, falls on uneven surface. (2) Indirect violence. Force applied along long axis of vertebral column, e.g. fall on feet, buttocks or head (diving into shallow water common cause of fracture of cervical vertebrae).

Types. (1) Crush fractures. Flexion force compresses vertebral bodies, most commonly at front, causing one to become wedge-shaped. Cord not usually involved and ligaments not torn, hence fracture is stable. (2) Angulation fracture and dislocation. Vertebral end-plates ruptured and intervertebral disc forced into vertebral body. Comminuted fracture results with various degrees of dislocation. Bony fragments may be driven into cord. If articular processes fracture or facet joints dislocate, one vertebra is forced into next below. (3) Various types of dislocation and subluxation. Vertebral bodies may be forced apart or displaced in forward direction.

Treatment. Aim: to avoid displacement and damage to cord.

FIRST AID. Patient kept lying flat and all movement avoided. Moving on to stretcher not attempted unless sufficient people available. Ideal is 5 persons — 1 to hold head, 1 to hold feet, 2 to support spine and roll patient, 1 to place blanket or stretcher under patient. All must work in unison and keep patient perfectly horizontal. Small hard pillows placed under natural curvatures.

DEFINITIVE. Depends on fracture site.

Cervical. (1) Massage and analgesics. Hyperextension in cervical collar — plaster, or, more commonly, plastic. (2) Skull traction. Various types of tongs available (Crutchfield's, Barton, Roger Anderson). Burr holes made in skull in parietotemporal regions and tips of tongs inserted. Weights suspended over pulley. 20—40 lb tolerated without discomfort when over-riding articular processes must be disengaged. Once reduction achieved 8—12 lb sufficient for maintenance. (Close observation necessary while heavy weight engaged as injudicious traction may cause damage to cord or medulla.) (3) Open reduction. Necessary if above measures fail or fracture unstable. Laminectomy and arthrodesis or plates and screws along spinous processes.

Thoracic. Stable fracture. No immobilization needed. Patient may rest in bed 3—4 weeks. Exercises to restore normal function started as soon as pain subsides. Surgical corset or brace may be worn to permit early ambulation. If pain severe, immobilization may be needed: plaster of Paris jacket from head to waist with openings for face and arms.

Lumbar. In older age group: bed rest for few days followed by brace. Younger age group: reduction by hyperextension then immobilization in plaster jacket. Open reduction and arthrodesis if damage to cord or cauda equina suspected.

Complications. Mal-, non- or delayed union. Arthritic changes. Damage to spinal cord causing paralysis (including diaphragm), paralytic ileus, bladder distension and stasis.

HERNIATED OR DISPLACED INTERVERTEBRAL DISC

So-called 'slipped disc'. Dislocation or extrusion of nucleus pulposus into neural canal through weakness or rupture of annulus fibrosus.

Signs and symptoms. CERVICAL. Pain: neck, shoulder, scapular region; made worse by straining or coughing. Paraesthesia into fingers. Restricted neck movements due to spasm of neck muscles. Weakness of muscles supplied by compressed nerve root.

LUMBAR. Episodic in back and/or leg. Aggravated by straining. Limp favouring affected leg. Pain accentuated by stretching sciatic nerve, e.g. by raising straight leg. Diminished knee and ankle reflexes. Varying sensory response: normal to complete analgesia of affected root.

Diagnosis. Confirmed by X-ray. Straight X-ray may show narrowed interspaces or arthritic changes. Myelogram records extent and level of damage. Discogram: radio-opaque dye injected directly into disc. Normal disc accepts not more than 0.5 ml, damaged disc may accept 2–3 ml. Injection frequently reproduces pain. Opaque dye demonstrates damaged disc.

Treatment. CONSERVATIVE — bed rest, analgesia. Traction — continuous halter traction for neck; bilateral pelvic or leg traction for back; to overcome muscle spasm. Physiotherapy after acute phase to strengthen muscles of back, abdomen and legs. Patient instructed in correct method of lifting to prevent further straining injuries. Support to area — plastic neck collar; corset for back.

SURGICAL — indicated when pain severe and unrelieved by above methods, or when signs are suggestive of neurological disturbance.

Laminectomy. Removal of laminae and excision of protruding nucleus pulposus adequate in most cases. Intervertebral fusion necessary in some cases.

INJURIES TO SPINAL CORD

Causes. Herniation of displaced intervertebral discs. Fracture or fracture-dislocation of vertebrae. Penetrating injuries, e.g. gunshot wounds.

Pathology. (1) Minor injury, e.g. disc lesion may cause compression of one or more nerve roots resulting in sensory changes in skin and weakness of muscles. (2) Spinal cord lesion. Depends on site: (a) Cervical – either complete or incomplete. Appears to bear no constant relation to severity of skeletal injuries. (b) Thoracic. Usually complete transection because force required to displace thoracic vertebra is always great. (c) Thoracolumbar (T12–L1). Mixed nerve lesion. May involve cord but more likely to damage nerve roots of cauda equina. (d) Lumbar. Cauda equina more resistant to injury than spinal cord, extent of damage less, and more likely to recover. (3) Spinal shock or concussion occurs following damage to cord. Total suppression of function below lesion. Complete sensory loss, flaccid paralysis and absence of visceral responses. May last days or sometimes weeks. As it passes off paralysis becomes spastic, exaggerated tendon and visceral reflexes, being unmodified by higher control. (4) Recovery. If cord only bruised and oedematous recovery of complete function achieved. If cord incompletely transected recovery of sensory and motor power usually good but limited. If cord completely transected reflex activity returns but sensation and control of voluntary movement lost permanently. If sheaths of nerves in cauda equina are intact they will recover in the same way as any peripheral nerves. Regeneration occurs at about 1 in per month.

Terminology. *Paraplegia*. Complete motor and sensory paralysis which includes both legs. Caused by injury or disease of lower spinal cord.

Tetraplegia. (Quadriplegia – old terminology, etymologically incorrect.) Complete motor and sensory paralysis which includes all 4 limbs. Cervical cord affected.

Paraparesis. Partial motor paralysis associated with varying degrees of sensory loss.

Monoplegia. Paralysis of one limb.

Hemiplegia. Paralysis of arm and leg on one side of body only.

Signs and symptoms. Flaccid paralysis below lesion. Sensory loss below lesion. Urinary retention. Paralytic ileus. Respiratory difficulty of lesion above C4. Lack of perspiration below lesion.

If brain injury present, cord injury may be difficult to detect and may be overlooked.

Definitive management. Best results achieved in units specializing in this care where high degree of skill available during initial stages; adequate facilities and personnel available for rehabilitation; mental depression and discouragement less likely to occur if patient associating with others in similar predicament.

Care. Aims — anticipate, prevent, recognize and treat complications.

Complications. (1) Further irreparable damage from careless unnecessary movements or from spreading of oedema and haemorrhage. (2) Urinary retention, retention with overflow, urinary stasis; leading to cystitis infection may spread to kidneys. (3) Paralytic ileus. (4) Respiratory paralysis. (5) Pressure sores due to impaired circulation, immobilization, incontinence, loss of sensation. Once formed these are very difficult to cure. (6) Impacted faeces due to diminished visceral movement, immobilization. (7) Contractures and atrophy from immobility. (8) Foot drop due to spinal injury, lack of muscle power and lack of support against gravity. (9) Inability to avoid injury, e.g. burns, due to loss of sensation and inability to move away from danger, e.g ray lamps. (10) Chest complications from prolonged recumbency and damage to nerve supply of chest. (11) 'Psychological' cripple from inability to accept condition and develop compensation.

Immediate care. Patient not moved until thorough examination performed including: neurological examination to establish level of injury and extent of functional loss; spinal X-ray; lumbar puncture — positive Queckenstedt test indicating total block. To ensure that no distortion of spine occurs, 4 to 6 people required to lift patient on to bed. Bed: mattress on rigid base to prevent sagging; divided mattress, 3–4 sections to permit alteration of pressure distribution. Position: patient supported on pillows and arranged so that neither contracture nor overstretching occurs; feet supported at right angles to leg to prevent foot drop; venous thrombosis must be prevented; 2-hourly change of position day and night essential to relieve pressure areas: adequate numbers of skilled staff, 4 in team, needed to ensure spine not distorted during turning. Bladder: patient asked to void and if ineffectual, indwelling catheter inserted under strict aseptic precautions. Polythene catheter, size 14–16 Fr, used and connected to underwater seal containing 40% formalin. Intermittent drainage, 2-hourly release of catheter, to avoid overdistension or 'shrinkage'

313

of bladder. Respirator, e.g. Bird's, at hand if lesion in cervical region above C4. Tracheostomy may be needed. Paralytic ileus: prevention and treatment, p. 28.

Surgery. Laminectomy. Indicated if (1) progressive neurological loss, (2) positive Queckenstedt test, (3) evidence of bone fragments compressed into spinal cord, (4) wound, e.g. gunshot.

Continuing care. PRESSURE SORE PREVENTION. Turn 2-hourly; scrupulous attention to bedmaking; protection against injury — bedcradle, no hot water bottles; scrupulous cleanliness; control of incontinence; regular, thorough examination of all pressure areas for evidence of redness.

DIET. Copious fluids to maintain bladder function, prevent urinary stasis and renal calculi, eliminate toxins; high protein to avoid muscle wasting. Encourage patient to eat with tempting meals according to his taste. Obesity avoided. Added vitamins and minerals may be necessary.

DRUGS. Morphia or pethidine during immediate post-operative period. Reduce to mild analgesics as soon as pain subsides, e.g. Panadol. None required after 4–5 days. Antibiotics may be used as prophylaxis against infection. Urinary antiseptics may be used to prevent urinary infection.

PHYSIOTHERAPY. Breathing exercises started immediately. Passive full range of movements of all paralysed limbs. Encourage patient to exercise all muscles not paralysed.

BLADDER. Aim to prevent retention and overdistension. After spinal shock (oliguria from kidney suppression during this stage) sphincters become contracted and catheterization necessary. Turning into prone position for short periods daily facilitates emptying. Catheter changed weekly. Tubing observed for kinking or blockage which is corrected at once. Amount and type of drainage observed and recorded. Signs of urinary infection reported at once and appropriate antibiotic or urinary antiseptic started.

Catheter removed 4–6 weeks after injury and patient evacuates urine by gentle supra-pubic pressure every 3–4 hours. Residual urine measured. Bladder must be completely emptied otherwise debris remains and predisposes to calculi and infection. If more than 270 ml residual urine catheter re-inserted for few days and procedure then repeated. Intravenous pyelogram to detect back pressure causing dilatation or renal calculi. If after 3 months residual urine still high, may be necessary to relieve bladder-neck obstruction by transurethral resection or division of pudendal nerve. This may result in partial incontinence but suitable rubber urinals can be worn and patient can engage in social activities. More important that there should not be any retention and distension.

BOWELS. Once on normal diet patient must learn routine for himself — digital examination of rectum each morning, if faeces present patient bears down and attempts evacuation. If unsuccessful, suppository inserted. Manual removal may be required. Enemata and aperients less reliable. High residue diet and regularity of attempt to defaecate essential to establish good result.

Psychological support. Independence encouraged as soon as possible, e.g. turn in bed, feed himself, wash, clean teeth and nails and do own hair. Later, dress himself, sit up, stand up and eventually walk if lesion permits. Patient must learn to accept permanent disability. Aided by frank explanation by doctor; realization that it is possible to lead full and active social life; early encouragement of above; contact with other paraplegics; contact with relatives and visitors; constant encouragement and recognition of small day-to-day achievements; training for occupation on discharge.

Rehabilitation. Aim: to discharge to home and family with good prospect of full employment and remuneration. Combined efforts of physiotherapist, occupational therapist and medico-social worker. On discharge patient must be able to control bladder and bowels and to prevent pressure sores on any part of body. Usually discharged in wheel chair but many are able to graduate to walking with support and crutches.

BRAIN AND SPINAL CORD DISORDERS

HYDROCEPHALUS

Enlargement of cerebrospinal fluid pathways as a result of increase of amount and/or pressure of fluid.

Causes. Decrease in normal c.s.f. absorption rate due to obliteration of subarachnoid space, e.g. following meningitis. Obstruction of communications between ventricles or opening into cisterna magna by congenital defect, blood clot, inflammation or tumour (internal hydrocephalus). Compression of brain causes external hydrocephalus. Overproduction of c.s.f. rare; due to papilloma of choroid plexus.

Pathology. Two forms. (1) *Communicating type:* c.s.f. passes through ventricular system but is obstructed at some point in subarachnoid space. (2) *Non-communicating type:* flow of fluid obstructed within ventricular system, e.g. at aqueduct of Sylvius; c.s.f. accumulates in ventricles causing distension. In child cranial sutures have not fused and skull is capable of expansion. In older child or adult symptoms not associated with increase in circumference of head but with increased intracranial pressure.

Signs and symptoms. Early: fontanelles tense and not pulsating; sutures wide; circumference of head greater than normal; frontal bosses prominent; visible distended scalp veins; sclera visible above iris due to down-turned gaze of eyes (pressure on thin orbital roofs displaces eyeball); increased intracranial pressure — irritability, increased drowsiness, vomiting, papilloedema, occasionally fits. In babies where skull capable of expansion signs of increased intracranial pressure are absent.

Investigations. Measurement of head circumference repeated frequently. Examination of c.s.f. through ventricular puncture of burr holes (site — lateral angle of anterior fontanelle or coronal suture well away from midline) for blood to exclude subdural haematoma, protein, to ensure c.s.f. sterile, pressure measured with manometer (child must be relaxed, crying increases pressure of c.s.f.). Dye injected into ventricles and lumbar puncture done. Dye should appear within 20 minutes, if not — hydrocephalus of obstructive type. Ventriculogram. Needle inserted into ventricle via anterior fontanelle, c.s.f. aspirated and equal amount of air injected. X-ray should show entire ventricular system and determines width of cerbral cortex (prognosis poor if less than 1 cm thick), establishes cause of hydrocephalus. Cerebral arteriogram.

Treatment. Tends to arrest spontaneously but enlargement of head may have caused permanent disability by time this occurs. Aim — to remove excess fluid.

1. Repeated lumbar punctures in communicating hydrocephalus.

2. Ventricular taps in obstructive type.

3. Surgery to drain c.s.f. into other parts of body. Ventriculo-atrial shunt most successful. Piece of silicone rubber tubing inserted into lateral ventricle via burr hole. Another piece inserted subcutaneously down neck into internal jugular vein and threaded into right atrium. Tubes connected to sensitive one-way valve which prevents blood passing from atrium to lateral ventricle (Spitz-Holter valve most successful). As long as pressure in ventricle greater than that in atrium c.s.f. will flow but if atrial pressure raised, e.g. by coughing or straining, valve closes and prevents backflow.

Complications. 1. As child grows, tubing comes out of atrium into superior vena cava and later into innominate vein. Blood clots tend to form around catheter. Treatment: lengthening of catheter when X-ray shows shortening or when tube blocked.

2. Blockage of ventricular end of catheter by ingrowths of choroid plexus tissue into holes of tube. Treatment: change tube.

3. Septicaemia. Micro-organisms tend to accumulate in valve and spread into blood stream. Treatment: remove system and replace new one.

4. Pulmonary emboli due to clotting around catheter in heart.

5. Changes in intracranial pressure. (a) Overdrainage, indicated by indrawn fontanelles. May result in respiratory or cardiac collapse. Treatment: posture child in head down position to retard drainage. (b) Insufficient drainage indicated by convex fontanelle instead of normal slight concavity. Treatment – posture, head of cot elevated on blocks; pump valve by rhythmical compression and release (approximately 100 compressions force 7 ml c.s.f. through).

SPINA BIFIDA

Congenital malformation of vertebral column in which neural arch fails to close over spinal cord. Spinous process is therefore double instead of single.

Spina bifida occulta. Neural arches of vertebrae fail to unite (usually sacrum or lumbar spine). Skin closes over neural canal instead of bone and muscle.

SIGNS AND SYMPTOMS. Usually none (hence 'occult' or hidden). Skin anomalies may be present, e.g. hair tuft, dimple,

317

abnormal pigmentation. As child grows cord and nerve roots may be pulled up and cease to function resulting in gradual onset of partial or complete paralysis of lower limbs and sphincters usually after age 5–6 years. May be associated with other abnormalities especially of feet, e.g. talipes (p. 292), pes cavus (p. 292).

DIAGNOSIS. Confirmed by X-ray findings, e.g. myelogram.

Meningocele. Protrusion of sac of meninges through defective neural arch. Sac covered with skin. No nerve involvement. (Rare condition.)

Myelomeningocele. Most common type. Also known as spina bifida cystica. Protrusion of sac of meninges containing c.s.f. and cord through bony defect. Shape varies from simple flat protrusion to huge sessile mass with significant portions of neural tissue exposed on surface. Site – most common in lumbar or lumbosacral region, but may occur anywhere along vertebral column or even in skull (encephalocele).

SIGNS AND SYMPTOMS. c.s.f. may leak from sac if ruptured – sac collapses and refills intermittently. Paralysis – motor and sensory. Varies from paresis in one or more muscles to total paraplegia – lower limbs, anal and urethral sphincters, occasionally lower trunk muscles also.

Myelocele. Complete failure of fusion of neural arches. Very little meningeal sac and lower part of cord lies open on surface.

SIGNS AND SYMPTOMS. Gross paralysis. Spinal column becomes increasingly more bent as there is no muscular support for it.

Complications

More likely with myelocele and myelomeningocele, less likely with meningocele and hardly ever with spina bifida occulta.

1. Associated hydrocephalus due to congenital malformation at base of brain or infection, meningitis, ascending via raw surface of sac.

2. Paralysis leading to malformations – talipes, extension of knee, flexion of hip (easily dislocates); anal sphincter leading to constipation and/or leaking of faecal contents; urinary incontinence – increasing risk of pressure sores.

3. Skin changes. Venous return from legs impaired due to paralysis. Become cold, cyanosed, subject to chilblains and

pressure sores. Infection may occur even to extent of osteo-myelitis.

Treatment

NURSING CARE. Aims: prevent infection by keeping area dry, clean and intact. Cover skin wih soft sterile dressing or tulle gras. Protective barrier devised between area and buttocks. Avoid pressure on area — nursing babe in prone position by building up pillows (ensure that mouth and nose are free). Padded bed-cradle over back. Avoid use of antiseptics because of danger to nerve cells.

SURGERY. *Indications.* Evidence that surgery will reduce paralysis; danger of sepsis, i.e. ruptured sac exposing neural plaques; cosmetic reasons.

Time. In urgent cases may be before 6 months but best left until sufficient skin covering lesion to give adequate closure.

Aims. Avoid damage to nerves. Obtain skin cover.

Method. Excise sac carefully preserving nerve tissue. Closure: if narrow cleft, close with dura mater and cover with muscle and fascia; if large defect, skin graft. Rotating skin flaps and relieving incisions or artificial devices such as polythene or rubber case.

COMPLICATIONS. Hydrocephalus may increase when sac removed and area repaired. Meningitis. Paralysis.

Treatment of spina bifida only in initial stage, later other conditions must also be corrected, e.g. incontinence — in females may be necessary to divert urinary stream to avoid continuous incontinence; deformities may need orthopaedic correction. Parents need special emotional support to assist them in their acceptance of deformed child.

INTRACRANIAL ABSCESS

Localized collection of pus within brain substance.

Cause. Direct spread from mastoid process, paranasal sinuses, middle ear. Spread via blood stream from septic focus, e.g. from lungs: bronchiectasis or lung abscess. Septicaemia.

Pathology. Usually originate in areas of least vascularity. At first infection not well sealed off but thick protective wall soon develops from reaction of neuroglia similar to fibrous tissue encapsulation of abscesses elsewhere.

319

Signs and symptoms. Inflammation and pus formation: general malaise, anorexia, irregular pyrexia, leucocytosis, tachycardia. Local: convulsions, increasing headache, visual disturbance, drowsiness, facial palsy. Chronic stage: signs and symptoms of increasing intracranial pressure due to space occupying lesion.

Diagnosis. Confirmed by air encephalogram or cerebral angiogram; examination of c.s.f. by lumbar puncture (never done in presence of papilloedema because of danger of coning of brain) may reveal elevation of cell count and protein.

Treatment. (1) Antibiotic therapy. (2) Drainage when suppuration localized. Burr holes made in skull, needle inserted into abscess and pus aspirated. Extent of cavity revealed by injecting radio-opaque dye and X-ray taken. Aspiration repeated when necessary and appropriate antibiotic given systemically. (3) Resection of abscess, intact if possible, or removal of part of abscess wall so that pus can drain on to skin surface.

NEOPLASMS

Cerebral tumours. May be malignant or benign, primary or secondary (metastatic).

Types. Glioma, meningioma, adenoma of pituitary gland, haemangioma, congenital tumour.

Signs and symptoms. GENERAL. Slowly increasing intracranial pressure — headache (worse in morning and relieved when standing up); nausea; vomiting; papilloedema (swelling at fundus of eye at point of entry of optic nerve); compensatory changes in pulse and blood pressure — pulse rate falls, blood pressure rises.

LOCAL. Depends upon site of growth, e.g. Frontal lobes: personality and mental changes, varying degrees of hemiparesis, convulsions. Parietal lobes: degrees of paralysis, visual changes. Occipital lobes: visual disturbances. Temporal lobes: convulsions, distorted perception of sounds, size and shape of objects. Cerebellum: ataxia, incoordination of arms and legs, nystagmus. Brain stem: cerebral nerve palsies. Pituitary gland: may press on optic chiasma causing visual changes, also hyper- or hyposecretion of various hormones.

Investigations. Air encephalogram, ventriculogram, cerebral angiogram, electroencephalogram, neurological examination.

Treatment. SURGICAL. Exploration through craniotomy or craniectomy, followed by total removal of tumour or decompression (palliative measure) by partial removal of tumour, or craniectomy to allow room for expansion; c.s.f. shunt from ventricles to cisterna magna if tumour blocking c.s.f. flow.

CONSERVATIVE. If tumour inaccessible X-ray irradiation sometimes used. Measures to overcome — headache, e.g. analgesics; nausea and vomiting, e.g. anti-emetics.

VASCULAR DISORDERS

Surgical disorders of brain (1) occlusion leading to ischaemia, (2) haemorrhage.

Cerebral ischaemia

Cause. Partial or complete blockage of extra- or intracranial vessel by atheromatous plaque, thrombosis or embolus.

Site. May involve any vessel but more common in carotid, cerebral and vertebral arteries.

Signs and symptoms. Loss of function of area of brain. Signs and symptoms vary with actual site and include paralysis, anaesthesia, blindness, aphasia.

Treatment. CONSERVATIVE. Nursing care to prevent complications of prolonged bedrest. Anticoagulant therapy.

SURGICAL. Depends on area. Extracranial portions of carotid and vertebral arteries may be treated by thromboendarterectomy or various bypass procedures.

Haemorrhage

Causes. Injury; spontaneous rupture in hypertension, aneurysm, haemorrhagic conditions.

Aneurysm. Commonest cause. Usually congenital. Occur in circle of Willis mainly at point of arterial bifurcation. Types — congenital 'berry' aneurysm, small, thin-walled, spherical, tend to rupture between ages 30 and 50 years especially when hypertension coexists. Most common cause of subarachnoid haemorrhage. Atherosclerotic — rare, seldom rupture, not related to arterial bifurcations. Occur outside subarachnoid space on carotid, basilar and vertebral arteries (carotid artery in cavernous sinus commonest site). Mimic signs and symptoms of intracranial tumour. Dissecting aneurysm and infective aneurysm may also occur but are rare.

Site. Subdural: rare. Subarachnoid: most common. Intracerebral.

Signs and symptoms. SUBARACHNOID HAEMORRHAGE. Sudden onset with severe headache but not necessarily loss of consciousness. Signs of cerebral or meningeal irritation — neck stiffness, photophobia, headache, irritability. Mortality high with first bleed 30–40%. Recurrence common within first 3 weeks and mortality rate rises with subsequent bleeding.

Diagnosis. Confirmed by lumbar puncture: reveals blood-stained fluid and raised pressure. If blood is old c.s.f. is yellow.

If aneurysm bursts into brain substance (intracerebral), neurological damage, e.g. hemiplegia, aphasia and unconsciousness, results.

CRANIAL NERVE PALSIES. Caused by pressure on adjacent structures; especially nerves 2, 3, 4, 5 and 6 affected. Signs and symptoms of ischaemia if partial obstruction occurs.

HEADACHE. Caused by pressure on pain sensitive structures; usually orbital or supra-orbital.

Treatment. CONSERVATIVE. Absolute bedrest. Control of headache and restlessness by analgesia. Maintenance of adequate fluid balance.

SURGICAL. If indicated, performed as soon as patient's condition permits: (1) Isolation of aneurysm by clipping its neck or by diverting blood round it through other branches of circle of Willis. (2) Subsequent haemorrhage averted by reducing pressure by ligation of carotid artery in neck when aneurysm is in wall of carotid artery. (Ineffective when aneurysm is in circle of Willis as collateral circulation maintains high pressure.)

BRAIN SURGERY

Burr holes and trephine. See p. 307.

Craniotomy. (Osteoplastic flap.) Opening into brain. Used to expose any area. Semicircular-shaped incision made in scalp, broad enough to ensure adequate blood supply to flap. Flap raised and 5 or 6 burr holes made. Dura mater separated from skull and Gigli saw passed between adjacent holes. Bone sawn through with outward bevel so that when area of bone replaced it does not sink below surrounding level. Bone at base of section partly divided and bent outwards. At end of operation, dura sutured, bone piece replaced with some sutures in pericranium, scalp sutured in two layers.

Lobectomy. Removal of frontal or right temporal lobe. (Partial removal only of left temporal lobe as it contains speech area and aphasia would result from total lobectomy.)

INDICATIONS. Tumour not enclosed in capsule. (Encapsulated tumours can be shelled out with blunt dissection.)

In majority of malignant tumours complete removal not usually possible. Subtotal or partial removal gives palliative relief of increased intracranial pressure.

Leucotomy. Interruption of nerve pathways from frontal lobes to main central relay nucleus, the thalamus.

INDICATIONS. Psychiatric conditions, e.g. chronic obsessive compulsive depression. Relief of pain, e.g. in inoperable cancer. Main effects — relieves severe anxiety, tension, remorse and recurrent thoughts of an undesirable nature. Analgesics can be withdrawn without distress. Appetite and sleep improve.

METHODS. Leucotome inserted through burr holes at junction of temporal crest and coronal suture. White matter in front of tip of anterior horn of lateral ventricle divided. Alternatively, fibres divided with instrument introduced through orbital roof.

Hypophysectomy — removal of pituitary gland.

INDICATIONS. (1) Tumour especially when compressing optic chiasma. (2) Palliative measure to control pain and rapid growth of some forms of cancer which are 'hormone dependent', e.g. breast (p. 197).

METHODS. (1) Transfrontal approach: frontal osteoplastic flap raised, tumour located and removed. (2) Trans-sphenoidal approach: through mouth in front of upper gum, exposing floor of nose and nasal septum. Submucous resection carried upwards through vomer to roof of nasopharynx. Anterior wall of sphenoidal air sinus removed with punch. Floor of pituitary fossa removed and gland removed, mainly by suction.

Removal of scar tissue. Scar tissue causing Jacksonian epilepsy removed from cerebral cortex or meninges. Osteoplastic flap, dura incised and scar tissue excised widely.

NURSING MANAGEMENT

Pre-operative care. Psychological: 'mystery' surrounds brain surgery. Nurse must create warm, accepting atmosphere for patient and allow him to voice his fears and apprehensions. Permission for anaesthesia must be given by patient where possible, or next-of-kin if patient irrational or unconscious. In females permission to cut hair and shave head must be carefully sought.

Visitors encouraged. Careful observations, over and above routine, for personality changes, twitching and fits. Hypothermia may be used in cerebral surgery.

Post-operative care. Specific.

OBSERVATIONS. Routine plus careful observation for increased intracranial pressure. Continued for 48 hours.

POSITION. Depends upon extent of surgery. Recumbent while unconscious. Gradually elevated to semi-upright when conscious to aid venous drainage and reduce cerebral oedema. Two-hourly changes of position to prevent pressure sores and pneumonia. (Patient may be prohibited from turning on operated side if large amount of basin tissue removed. Shifting of brain dangerous until non-operated side has compensated and filled gap.)

RESTLESSNESS. Heavy sedation contra-indicated. Tends to cloud post-operative signs and symptoms, e.g. conscious state. Light restraint may be needed to prevent patient from removing dressings from head. Padded cot sides may be needed. Headache may be due to cerebral oedema. In addition diuretic drugs such as Ureaphil or Mannitol may be given intravenously (they have low potential for sodium retention thus increasing urinary output and lessening oedema.) Mild analgesics, e.g. Panadol, calcium aspirin may be given.

HYPERPYREXIA. Surgical intervention may disturb heat regulating centre.

FLUIDS AND DIET. Started when patient ready — normal requirements.

WOUND. Inspected within 24 hours to exclude possibility of haematoma. Sutures removed fifth—seventh day. Skull cap usually applied until hair grows.

BOWELS. Straining must be avoided. Aperients from first post-operative day to ensure soft motions.

Rehabilitation. May be slow — depends on brain involvement. Teamwork essential and may involve nurse, relatives, friends, physiotherapist, occupational therapist, speech therapist and medico-social worker.

SPINAL CORD SURGERY
Laminectomy
Removal of spinous process and laminae from one or more vertebrae.

Indications. Relieve pressure on spinal cord: (1) prolapsed intervertebral disc; (2) vertebral fractures; (3) spinal tumours.

Method. Patient in prone or lateral position. Centre of table raised for lumbar operation so that normal concavity is levelled. Head rest needed for cervical operation.

Paramedian incision 15–20 cm. Supra- and intraspinous ligaments divided. Spinous process removed with bone shears. Laminae removed. (Initial opening into vertebrae may be difficult. May be done with trephine or burr tool.) Dura opened and cord inspected if necessary. Not opened if disc to be removed. Disc curetted after small opening made in annulus fibrosus. Intervertebral fusion may be done with bone graft from tibia or by bone chips inserted between spinous processes. Necessary if patient has osteoarthritic changes.

Cordotomy
Division of spinothalamic tract (transmitting pain and temperature sensations from periphery to brain).

Indications. Intractable pain involving lumbosacral or brachial plexus, e.g. in malignancy.

Method. Spinothalamic tract lies in anteriolateral segment of cord. (Controversy over actual site so operation not standardized.) Upper thoracic region for lower limbs and high level in cervical section for upper limbs.

Complications. Rare. Sphincter disturbance. Motor weakness. Pressure sores. Diaphragmatic paralysis.

Pre-operative care. Routine. Nil specific.

Post-operative care. Specific.

POSITION. Recumbent or lateral with spine well supported and in good alignment. Turned 2-hourly. After 48 hours patient may be able to roll himself without pain.

ANALGESIA. Pethidine or morphia 4-hourly, 48 hours. Milder analgesics until fourth—fifth day when pain should be negligible.

OBSERVATIONS. Usual post-operative. Legs and feet examined 1—2 hourly for changes in temperature, sensation and movement.

FLUIDS. On demand, increasing to copious (2½—3 litres daily).

DIET. Light; started as soon as oral fluids are tolerated.

PHYSIOTHERAPY. Breathing and leg exercises on recovery from anaesthetic. Third—fourth day back exercises started and continued until discharge.

BLADDER. (1) Psychological, overcome with nursing measures. (2) Sphincter disturbance, usually temporary. Catheterize for 2—3 days. Incontinence may occur from sphincter damage, usually temporary.

BOWELS. Patient often afraid to defaecate because of back pain. Females taught in pre-operative period how to use special urinal or kidney dish. Suppositories on third—fourth day to initiate first bowel action.

SUTURES. Removed 7—14 days.

AMBULATION. Usually not allowed out of bed until wound healed. Must be well supported when sitting. Graduated exercises until fully ambulant. Discharge 2—4 weeks. Advice given on methods of lifting and how to avoid strain and further prolapse of discs.

SPECIAL INVESTIGATIONS
Air encephalography

X-ray of ventricles of brain following introduction of air into subarachnoid space.

Indications. Cerebral tumour especially tumour of pituitary gland; cerebral ischaemia; in absence of localizing symptoms; hydrocephalus.

Contra-indications. Raised intracranial pressure.

Preparation. Premedication — barbiturate, e.g. Nembutal 100—200 mg, to allay anxiety and gain cooperation. Explanation of the procedure. (General anaesthetic may be used.)

Method. Position as for lumbar puncture (p. 330) or cisternal puncture (p. 331). X-ray taken after c.s.f. removed and 5 ml air introduced; further 5 ml c.s.f. removed and further 10 ml air introduced, X-ray taken. Procedure repeated until 25–30 ml air introduced. Patient postured to encourage air to enter all parts of ventricles.

Complications. Severe headache. 'Coning' of brain (p. 331).

Aftercare. Lateral position for 48 hours. Turned 2-hourly from side-to-side. Oxygen given by intranasal tube (reduces incidence and severity of headache).

ANALGESIA. Pethidine or codeine.

OBSERVATIONS. Blood pressure and pulse. Taken hourly for 8 hours, 2-hourly for 10 hours, 4-hourly for remaining 48 hours. Some degree of shock accompanies procedure. Slowing of pulse and increasing blood pressure indicate increasing intracranial pressure. Slight pyrexia often present. Hyperpyrexia may indicate brainstem damage. Voluntary movements: e.g. hand grip, ability to move all 4 limbs. (If coning of brain present patient will be unable to respond.) Pupil reactions (p. 302). Respirations – (Cheyne-Stokes respirations indicate raised intracranial pressure). Fluid intake and output, especially for bladder dysfunction.

Ventriculography

X-ray of ventricles of brain after direct introduction of air or dye via needle inserted through burr hole in skull.

Indications. Papilloedema or other signs of raised intracranial pressure when no localizing symptoms present. Hydrocephalus: dye can be induced to fill third and fourth ventricles from lateral ventricles and help to elucidate cause of internal hydrocephalus.

Disadvantages. Surgeon committed to perform immediate surgery, therefore must have facilities available (dangerous procedure unless surgery performed to relieve hydrocephalus): 'coning' of brain (p. 331).

Preparation. Routine for general anaesthesia. Scalp shaved.

Method. Burr holes either side of midline in occipital region. Cannula inserted through brain substance into posterior horn of lateral ventricle. (Each ventricle normally contains 10 ml c.s.f.; withdraw a little at a time and replace with air.) 1–2 ml oily contrast medium may be injected.

Complications. As for encephalography.

Cerebral angiography

X-ray of cerebral blood vessels after injection of radio-opaque dye into carotid or vertebral arteries.

Indications. Space occupying lesions: neoplasm, abscess, haematoma. Vascular lesions: intracranial aneurysm, stenosis of carotid artery.

Advantages. Localizes lesion. Reveals exact nature. Enables carefully planned surgery.

Preparation. Cross circulation in circle of Willis tested by compressing alternately both common carotid arteries. Routine preparation if to be done under general anaesthesia. If under local — patient's cooperation necessary hence — careful explanations. Sedation — e.g. barbiturates, Nembutal 100—200 mg to allay anxiety, half-hour beforehand.

Method. Position: recumbent.

CAROTID APPROACH. Dye, e.g. Diodine, rapidly infused into internal carotid artery (common carotid may be used if there is difficulty getting into internal). Series of X-rays taken as dye travels into all branches. Patient will feel a warm but not unpleasant sensation and should be warned of this.

VERTEBRAL APPROACH. Similar but more difficult technique as vertebral arteries traverse bony canals in transverse processes of cervical vertebrae.

Complications. Haematoma of neck. Transient motor or sensory paralysis, e.g. hemiplegia on contralateral side; dysphagia; difficulty in finding appropriate words to express thoughts and feelings. Visual disturbance (vertebral angiogram). Danger of further haemorrhage if patient has berry aneurysm.

Aftercare. Recumbent position 48 hours. Observe as after encephalogram. Observe for dysphagia: haematoma — apply cold applications, give analgesics.

Myelography

X-ray of spinal cord after injection intrathecally of radio-opaque substance.

Indications. Obstruction of subarachnoid space — neoplasm, prolapsed intervertebral disc, fractured vertebrae.

Preparation. As for air encephalogram. Patient asked about sensitivities and allergies especially to iodine.

Method. Patient prepared as for lumbar or cisternal puncture. Some c.s.f. removed and dye 1–3 ml injected. Observed under fluoroscope. Dye has a high specific gravity and moves up or down the subarachnoid space according to position of patient. X-rays taken at different levels to reveal affected area and its cause.

Aftercare. Patient remains flat for 24 hours.

Electro-encephalography

Recording on graph paper of electrical emissions, greatly amplified, from brain.

Indications. Space occupying lesions of brain; fits – epileptic, Jacksonian.

Preparation. Explain procedure. Reassure patient that it does not hurt. Wash hair. Sedation may be necessary for children. Inform investigator if patient is receiving anticonvulsant drugs.

Method. Electrodes attached to scalp at various points. Electrical emissions amplified and made to trace a line on moving graph paper.

Aftercare. Hair may need to be washed to remove electrode paste.

Lumbar puncture

Removal of c.s.f. by means of needle placed into pool of c.s.f. lying below tip of spinal cord (L1) in subarachnoid space (spinal theca).

Indications. DIAGNOSTIC. Infections – meningitis, encephalitis, poliomyelitis, neurosyphilis. Subarachnoid haemorrhage. Cerebral and spinal tumours. Multiple sclerosis. Polyneuritis. Carcinoma. Radiological investigations, e.g. myelogram.

THERAPEUTIC. Introduction of drugs directly into theca, e.g. antibiotics, steroids, spinal anaesthetics. Relief of intracranial pressure in hydrocephalus.

Contra-indications. Raised intracranial pressure evidenced by papilloedema.

Normal c.s.f. Pressure: 60–120 mm water. Total protein: 15–40 mg/100 ml. Sugar: 45–80 mg/100 ml. Chlorides: 700–760 mg/100 ml. Lymphocytes: 0–4 per cu. mm. Globulin: almost absent. Appearance: clear, colourless.

329

Pathological changes. PRESSURE. Raised, e.g. 400–500 mm in space occupying lesions (tumour) and in hydrocephalus. Queckenstedt's test: c.s.f. pressure measured with manometer and while still in situ, jugular veins compressed. Normally pressure in manometer rises. Abnormal if pressure does not rise and indicates blockage in subarachnoid space. (Must never be done if intracranial lesion suspected.)

CYTOLOGICAL. Red blood cells – intracranial or spinal haemorrhage. Inflammatory cells or pus – infection. Microorganisms may be isolated. Malignant cells (special staining techniques).

BIOLOGICAL. (Examples only, too numerous to list completely.) Protein content raised in tubercular meningitis. Chlorides decreased in dehydration. Globulins, enzymes, immunological bodies – multiple sclerosis, motor neurone disease.

Preparation. Trolley set under strictest aseptic precautions. Careful explanations to patient to obtain full cooperation. Privacy ensured. Bedpan offered if necessary. Lateral position with spine flexed to separate vertebral spinous processes. Spine must be horizontal and near edge of bed. Mattress should be firm with no hollow. Knees and neck flexed so that patient is 'C' shaped. No restraint used as it raises intracranial pressure. Sedation may be required. Alternatively, if patient unable to lie down, may sit on edge of bed with back facing doctor. Instructed to bend the back and clasp hands under the knees. Baby supported on nurse's knee.

Procedure. Strict aseptic technique. Skin cleansed with antiseptic lotion. Local anaesthetic infiltrated. Needle inserted between L3–4 or betweeen L4–5. First drops of c.s.f. allowed to run out and then specimen collected into sterile test tube. Pressure may be measured and Queckenstedt's test performed. Further 2 specimens may be collected to compare colour and clarity. Drugs introduced if necessary. Needle withdrawn and small dry dressing applied.

Complications. 1. Headache due to lowering of c.s.f. pressure which causes dilation of intracranial venous sinuses and pull on sensitive structures, e.g. sinuses, dura mater, arteries, base of brain. Prevented by patient lying flat for 12–24 hours which reduces traction by gravity and allows c.s.f. pressure to return to normal.

2. Introduction of infection. Meningitis most commonly but also extradural abscess, infected disc, osteomyelitis of vertebral bodies.

3. Damage to intervertebral disc which may cause prolapse.

4. Damage to nerve roots by needle, blood clot or drug may result in paraesthesia or paralysis.

5. 'Coning' of brain. Sudden lowering of pressure below foramen magnum while intracranial pressure is high may cause herniation of temporal lobe into tentorial opening or herniation of cerebellar tonsils into foramen magnum thus compressing medulla oblongata causing respiratory and cardiac dysfunction or even arrest.

Cisternal puncture

Removal of c.s.f. by means of needle inserted into cisterna magna (dilated portion of subarachnoid space between inferior surface of cerebellum and posterior surface of medulla oblongata).

Indications. To clarify doubtful findings from lumbar puncture, e.g. Queckenstedt's test. Patient unable to have lumbar puncture, e.g. spondylitis. Therapeutic, e.g. to introduce drugs in basal meningitis. Myelography, encephalography.

Preparation. Back of head and neck shaved. Position: lateral or sitting on chair. Neck flexed with chin on manubrium to open up space between occiput and atlas.

Method. Skin prepared. Anaesthetic injected. Needle inserted in midline at back of neck where it is bisected by line between mastoid processes. Needle passes through foramen magnum into widest part of cisterna magna. Then as for lumbar puncture.

Complications. Piercing of medulla oblongata. (Causes respiratory and cardiac collapse.) Otherwise as for lumbar puncture.

Chapter 11

GENITO-URINARY TRACT

CONDITIONS OF THE KIDNEYS AND URETERS

CONGENITAL ABNORMALITIES

Polycystic disease

Abnormal development of collecting tubules which do not link up with nephrons. Urine manufactured and forms multiple cysts which gradually impair function of kidney.

Pathology. Exact process not known. Familial incidence. May manifest at birth and prove fatal in infancy. May not exhibit until adult life usually between 30 and 60 years. Collecting tubules form but do not join successfully with nephrons. Cysts form with normal tissue between them. Enlargement of cysts gradually destroys normal tissue. Kidney becomes grossly enlarged. Always bilateral though one kidney more affected than the other.

Prognosis. Slowly progressive with renal hypertension and renal failure within 5–10 years.

Signs and symptoms. INFANTS. Stillborn; death within 24 hours; may survive to 12 months and die from uraemia.

ADULTS. Loin pain, aching in nature (due to weight of kidney). Haematuria (damage to normal tissue). May present with symptoms of renal failure — headache, nausea, vomiting, weakness, weight loss. Hypertension. Pyelonephritis. One or both kidneys may be palpable. Urine may show albumin and blood.

Diagnosis. Confirmed by retrograde or intravenous pyelogram (renal outlines enlarged, pelvis almost obliterated, calyces elongated, narrowed and distorted). Renal function tests show impairment. Blood urea raised.

Treatment. Control pyelonephrosis. Treat chronic renal failure. Surgical: exposure and pricking of large cysts — may relieve tension and delay uraemia temporarily.

Agenesis of kidney

Failure of kidney to develop. Usually associated with absence of ureter and partial development of trigone (hemitrigone).

Incidence. Bilateral rare. Unilateral not uncommon.

Signs and symptoms. Usually none. Full investigation of renal tract must be performed before any operation on kidneys contemplated.

Investigations. Plain abdominal X-ray. Intravenous pyelography. Cystoscopic examination to show hemitrigone. Renal arteriogram to show absence of renal vessels.

Duplex kidney

Duplication of kidney with double pelvis and blood supply. Common capsule envelops both structures.

Pathology. Embryologically kidney develops in 2 segments. These fail to unite. Demarcation varies from almost imperceptible sulcus to deep cleft. Smaller upper portion often functionless and may develop hydronephrosis, pyelonephrosis or calculi. Double ureters may be complete and both enter bladder independently, or may join before entry to bladder.

Signs and symptoms. None until above complications occur.

Diagnosis. Confirmed by intravenous or retrograde pyelography.

Treatment. Partial nephrectomy – removal of non-functioning portion.

Horseshoe kidney

Fusion of right and left kidneys at lower poles across lumbar vertebrae.

Pathology. Pelves face anteriorly and ureters pass anteriorly to fused poles and are closer than normal to the midline. Blood supply may come from internal iliac artery.

Signs and symptoms. None unless infection, hydronephrosis or calculi form.

Treatment. Non-specific. Treat complications.

Ectopic kidney

Kidney develops in abnormal position anywhere from true pelvis to upper abdomen.

Site. Commonly iliac fossa, pelvic brim, convexity of sacrum.

Signs and symptoms. Vague abdominal pain. Tender mass in lower abdomen or pelvis. Often asymptomatic unless complicated by hydronephrosis, infection or calculi.

Treatment. Of complications only.

RENAL INJURY

Uncommon because of protection from lumbar vertebrae, lower ribs and lumbar muscles. Potentially serious and usually complicated by other injuries.

Types. Open: penetrating wound, e.g. bullet. Closed: crushing injuries of trunk; direct blow on loin, e.g. during road traffic accident or kick during football match — most common causes.

Effect. Range from mild bruise, contusion, laceration to rupture. (Small tears usually heal without surgical repair.)

Signs and symptoms. PAIN IN LOIN. May be severe even with slight damage. Due mainly to bruising and spasm of lumbar muscles. Often obscured by associated injuries.

HAEMATURIA. Usually present and occasionally the only sign. May not be revealed until shock has been treated and urinary output returns to normal. Length and severity do not seem to have any direct bearing on severity of damage to kidney.

RENAL COLIC. Occurs as clots are passed down ureter. Shock and haemorrhage. Signs and symptoms may be present to greater or lesser degree depending on severity of injury. Bruising of loin. Palpable mass in loin; may be haematoma or extravasated urine. Paralytic ileus may occur because of bleeding retroperitoneally and interference with nerve supply to bowel.

Investigations. Plain abdominal X-ray — loss of psoas shadowing if blood or urine present. Intravenous pyelogram after shock passed to demonstrate injury and function of other kidney in case nephrectomy is necessary. Retrograde pyelogram — seldom necessary and contra-indicated during acute phase because of danger of perinephric abscess.

Treatment. CONSERVATIVE. Treat shock. Observe pulse, respirations and blood pressure to assess state of shock and continuance of haemorrhage. Urine. All specimens saved and labelled with date, time of passing. Arranged serially so that direct comparisons may be made to assess improvement or otherwise of state of kidney. Fresh bright red blood indicates recent and continuing haemorrhage. Brown urine indicates old blood and control of bleeding vessels by clotting. Rest should be complete for up to 14 days. Antibiotics as prophylaxis because of danger of infection of haematoma and urinary infection.

SURGERY. *Indications.*(1) Persistent severe bleeding not responding to above measures. Blood transfusion may be needed pre operatively. May not be time to investigate function of other kidney so during operation surgeon palpates other kidney to make sure of its presence. (2) Complications. Perinephric infection may require drainage. Later — ureteric stenosis with hydronephrosis; atrophy of kidney due to injury or thrombosis of renal artery.

Types. (1) Suturing of laceration. (2) Partial nephrectomy. (3) Nephrectomy.

NEOPLASMS
Benign

(1) Papilloma. Commonest form. May manifest by painless haematuria. Should be treated surgically because of danger of seeding and malignancy. (2) Other tumours may occur, e.g. adenoma, fibroma, lipoma, angioma. Rarely require surgery as growth slow.

Malignant

Embryoma. (Wilms' tumour; nephroblastoma.) Rare condition seen in children under 7 years. Type. Mixed cell tumour (consisting of endodermal and mesodermal cells, muscle fibres, cartilage, teeth, bone and glandular tissue). Highly malignant. Occasionally bilateral. Metastasizes readily, because of rich blood supply, to lungs, liver and brain.

SIGNS AND SYMPTOMS. Do not usually manifest until tumour of large size. Mass in flank. Hypertension. Late symptoms of metastases. Haematuria is rare.

INVESTIGATIONS. Intravenous pyelography. Kidney enlarged and calyces distorted.

TREATMENT. Irradiation may reduce size considerably before surgery. Nephrectomy followed by further irradiation. Cytotoxic drugs, e.g. actinomycin D, may be of value.

335

Carcinoma. *Adenocarcinoma.* (Grawitz's tumour; hypernephroma.) Commonest form of renal malignancy. Occurs most commonly in males. Types. Arises from nephrons. Grows rapidly and spreads readily. Metastasizes to lungs, bones, liver and brain. Often grows directly into inferior vena cava.

Epithelioma. Occurs in renal pelvis but rarely produces large tumour.

SIGNS AND SYMPTOMS. Do not usually appear until late. Painless haematuria, often intermittent. Swelling in loin — may not be palpable in obese or muscular patient or if tumour in upper pole. Pain, very late feature, dull and aching. Indicates extrarenal spread. Occasionally renal colic from blood clot.

INVESTIGATIONS. Plain abdominal X-ray shows enlarged kidney and occasionally calcification of tumour. Intravenous pyelography demonstrates filling defect and space occupying tumour. Cystoscopy excludes bladder and urethra as cause of haematuria and if performed during haematuria blood may be seen coming from ureteric orifice.

TREATMENT. Nephrectomy in absence of metastases. Irradiation may be used pre- and post-operatively or as palliative measure. Nephro-ureterectomy if growth occurs in pelvis or ureter.

RENAL CALCULI   sulphonamides can cause crystals in kidne

Precipitated crystalloids clump in renal tubules and are bound by a cement-like substance.

Composition. Usually mixed. May contain any of following.

MINERALS. Calcium, phosphate, magnesium, carbonate — relatively insoluble so precipitate easily. Colour varies from white to mulberry or may be stained black by blood pigments. Usually hard and sometimes branched.

ACIDS. Oxalic, phosphoric and uric — from metabolic disorders. Various colours and consistency. Oxalic stones when combined with calcium may be hard and covered with sharp crystals. Calcium stones may be smooth.

AMMONIA. Produced from (a) amino acid breakdown, (b) from urea by certain micro-organisms, e.g. Staphylococci. Soft friable stones.

CYSTINE. Hereditary metabolic disease in which patient

unable to break down cystine (an amino acid) and hence excretes large amounts. It is relatively insoluble and precipitates readily in renal tract forming smooth waxy stones.

SULPHONAMIDES. May crystallize out in tract. Muddy in appearance.

Causes. IDIOPATHIC. Little known about stone formation. Following factors may contribute (1) Climate. Hot dry tropical or subtropical climate may result in diminished urinary output and more concentrated urine in which stones precipitate more readily.

RACE AND SEX. Rare in negroid people. Males more commonly affected than females.

STASIS. Allows sedimentation of crystals and predisposes to infection. Minor deformity of single calyx may interfere with drainage and cause calculi. Prolonged recumbency especially if bone disease present. Maintenance of one position for a long time results in calculi in dependent calyces.

INFECTION. Raises pH (more alkaline) by breaking down urea, and increasing tendency for uric acid, cystine, oxalates and minerals to be deposited. Also debris from chronic infection may form central focus on which crystals may aggregate.

HYPERPARATHYROIDISM. (p. 190.) Results in increased calcium in blood and urine and is common cause of calculi.

DIET. Some people cannot increase calcium output in urine despite dietary indiscretions, others can. Vitamin A deficiency appears to predispose in some cases. Hypervitaminosis D also appears to play a part.

Possible results of stone formation. OBSTRUCTION. Calyx, pelvi-ureteric junction, ureter. Predisposes to infection and malignancy from chronic irritation.

Signs and symptoms. Sudden onset of smaller stones causes renal colic — severe stabbing pain extending from twelfth rib to hypochondrium. Fixed dull ache in loin between attacks. Ureteric colic: pain extends round flank towards inguinal ligament and into scrotum or labia majora. Nausea and vomiting between attacks. Patient cold, sweating, pale, restless. Pulse rate increased. Haematuria may be gross. Larger stones remain 'silent' until infection occurs. Tenderness may be marked over kidney area.

Investigations. Straight abdominal X-ray may reveal opaque

337

stones. Intravenous pyelography, after pain has subsided – locates stone and depicts extent of kidney damage or obstruction caused by stone. Urinalysis. Red blood cells in sterile urine. White cells and organisms if infected. Crystals of oxalate, phosphate, uric acid or cystine may be present. Investigations of cause of stone, e.g. urinary calcium excretion test, renal function tests, fasting serum calcium, phosphorus and proteins, serum uric acid. Cystoscopy. Rarely necessary unless relationship of calculi not clearly depicted by X-rays.

Treatment. CONSERVATIVE. During attack of colic – antispasmodics, e.g. pethidine, Buscopan, atropine. Ureteric stones usually voided. Urine must be strained to ascertain presence of stone fragments (gravel). Preventive measures to prevent further stone formation, or enlargement of existing stones (see later).

SURGICAL. Avoided as much as possible. Entire stone removed. Remaining fragments enlarge. Recurrence common.

Indications. Persistent pain. Obstruction. Infection.

Types. (1) Nephrolithotomy: removal of stone from kidney substance. (2) Pyelolithotomy: removal of stone from pelvis of kidney. (3) Ureterolithotomy: removal of stone from ureter. (4) Nephrectomy: if extensive damage by stone and other kidney is normal. (5) Nephrostomy: drainage of kidney via skin. Massive calculi, sometimes bilateral, with renal failure caused and complicated by obstruction and infection. Attempts may be made to dissolve stones (especially large staghorn calculi, so named because of their multiple branches). Continuous or intermittent irrigation with a mixture of citric acid, anhydrous magnesium oxide and anhydrous sodium carbonate.

Prevention. (1) High fluid intake. Prevents stasis and concentrated urine. More than 3 litres daily and ½ litre on retiring and immediately on rising to ensure that water is passing through kidneys while sleeping. (2) Specific measures. Calcium stones – exclude hyperparathyroidism. Avoid milk and cheese. Phosphate stones – ensure acid urine to increase solubility of calcium and magnesium ammonium phosphate. Oxalate stones – low oxalate diet. Metabolic stones – special diets low in cystine, protein and oxalates. Urine kept alkaline as cystine and uric acid insoluble in acids. (3) Eliminate all urinary tract infections.

338

Antibiotics given to sterilize urine after stone removal and in cases of obstruction.

RENAL ARTERY STENOSIS

Narrowing of renal artery causing hypertension.

Cause. Atheroma most common cause. Congenital hypertrophy of muscle coat.

Pathology. Site of stenosis varies but more common near origin of renal artery. Infarction or partial infarction of kidney distal to stenosis. Renal pressor mechanism: release of renin to produce angiotensin after acting on substrate in plasma (angiotensinogen). Causes rise in general blood pressure. Mechanism activated by kidney ischaemia and continues until obstruction removed. Prolonged infarction results in renal failure.

Signs and symptoms. Suspected in any of the following: (1) unexplained hypertension in under 30-year age group. (2) Severe hypertension without family history. (3) Hypertension following recent episode of loin pain or haematuria. (4) Hypertension associated with evidence of atherosclerosis especially when hypertension suddenly becomes more severe. Bruit may be heard over renal artery. Occasionally polyuria.

Investigations. INTRAVENOUS PYELOGRAM. May be (1) normal, (2) show difference in size between 2 kidneys, (3) show impaired function.

Aortogram. Injection of radio-opaque dye into aorta at level of renal arteries either directly or from catheter introduced through femoral artery.

Divided renal function tests. Catheters passed into both ureters and urine collected separately. May show differing results to stimulation of renal function. Often as much as 50% reduction in affected kidney. (Ineffective if urine leaks around catheter into bladder.)

Treatment. CONSERVATIVE. Measures to lower blood pressure if patient atherosclerotic over 50–60 years.

SURGICAL. Treatment of choice (1) removal of stenotic area, e.g. resection of area and end-to-end anastomosis; endarterectomy if atherosclerotic; anastomosis of splenic artery to area of kidney distal to occlusion (left kidney only); arterial graft. (2) Nephrectomy if other kidney normal and above measures cannot be attempted.

339

INFECTION
Pyelonephritis
Inflammation of kidney pelvis and parenchyma.

Causes. VARIETY OF MICRO-ORGANISMS. *E. coli, Proteus vulgaris; Staph. aureus; Strep. faecalis; Pseudomonas pyocyanea.*

Routes of spread. (1) Ascending infection following catheterization. (2) Blood stream, e.g. acute bacterial endocarditis. Catheter fever − instrumentation of patients with urinary tract infection resulting in septicaemia and bacteraemia. (3) Lymphatic spread − very little supporting evidence that kidney infected by this route.

Predisposing factors.

1. Obstruction, e.g. congenital abnormalities, previous scarring from infections, calculi, bladder neck obstruction, prostatic enlargement, urethral stricture.

2. Stasis − neurological bladder disorders, pregnancy (enlargement of pelvis and ureter occurs naturally).

3. Ureterovesicular reflux.

4. Lowered body resistance, e.g. in diabetes mellitus (higher incidence proved but cause unknown).

5. Drugs, e.g. phenacetin taken in excess over long periods causes damage to kidney. Infection may be caused by or due to effects of damage.

Pathological changes. Due to multiplication of organisms, fibrosis as a result of inflammatory changes, hypertension due to secretion of renin as increasing fibrosis impairs blood supply. Usually bilateral but can be unilateral.

Signs and symptoms. ACUTE. Sudden onset of pyrexia, rigors, sweating, nausea, vomiting. Pain and tenderness over kidney area. Frequency, dysuria and lower abdominal pain associated with inflammation of bladder. Urine − cloudy, offensive and contains albumin and blood.

CHRONIC. Nil specific except at times of exacerbation, e.g. pyrexia, back pain, dysuria and frequency (latter from bladder irritation). May present as (1) symptomless proteinuria; (2) inexplicable anaemia; (3) renal failure; (4) hypertension.

Investigations. RENAL FUNCTION. Interference varies from mild to severe according to extent of inflammatory process. Acute renal failure in severe cases. As infection subsides renal function improves. In chronic disease tubules more affected than glomeruli at first, causing marked reduction in concentrating power. Usually there is small reduction in creatinine clearance, blood urea remains within normal limits. Disease is usually bilateral but divided renal function tests may show that one kidney is more affected than the other. Between acute attacks urine may be sterile.

URINALYSIS. White blood cells, micro-organisms, red blood cells, albumin. Casts and clumps of white cells diagnostic of infection of renal parenchyma.

BLOOD TESTS. Full blood examination may show moderate leucocytosis, lowered haemoglobin. Blood urea may be normal until considerable renal damage has occurred.

X-RAYS. Intravenous pyelography. Fibrosis causes significant changes — clubbing and distortion of calyces, narrowing of areas of parenchyma. Obstructive lesions may also be seen. Voiding cysto-urethrogram — may be normal or may show ureteric reflux.

CYSTOSCOPY. May show changes due to inflammation or cause of infection e.g. stones, bladder neck obstruction, abnormalities of ureteric orifices.

RENAL BIOPSY. Difficult in small fibrous kidney. If infection is localized biopsy may reveal nothing abnormal. Occasionally culture of tissue may grow organisms not present in urine — valuable aid to treatment.

Treatment. Acute stage — bedrest until symptoms subside. Copious fluid intake — at least 3 litres daily. Antibiotics vary according to type and sensitivity of organisms, e.g. sulphadimidine, 2 g statim and 1 g, 6 hourly, tetracycline 250 mg, 6-hourly. Drugs continued for 3 weeks. Urine cultured 48 hours after drugs discontinued. If still infected drugs recommenced for further 3 weeks. When urine is sterile drugs discontinued but urine examined monthly for 12 months. Alternatively, maintenance doses of drugs continued to keep urine sterile, e.g. sulphadimidine 0.5 g twice daily.

Treatment of causes, e.g. correction of obstruction, removal of badly damaged kidney, gout and other causes of calculi.

Prevention. Aseptic catheterization especially during pregnancy; avoidance of obstruction and stasis improvement of general health in patients with acute attacks to prevent condition becoming chronic.

Pyelonephrosis

Low grade infection in pelvis of kidney due to obstruction in ureter.

Cause. Pyelonephritis associated with calculi of ureteropelvic junction or ureter.

Signs and symptoms. Of hydronephrosis and pyelonephritis.

Treatment. Surgical. Nephrostomy or nephrectomy if kidney too damaged.

Complications. Untreated case may rupture and involve perirenal fat and persist as perirenal abscess.

Hydronephrosis

Distension of renal pelvis due to blockage of urinary outflow. Blockage may be partial or complete, continuous or intermittent. If ureter also distended condition called hydro- or mega-ureter.

Cause. Obstruction: (1) Congenital. (2) Acquired, e.g. calculi; stricture; stenosis; aberrant arteries (may exaggerate obstruction already present or may cause kink in ureter); ureterocele (prolapse of ureter into bladder with dilation of ureter distal to prolapse); pressure from outside, e.g. tumours of cervix, colon, bladder; uncoordinated persistalsis of ureter and pelvis of kidney; bladder neck obstruction; enlarged prostate gland; occasionally ureter may be accidentally ligated during pelvic surgery.

Pathology. With obstruction, e.g. stone in ureter, ureter attempts to dislodge stone by powerful peristalsis causing renal colic. If this fails ureter above obstruction becomes dilated. Long-standing dilatation of ureter results in atony of its walls and ureters become tortuous as well as dilated. As pressure builds up pelvis becomes dilated and glomerular filtration is greatly reduced. Eventually cortex and medulla are destroyed and kidney becomes a thin-walled bag of fluid. Stagnant urine quickly becomes infected, pyelonephritis develops and fluid in pelvis becomes purulent.

Signs and symptoms. Pain occurs early. May be intermittent. Later becomes continuous ache in upper abdomen. Not referred to loin. Intensity of pain varies with degree of obstruction. Made

342

worse by anything which produces a diuresis. Haematuria may occur. Signs and symptoms of infection or renal failure may be present.

Diagnosis. Confirmed by intravenous pyelography which shows variations in size and shape of calyces, pelvis and ureter; delayed emptying time. Reveals functional ability of other kidney.

Retrograde pyelography best avoided because of risk of infection and intensification of obstruction due to oedema. May be unavoidable if concentration of intravenous contrast medium is insufficient to reveal condition. May also be used to demonstrate that obstruction is at pelvi-ureteric junction.

Treatment. Mild cases discovered accidentally may need no treatment except removal of cause.

SURGERY. 1. Pyeloplasty — repair of dilated pelvis of kidney by excision of a portion, and anastomosis with remaining portion and ureter. Cause of obstruction must also be removed. This method performed only if there is still adequate kidney function.

2. Nephrectomy if there is gross impairment in one kidney only. (Risk of subsequent hydronephrosis in remaining kidney.)

3. Permanent nephrostomy. May be of value in poor anaesthetic risk patients. Subsequent management difficult and tube needs changing every 2 weeks.

4. Ureteric transplantation, e.g. via ileostomy, makes external drainage easier to manage and lessens risk of subsequent infection (see later).

ACUTE RENAL FAILURE

Sudden severe impairment or total loss of renal function resulting in oliguria and anuria, leading to uraemia. Oliguria — less than 400 ml urine in 24 hours, i.e. insufficient excretion to maintain life. Anuria — no urine produced in 24 hours. Catheterization reveals none in bladder.

Causes. PRE-RENAL. Due to fall in systemic blood pressure, e.g. in oligaemic shock due to burns, severe blood loss, acute dehydration.

RENAL. Reduction of glomerular flow, e.g. in incompatible blood transfusion, crush syndrome, acute inflammatory

343

conditions, e.g. pyelonephritis, overwhelming infections, e.g. septicaemia due to septic abortion, drugs, e.g. barbiturates, aspirin and heavy metal poisoning.

POST-RENAL. Mechanical obstruction, e.g. calculi strictures, tumours, pressure from outside.

Phases. OLIGAEMIC. May last hours, days or weeks. Results in death if not treated. Dangerous effects — overhydration; electrolyte imbalance especially potassium which can result in sudden death from cardiac muscle arrest; rise in blood urea; fall in serum bicarbonate resulting in acidosis; anaemia due to cessation of haemopoiesis and haemolysis; lowering of resistance to infection.

DIURETIC. Lasts a few days. Indicates improvement. Production of steadily increasing amounts of dilute urine. Slow return of concentrating power. Danger of dehydration.

RECOVERY. Ability to concentrate urine gradually returns. Improvement may be rapid for 1—2 weeks then more gradual over several months.

Investigations. Catheterization to obtain specimen and ensure that bladder is empty. Cystoscopy and ureteric catheterization to ensure patency of ureters. Blood examined for serum electrolytes, urea, haemoglobin, serum proteins. Urine tested for specific gravity, albumin and blood. Weight is guide to fluid replacement.

Treatment. Aims: prevent irreversible kidney damage and rest kidney to allow time for recovery.

1. FLUIDS. 500 ml (amount of insensible loss) plus amount of previous day's output: urine, vomit, diarrhoea, etc. Given orally if possible to keep mouth clean and allay thirst. Intravenously if patient unconscious or unable to tolerate oral administration. Types: electrolyte fluid according to serum electrolyte estimations; blood to maintain haemoglobin above 60%, packed cells used to prevent overhydration or circulatory overloading; calories, if peritoneal dialysis available 1,260 calories may be given intravenously and may include 100—200 in form of first-class protein. Protein restricted if dialysis not available.

2. DRUGS. (a) Anabolic hormones, e.g. Durabolin, Anabol, given to patients with excessive protein katabolism. (b) Mannitol, a carbohydrate given by infusion, 200 ml 25% solution rapidly twice daily. Produces osmotic diuresis and prevents tubular necrosis in early cases.

344

3. DIALYSIS. Process whereby osmotic exchange of colloid particles for particles in true solution occurs across a semi-permeable membrane.

Indications. Blood urea 350 mg% or over; gross overhydration; serum potassium high (7 mEq or higher); bicarbonates low (14 mEq or less).

Types. (a) *'Artificial kidney' Haemodialysis.* Large tank prepared with coils of cellophane providing the semipermeable membrane. Inside the coils the patient's blood is conducted via a cannula inserted into an artery: radial, brachial or femoral. Outside the coils is the dialysing fluid containing dextrose and salts which attracts to itself metabolic wastes and poisons that are not being excreted. Exchange of water and electrolytes to the patient's blood or from it can be arranged by varying the concentration of the solutes in the dialysing fluid. Blood is returned to the patient by another cannula placed into a vein. (Patients needing repeated haemodialysis can be fitted with Teflon or siliconized rubber 'shunts' connecting an artery and a vein. When not in use for dialysis the tubes are connected to each other.) The machine needs to be filled with compatible blood and heparin must be added to prevent coagulation.

(b) *Peritoneal dialysis.* Patient's own peritoneum provides the semipermeable membrane and the peritoneal cavity is filled and drained intermittently with the dialysing fluid. Advantages over haemodialysis: minimal preparation of patient or apparatus; minimal space required; low operating cost and maintenance; less danger of haemorrhage and acute electrolyte imbalance (in haemodialysis cerebral oedema and convulsions may occur due to slow rate of urea clearance from brain in comparison with rapid clearance from other tissues; slow, even clearance occurs with peritoneal dialysis).

Method of insertion. Patient voids urine or is catheterized to avoid damage to bladder. Under local anaesthesia, trocar and cannula inserted through anterior abdominal wall just below umbilicus in midline. Nylon or Teflon catheter with many small holes (often over 100) is inserted through cannula and placed in pouch of Douglas. Cannula withdrawn and catheter stitched to skin. Dialysing fluid run in from suspended bottles. (Standard isotonic fluid: per litre, dextrose 13.6 g, sodium lactate 5 g, sodium chloride 5.6 g, calcium chloride 0.39 g, magnesium chloride 0.15 g, heparin 12.5 units, tetracycline 125 units. May be made hypertonic by increasing dextrose to 63.6 g per litre.)

Management of cycle. Patient sits in semi-recumbent position. 1½ litres fluid run in rapidly in 10 minutes. Inlet and outlet clamped for 10 minutes then fluid drained off into container on floor. Drainage takes 10–15 minutes. Fresh fluid inserted and cycle may be repeated for 48 hours. Dialysis may be repeated as often as necessary but new catheter inserted each time. Originally a button device was used but rate of infection was high.

Main complications. Peritonitis; leakage of fluid around catheter; pain and discomfort for which sedation and analgesia may be used.

4. RENAL TRANSPLANT. May be indicated.

5. **Nursing care.** All measures to prevent pressure sores. Scrupulous care of mouth. Minimizing possibility of cross infection; patient barrier nursed in single room. Observations of vital signs for onset of infection; circulatory overloading (full and bounding pulse, increased pressure in jugular vein, rising blood pressure, pulmonary oedema with dyspnoea, frothy sputum, cough and occasionally haemoptysis); improvement or otherwise in general condition. Fluid balance chart kept meticulously. Patient weighed regularly; useful guide to oedema. In peritoneal dialysis frequent examination for kinking and airlocks in tubing; interference in flow reported; leakage round catheter reported; all outflow measured; fluid may be needed for laboratory investigation.

Care of catheter; perineal or penile toilets necessary.

Psychological support. When blood urea is high various forms of mental disturbance may occur, e.g. lassitude, poor memory, unconsciousness, delirium, convulsions, depression, overactivity, aggressiveness or even paranoia. Nurse must (a) understand that changes are due to the disease process; (b) prevent patient from hurting himself; (c) give relevant explanations and support to relatives.

(Chronic renal failure not dealt with here as it is more a medical than a surgical condition.)

TYPES OF SURGERY TO KIDNEY AND URETER
Nephrectomy

Removal of a kidney.

Indications. Damage or disease of kidney which endangers life, e.g. laceration or complete tear of renal cortex, neoplasm, non-functioning kidney due to chronic infection, e.g. tuberculosis, pyelonephritis; obstruction, e.g. hydronephrosis. Multiple calculi or single staghorn calculus which has damaged kidney extensively. Abnormalities, e.g. ectopic kidney, aberrant arteries, renal artery aneurysm. Renal hypertension due to stenosis of renal artery (p. 339).

Pre-operative preparation. *(Specific.)* Emergency for injury. Prepare for theatre. Observe and save all urine specimens. Evidence of heavy continuous bleeding — patient taken to theatre without delay. Blood taken for grouping and crossmatching (in severe injury, no time to assess function of other kidney).

Ryle's tube may be needed to empty stomach, prevent vomiting and paralytic ileus from accompanying shock. Elective. Efficiency of other kidney ensured by intravenous pyelography, renal function tests, cystoscopy and retrograde pyelography, blood urea estimation. Copious fluids given. Physiotherapy, especially for chest as incision made in area of lower ribs and may restrict respirations. Urinary tract sterilized with antibiotics and/or urinary antiseptics. Urine observed especially for calculi, blood, albumin and pus.

Operation. POSITION. Varies with actual operation; most commonly, patient lies on unaffected side with kidney bridge in loin so that kidney area is raised. Pelvis fixed with strap encircling patient and table. Upper leg straight. Lower leg slightly flexed. Sandbag between legs. Arm rest takes full weight of upper arm so that shoulders are vertical. Various supports fitted to table so that shoulders and thorax do not move.

INCISION. Depends on reason for surgery: (1) parallel to and below twelfth rib extending to abdominal wall, exposes lower pole of kidney; (2) higher incisions through tenth or eleventh rib; (3) thoraco-abdominal incision through ninth rib, and diaphragm split; (4) parallel to vertebral column, twelfth and/or eleventh rib divided and incision brought round to abdomen. Abdominal muscles divided in line of incision and perirenal fascia divided

347

with scissors. Kidney then exposed and separated from perirenal fat.

PEDICLE. Ideally, renal arteries and veins ligated, tied and divided separately. If gross inflammation present may be necessary to use pedicle clamp, divide and ligate after kidney removed.

CLOSURE. In layers. Precautionary drain tube in perinephric region to detect haemorrhage early and to prevent infection from accumulation of serum.

Post-operative care. POSITION. Gradually raise to semi-upright position as condition permits, slightly leaning towards affected side to assist drainage and to ensure maximum lung expansion.

ANALGESIA. Pain usually severe because of involvement of thick abdominal muscles. Adequate analgesics must be given.

PHYSIOTHERAPY. Deep breathing started as soon as conscious and repeated at frequent intervals. Adequate analgesia before exercises. Leg exercises to prevent vascular complications. Trunk exercises to strengthen abdominal wall as soon as sutures removed.

DRESSING. Careful inspection to detect haemorrhage.

DRAIN TUBE. Shortened daily and removed when drainage ceases, usually in 3–4 days, but often longer.

URINE. Carefully observed for quantity and quality, abnormalities reported at once. Guide to assessment of kidney function. Haematuria usually present. Specimens set up serially for comparison.

FLUIDS. Oral fluids commenced carefully as paralytic ileus occurs occasionally (if large autonomic nerves of mesentery bruised during operation). Increase to copious fluids to ensure adequate functioning of remaining kidney.

DIET. Gradually increased to normal.

SUTURES. Removed 7–10 days.

AMBULATION. Usually patient sat out of bed second day. Exercises gradually increased to full ambulation on third-fourth day. Care taken in handling patient to remember that suture line is usually long and avoid placing hand on same during movement of patient.

DISCHARGE. Usually 10–12 days.

Complications. Shock because of extent of surgery. Haemorrhage — rare. Paralytic ileus — as above. Chest complications — lung collapse, pneumonia. Failure of other kidney. Infection — perinephric abscess, wound infection. Fistulae — from damage to bowel or duodenum during surgery.

Nephro-ureterectomy

Removal of kidney and ureter.

Indications. Neoplasm of pelvis or ureter. Tuberculosis of kidney as infection may occur if stump left behind. Gross hydro-ureter.

Pre-operative preparation. As for nephrectomy.

Operation. Second incision necessary in supra-pubic region or iliac fossa to gain access to lower end of ureter.

Post-operative care and complications. As for nephrectomy.

Partial nephrectomy

Removal of one pole of kidney.

Indications. Calculi in distal calyx. Localized tuberculosis of kidney.

Operation. Renal vessels clamped and kidney substance divided (clamps must not be left on for longer than 15 minutes). Vessels on cut surface of kidney ligated and calyx sutured. Piece of muscle, fat or absorbable haemostatic gauze (gel foam) sutured to raw area or deep suture of catgut run through kidney substance with atraumatic needle.

Complications. Haemorrhage. May necessitate reopening of wound and total nephrectomy. Extravasation of urine from kidney. Urinary fistula.

Nephrolithotomy

Opening into kidney substance to remove a stone.

Operation and complications: as for partial nephrectomy.

Nephrostomy

Drainage of kidney via tube brought out on to skin.

Indications. Emergency measure: ureteric obstruction with renal failure especially in solitary kidney. May be able to pass substance via tube which will dissolve stone especially with solitary staghorn stone.

Operation. Exposure of kidney, self-retaining catheter (e.g. Malecot) inserted through kidney substance (trocar and cannula may be needed to guide catheter into renal substance although with gross swelling no difficulty in insertion into thinnest part of cortex). Catheter stitched to skin and tubing anchored with strapping and connected to closed underwater seal drainage to prevent ascending infections.

Post-operative care. Careful measurement of any drainage from tube as well as any urinary output. Tube may need to be changed in 2-3 weeks. Under general anaesthesia a Harris or St Peter's catheter inserted along tract formed by original drainage tube and fitted with a flange to retain catheter in position. A nephrostomy belt is fitted with a collecting bag attached to patient's leg. Irrigation performed only if renal pelvis dilated otherwise fluid will produce distension and pain. Accidentally dislodged tube must be replaced within 24 hours as tract quickly closes.

Nephropexy

Fixation of kidney.

Indications. 'Floating' or movable kidney. Occurs when there is very little perirenal fat, e.g. in emaciated and very thin females. Ectopic kidney. Nephropexy only required if complications occur, e.g. kinking of ureter and hydronephrosis.

Operation. Kidney exposed and immobilization achieved either by stitching to quadratus lumborum or psoas muscle or by making a sling of perirenal fascia.

Renal transplant

Grafting a donor kidney (human) into pelvis of recipient.

Indications. Terminal renal failure where measures fail to control hypertension, nausea and vomiting.

Pre-operative care. Specific. DONOR — identical twin ideally or voluntary living donor or recently deceased donor. Written consent for operation necessary. Dangers of nephrectomy explained.

PSYCHOLOGICAL SUPPORT. Outcome of operation uncertain and yet patient will die without it. Nurse must be aware of patient's apprehension and encourage him to talk about it.

350

Diversional therapy essential to keep patient's mind occupied. Nurse must remember that patients in isolation quickly become depressed and must do all she can to prevent it.

FLUID AND ELECTROLYTE IMBALANCE. With uraemia patient may be permitted restricted fluids only. Amount depends on previous day's output. Patient and relatives must be aware of this so that their cooperation can be gained. Fluids given orally unless uraemic nausea and vomiting are troublesome. Haemodialysis may be used for acidosis or alkalosis or if water retention is acute. Several dialyses may be needed.

NURSING OBSERVATIONS. Weighed daily at same time, on same scales, wearing same clothes and immediately after voiding urine. Fluid balance chart. Evidence of electrolyte imbalance — diarrhoea, muscle cramps and spasms, bradycardia weak and irregular pulse, hypotension. Regular serum electrolyte estimations especially bicarbonate, chloride and potassium levels. Patient observed carefully for signs of deterioration in remaining kidney function, e.g. nausea, vomiting, mental changes, electrolyte imbalance.

BLOOD TRANSFUSION. If haemoglobin low or blood loss anticipated.

DIET. Varies according to degree of renal failure. Protein and potassium intake usually restricted, carbohydrates and fats increased to ensure normal calorie intake.

SKIN CARE. In uraemia, patient may excrete urea through skin and need frequent cleansing with non-irritant agent, e.g. pHisoHex, to prevent infection. Pressure area care essential as patient's general body condition is poor.

MOUTH CARE. 2–4 hourly cleansing because of restricted fluids and thick coating of tongue usual with uraemia.

PREVENTION OF INFECTION. Patient usually 'reverse barrier' nursed 48–72 hours before operation, i.e. isolated in as sterile an atmosphere as possible to prevent any infection reaching him from exogenous source. Precautions include sterile bedlinen; attendants wear gowns, caps, masks, gloves and shoe coverings. Necessary because (1) uraemia lowers his resistance, (2) immunosuppressive drugs given in massive doses lower resistance still further. Frequent white cell counts and haemoglobin estimations necessary. Prophylactic antibiotics given, especially those to which his own organisms from skin, pharynx and stools are sensitive.

Operation. DONOR. Nephrectomy (p. 347) usually performed in adjoining theatre. Renal artery and vein divided as close as possible to aorta and inferior vena cava.

RECIPIENT. Upper midline incision and bilateral nephrectomy and splenectomy (to further suppress immunological response). Oblique lower abdominal incision made and new kidney transplanted in pelvis. Renal artery anastomosed to internal iliac artery and vein to common iliac vein. Ureter implanted into bladder. 30–50 minutes anoxia does not appear to be harmful to kidney but a degree of hypothermia during surgery may be used as precautionary measure.

Post-operative care. Specific. PREPARATION. Sterilized room with supply of gowns, caps, masks, gloves and overshoes for attendants. Gastric aspiration tray. Urinary drainage apparatus.

OBSERVATIONS. Routine for shock and haemorrhage. Urinary output: indwelling catheter in situ. No way of accurately predicting kidney function. May produce almost immediate diuresis with danger of dehydration and electrolyte imbalance, or it may be several days before kidney functions. In latter case dialysis may be necessary as temporary measure. Any decrease in output must be reported. All urine pooled as 24-hour specimens and a 30-ml sample sent to laboratory each day for electrolytes and quantitative protein evaluation.

Homograft rejection may occur at any time after surgery up to weeks or months later. Signs and symptoms: soreness in pelvic area, rising temperature, decrease in urinary output, malaise and vague uneasiness, rise in blood urea, rising blood pressure, weight gain without increase in appetite, increase in renal size felt on palpation.

GASTRIC ASPIRATION (danger of paralytic ileus). All aspirant saved and sent to laboratory for electrolyte estimation.

ISOLATION. May need to be continued if white cell count is low. Immunosuppresive drugs continued probably for rest of patient's life. (Missed doses of Imuran have been known to trigger off rejection.) Meticulous barrier nursing continued until white cell count has risen sufficiently. Some surgeons require sterilization of food and drink, sterilization of drugs, sterile perineal toilets after use of bedpan.

FLUIDS. Given intravenously until danger of paralytic ileus is passed. Amount and type according to electrolyte estimation and urinary output. Fluids given orally when bowel sounds heard. Milk alternating with antacids given hourly for indefinite period to prevent steroid-produced gastric ulcers.

DIET. Commenced when oral intake and urinary ouput satisfactory. Varies according to kidney function. Sodium may need to be restricted or increased.

AMBULATION. Encouraged third day.

TESTS. Daily white cell count; blood urea; serum creatinine; electrolyte estimation; urine for specific gravity, protein, blood and electrolytes; urine cultures every 2—3 days.

Routine and specific care as for nephrectomy.

Complications. Rejection of graft and uraemia. May occur months after operation. Haemorrhage. Paralytic ileus. Overwhelming infections. Effects of drugs — agranulocytosis, diabetes, gastro-intestinal bleeding. Hypertension due to ischaemia of kidney. Chest and vascular complications.

Pyelolithotomy

Removal of stone through incision made in pelvis of kidney.

Pre-operative preparation. Chemotherapy to sterilize urine. Plain abdominal X-ray on morning of operation to ensure that stone has not moved.

Operation. Upper ureter and pelvis exposed and stay sutures placed in wall of pelvis. Small incision made in pelvis. Stone-grasping forceps used. Various patterns with different angulations available. Pelvi-ureteric junction examined for obstruction which may have caused calculus formation, and if present corrected by plastic repair. Precautionary drain tube inserted.

Post-operative care. Haematuria may be heavy for 48 hours. Colicky pain from passage of clots down ureter. Drain tube removed after shortening daily for 3—4 days but must not be removed as long as drainage from urinary fistula remains.

Complications. Urinary fistula may persist 4—6 weeks due to oedema at pelvi-ureteric junction.

Pyeloplasty

Removal of excessive portion of renal pelvis and reconstruction of same after relief of obstruction.

Indications. Hydronephrosis.

Operation. Various techniques whereby large portion excised and pelvis partly sutured together. Ureter anastomosed into remaining portion. Nephrostomy catheter used in case of excessive oedema. Fine polythene tube may be used as 'splint' for site of anastomosis.

Post-operative complications. Urinary fistula as above.

Ureterolithotomy

Removal of stone from ureter.

Operation. (Plain abdominal X-ray taken before operation to make sure stone still present.) Commonest site for blockage to occur — last 5 cm of ureter. Ureter slit longitudinally and stone shelled out. Ureter sutured.

Complications. As above.

Ureterostomy

Considered with transplant of ureters, p. 362.

BLADDER CONDITIONS

INJURY

Causes. Complications of fractured pelvis. Sudden blow on lower abdomen while bladder full. Damage during surgery, e.g. hernia repair, transurethral resection, hysterectomy.

Signs and symptoms. Haematuria, often gross, or acute retention of urine with palpable distended bladder. Supra-pubic pain. Supra-pubic and rebound tenderness on palpation (due to peritoneal irritation). Rectal examination reveals large boggy mass over prostate.

Investigations. Blood found in micro-examination of urine. Plain abdominal X-ray may reveal fractured pelvis and grey shadow in bladder area. Intravenous pyelography for damage. (Catheterization contra-indicated in case incomplete rupture may be made complete.) Cystogram   reliable test as to degree of injury. Frank extravasation of urine may be demonstrated. Some surgeons do not advocate this investigation for reasons given above.

Treatment. (1) Treat shock and haemorrhage. (2) Observations – urinary output for haematuria and/or retention, increasing signs of peritoneal irritation (p. 108). (3) Surgery – exploration. Extraperitoneal rupture – supra-pubic cystotomy. Peritoneum opened and organs explored. Bladder repaired and indwelling catheter inserted.

Intraperitoneal. Tear closed transperitoneally if possible. Indwelling urethral catheter and supra-pubic tube inserted. Drainage continued until tear has healed.

Complications. Haemorrhage. Infection.

NEOPLASM

(1) **Benign** – papilloma.

(2) **Malignant** – carcinoma (transitional cell; epithelioma; adenosarcoma). Appearances – papillary or solid or ulcerated. Spread – invasive infiltration into bladder wall; lymphatic; blood stream to bones, lungs. Prognosis. Untreated. Urinary infection, obstruction, chronic renal failure.

Incidence. Relatively common (2% of all cancers). Males 3: female 1. 75% males over 50 years.

Cause. Unknown. Increasing evidence of carcinogens in urine, e.g. dye workers – alpha- and beta-naphthylamine and benzidine.

Signs and symptoms. Haematuria – painless, intermittent, fresh blood passed terminally. May be accompanied by clots in later stages. Secondary haemorrhage – painful. Frequency. With spread – supra-pubic pain. Palpable tumour on abdominal and rectal examination when tumour has reached advanced stage.

Investigations. X-Rays – intravenous pyelography may show ureteric obstruction, dilatation of ureter, primary renal tumour. Cystogram may show space occupying lesion. Cystoscopy ensures diagnosis and denotes size and shape of tumour. Biopsy to differentiate between papilloma and carcinoma. Bimanual examination under general anaesthesia determines size of tumour, whether soft and mobile. Urinalysis. If bleeding intermittent micro-examination necessary to detect red blood cells. Secondary infection common.

Treatment

1. BENIGN AND MALIGNANT SHOWING NO SPREAD. (a) Diathermy via cystoscope. (b) Transurethral resection — removal of tumour in small pieces via resectoscope using diathermy cutting current. (c) Partial cystectomy.

2. MALIGNANT WITH SUSPICION OF SPREAD TO BLADDER WALL. (a) Irradiation by implantation of radon or gold seeds directly into tumour. (b) Deep X-rays (effects satisfactory but not as good as direct implantation). (c) Total cystectomy with transplant of ureters into colon, loop of ileum or skin.

3. SPREAD BEYOND BLADDER WALL. Palliative measures, irradiation to control haematuria, diversion of urinary stream past obstruction — supra-pubic cystotomy or transplantation of ureters as above.

Complications. Without treatment — infection, cystitis, pyelonephritis, retention of urine, ureteric obstruction with hydronephrosis or pyelonephrosis, renal failure.

Post-operative. See below. Recurrence common.

VESICAL CALCULI

(See renal calculi, p. 336.)

Causes. (1) Migration from kidney. (2) Urinary stasis (especially residual urine) infected by urea-splitting organisms. (3) Prostatic calculi released into bladder.

Signs and symptoms. Pain — radiates down urethra and referred to tip of penis (stone rolling on to bladder neck). Haematuria — slight, at termination of micturition. Frequency, less noticeable at night unless there is infection (stone not pressing on trigone when patient recumbent). Micturition may suddenly cease in midstream (stone blocks urethral outlet). Retention follows.

Investigations. Plain abdominal X-ray may show opaque stone. Catheterization — may be arrested in urethra by stone or may measure high residual urine. (Normal bladder, after micturition, contains small amount of urine — 10–30 ml. 100 ml upper limit of normality.) Passage of urethral metal sound may 'click' when it touches stone. Cystoscopy visualizes stone, and may detect primary cause of stone.

Treatment. Treat cystitis. Surgery — (1) small soft stones —

lithopaxy. (2) Hard solitary stones — supra-pubic cystotomy. Recurrence rare if preventive measures instituted.

CYSTITIS

Inflammation of bladder.

Causes. (1) Spread: (a) from kidneys via ureter — tuberculosis, pyonephrosis; (b) from urethra — urethritis, instrumentation especially catheterization, coitus in female; (c) from adjacent structures, e.g. vulvitis, vaginitis, vesicocolic fistula.

(2) Bladder outlet obstruction producing high residual urine, congenital hypertrophy, stricture, prostatomegaly, balanitis.

(3) Within bladder — tumour, calculus, foreign object.

Common organisms. *Escherichia coli, Staphylococcus aureus, Streptococcus faecalis, Bacillus proteus, Pseudomonas pyocyanea.* May result from cross infection.

Pathology. Normal bladder epithelium highly resistant to infection but once micro-organisms gain entry multiplication is rapid. Women more prone than men because of shorter urethra and proximity to vagina and anus. Congestion and oedema of mucosa. If trigone involved, frequency occurs. Bladder lining appears swollen, red and cloudy. Urine mucopurulent or blood stained. If condition becomes chronic mucosa thickens, muscle atrophies and becomes fibrosed with eventual reduction of bladder capacity.

Signs and symptoms. ACUTE. Frequency (passing of small amounts of urine at short intervals. In acute severe cases, at few-minute intervals). Usually worse in morning and improves during day with increased fluid intake. Dysuria, during micturition there is burning pain which persists at external meatus after cessation of flow. Urine. Cloudy, offensive (has 'fishy' odour) with occasional haematuria at termination of micturition. General signs of infection heralded by rigors in severe cases.

CHRONIC. Prolongation of above signs and symptoms which are less severe but urine may become frankly purulent. 'Irritable' bladder may follow acute attack. Frequency and dysuria may persist but urine is sterile (thought to be due to residual oedema and spasm of detrusor muscle).

Diagnosis. Confirmed by urinalysis and cystoscopy.

Investigations. Done to eliminate any underlying pathology (see causes above).

Treatment. ACUTE. (1) Rest in bed until signs and symptoms subside. (2) Copious fluids to prevent stagnation. (3) Drugs — sulphadimidine commenced pending culture of midstream specimen of urine then one of wide range of urinary antiseptics given according to sensitivity, e.g. streptomycin 0.5–1 g daily, tetracycline 250 mg, 6-hourly, nitrofurantoin (Furadantin) 5–10 mg per kg body weight daily, Kanamycin 1–2 g daily. (4) pH changing — acidification of urine may help arrest growth of micro-organisms by making environment unfavourable to them. (Former practice of making urine alkaline to enhance effect of drugs such as streptomycin considered dangerous in presence of renal failure as it causes further rise of serum calcium.) (5) Antispasmodics, e.g. hyoscyamus, Buscopan. (6) Treat underlying cause.

CHRONIC. (1) Copious fluids. (2) Appropriate antibiotic. (3) Removal of cause. (4) Bladder washouts, e.g. chlorhexidine 0.05%.

RETENTION OF URINE

Inability to pass urine from bladder (differentiated from suppression of urine where no urine is being secreted from kidney).

Causes. (1) Psychological: (a) Fear — modesty in micturating in presence of others; pain, especially after abdominal operations. (b) Abnormal position for micturition.

(2) Obstruction: (a) Bladder — calculi, tumour, injury, blood clots, congenital bladder neck obstruction. (b) Urethra — calculi, tumour, injury, blood clots, congenital or acquired stricture, foreign objects, phimosis. (c) Prostate gland — hypertrophy, carcinoma, infection, abscess. (d) Outside urinary tract — impacted faeces, tumour of uterus or ovaries, retroverted uterus.

(3) Lesions of central nervous system.

Types. (1) Acute. Patient suddenly unable to pass urine in previously normal functioning bladder.

(2) Chronic. Failure to empty bladder at each act of micturition. May produce retention with overflow — bladder grossly distended and patient passes only few millimetres at a time and some excess urine dribbles away without control.

358

(3) Acute on-chronic — sudden complete blockage in patient with chronic retention.

Pathology. With an obstruction patient tries to force urine out of bladder. Raised intravesicular pressure causes trabeculae to deepen. One or more of these may pouch to form diverticulum into middle and outer coats. Urine may collect in these and become infected. If compensatory mechanism of bladder fails to overcome obstruction, muscle wall becomes hypotonic and bladder fails to empty completely (i.e. high residual urine). Bladder gradually fills painlessly and can be felt supra-pubically. Stagnant urine predisposes to infection — cystitis, pyelonephritis, or may spread to testes (orchitis) via vas deferens. Also predisposes to calculi.

Signs and symptoms. Acute. Sudden inability to pass urine from a distended bladder. May be precipitated by diuretic drugs, bronchodilators (contain ephedrine which inhibits bladder muscles), alcoholic bout. Pain — lower abdominal. Distended bladder palpable as tender supra-pubic mass.

Chronic. May present in any of the following ways: (1) Frequency and urgency. (2) Poor urinary flow with dribbling after micturition. (3) Nocturia (may be due to chronic renal failure with poor concentrating power of kidneys, or mild congestive cardiac failure). (4) Overflow incontinence. (5) Cystitis. (6) Abdominal distension and discomfort. (7) Chronic renal failure with anorexia, nausea and vomiting, anaemia, heart failure.

Treatment. (1) NURSING MEASURES. (Psychological causes only. Dangerous if obstruction present.) Ensure privacy by screening bed properly. Position of comfort — females, commode if permissible, otherwise swing legs over side of bed and support them on bedside chair; males, stand out of bed if permissible or sit on edge of bed. Help patient to relax by not over-dramatizing situation. Turn on neighbouring tap or pour water from one jug to another — sound of running water may help. Less frequently used measures — warm compress to lower abdomen, warm bath if practicable, small enema.

(2) DRUGS. To stimulate contraction of bladder, e.g. intramuscular, Carbachol 0.25 mg.

(3) CATHETERIZATION. *Urethral.* Strictly aseptic technique with sterile equipment. Types of catheters vary greatly. Present

359

one of choice — Gibbon — small lumen polythene catheter with straps than can be attached to penis to prevent dislodgement. Small diameter and polythene minimize risk of urethritis. Other advantages — clear material allows easy detection of urine. Length allows direct connection with drainage bag or bottle without connecting pieces and additional tubing.

When catheter in bladder not more than 600 ml urine withdrawn at first because of danger of bladder muscle atony and immediate suppression of urine. Cystitis may develop with sudden compression, due to congestion of bladder. Intermittent drainage preferable to continuous to retain tone of bladder wall.

Closed drainage preferably into disinfectant, e.g. 40% formalin to prevent ascending urinary tract infection. While catheter in situ — thorough cleansing of meatus and glans penis with antiseptic, e.g. pHisoHex or aqueous chlorhexidine 0.05% or hydrogen peroxide 25%, 2–3 times daily to prevent infection.

In cases of acute retention urethral catheterization may be found to be impossible, because of urethral obstruction.

(4) CATHETERIZATION. *Supra-pubic.* (a) Trocar and cannula may be inserted through lower abdomen into bladder and catheter, e.g. Malecot or de Pezzer self-retaining supra-pubic catheter. (b) Small needle, e.g. lumbar puncture needle, may be inserted into bladder. Has advantage of slower decompression. (c) Supra-pubic cystotomy — incision made into bladder and drain tube inserted.

(5) TREAT CAUSE OF OBSTRUCTION. (See separate sections.)

(6) TREAT AND PREVENT COMPLICATIONS — infection, calculi, hydronephrosis, renal failure.

SURGERY OF BLADDER
1. Lithopaxy
Crushing of small soft calculi by means of a lithotrite passed into bladder via urethra and flushing out of fragments by means of a special evacuator.

Indications. Small soft calculi especially in elderly patients who are poor anaesthetic risks.

Contra-indications. Obstruction. Infection.

Operation. Spinal anaesthesia. (Occasionally general anaesthesia.) Preliminary dilatation of urethra and cystoscopic examination. Lithotrite introduced and pressed into hollow above trigone — most dependent part — so that stones will gravitate between jaws. Stone then crushed by screwing jaws together. (It is ensured that mucosa is not caught between jaws before this manoeuvre attempted.) Lithotrite withdrawn and evacuating cannula inserted. Current of water swirled into bladder and aspirated with attached rubber bulb. Process repeated until bladder free from debris. Cystoscopy repeated to ensure bladder free from stones and debris.

2. Supra-pubic cystotomy

Opening into bladder via supra-pubic incision.

Indications. Vesical calculi. To approach diverticula, neoplasms, prostate gland, implantation of radium.

Operation. Bladder emptied pre-operatively. Incision — midline, size depending on reason for operation; transverse 5 cm above pubis — more time consuming but less danger of post-operative hernia. Bladder exposed after filling with air or fluid for ease of identification and to raise peritoneum. Bladder wall fixed with stay sutures, emptied by needle aspiration, opened with vertical or transverse incision and any further fluid removed by suction. Necessary procedure performed (see indications). Bladder closed completely if urine sterile (care taken to ensure that suture material does not penetrate mucosa as unabsorbed material may form focus for calculi). Precautionary drainage tube left in retropubic space. If urine infected supra-pubic tube left in bladder (supra-pubic cystotomy).

3. Supra-pubic cystostomy

Bladder opened and kept open for purpose of diversion of urinary stream from urethra.

Indications. Obstructing of urethra where passage of urethral catheter impossible.

Operation. Cystotomy performed as above and Malecot or de Pezzer catheter inserted, or trocar and cannula introduced. Drainage into underwater seal by gravity or by gentle suction.

4. Partial cystectomy

Removal of segment of bladder wall in its entirety.

Indications. (a) Solitary mobile tumours (curative). (b) Widespread malignant infiltration (palliative), to prevent miseries associated with condition.

Operation. Supra-pubic cystotomy. Tumour and healthy 2–3 cm around it removed. Any attached peritoneum also removed. Defect closed either completely or round cystostomy tube. Ureter may have to be excised and remainder re-implanted into bladder wall.

SPECIAL POST-OPERATIVE CARE IN 1 TO 4 ABOVE

(1) **Observations.** (a) Amount, colour and consistency of urine passed via urethra and supra-pubic cystotomy tube. (2) Onset of complications — chest, vascular, urinary tract infection, supra-pubic fistula. haemorrhage. clot retention, extravasation of urine, incontinence. (3) Copious fluids to ensure flushing of bladder. (4) Drain tube in retropubic space removed after 48 hours, supra-pubic tube according to drainage. usually 36 – 48 hours; urethral catheter 5 days after supra-pubic wound is completely dry.

5. Total cystectomy

Removal of bladder, seminal vesicles and prostate gland, and subsequent diversion of urinary stream.

Indications. Bladder tumour with infiltration. (Urinary diversion may be done with or without cystectomy in following conditions — congenital malformation of bladder; paralysis, e.g. associated with spina bifida and myelomeningocele.)

Operation. Bladder exposed by supra-pubic approach. Peritoneum stripped without being opened. Ligation of blood supply to bladder. Vas deferens and ureters diverted. Urethra divided below apex of prostate gland. Bladder, seminal vesicles and prostate gland removed *en bloc*. Pelvic tissues drained with tube. Urinary diversion achieved by one of following:

(a) NEPHROSTOMY. Rarely used unless patient unable to withstand further surgery and then as temporary measure only.

(b) PYELOSTOMY. Danger of infection and stone formation with both these measures.

(c) URETEROSTOMY. (i) *To skin* — (usually emergency measure only and replaced by (ii) and (iii) below). Both ureters brought out through small lateral wounds. Fascial sheath sutured

362

to wound margins so that it projects 2–3 cm beyond skin surface. Drainage collected into special appliance similar to ileostomy apparatus (p. 135). Various 'spout' arrangements have been devised to protect skin. e.g. 'nipple' ureterostomy where ureters drawn into cutaneous pedicle tube (rarely successful). Usually patient has to resort to some form of indwelling catheter which produces complications, e.g. infection and calculi formation.

(ii) *Ureterosigmoidostomy.* Ureters isolated usually trans- or extra-peritoneally, and distal end checked for viability. Right ureter implanted into distal part of sigmoid colon and left into proximal end. Attempt made to reproduce valvular action of ureters by burying end of ureter obliquely within muscle wall in a tunnel formed by blunt dissection.

Complications. (a) Electrolyte imbalance – hyperchloraemia – chlorides absorbed from bowel while urine stored. Acidosis develops quickly. Counteracted by oral alkali, e.g. sodium bicarbonate, copious fluids, frequent evacuation of bowels (at least 3-hourly) during day and indwelling rectal tube at night.

(b) Pyelonephritis. Reflux of fluid up ureter (largely prevented by above method of surgery).

(c) Fibrosis of anastomosis. Hydro-ureter and hydronephrosis may develop (avoided by side-to side anastomosis but this encourages reflux and infection).

(iii) *Ileal loop conduit.* Loop of terminal ileum, 15–30 cm isolated with blood supply carefully preserved. (Continuity of rest of ileum achieved by end-to-end anastomosis.) Proximal end of loop closed and ureters implanted at convenient points. Distal end brought out on to skin as ileostomy (p. 134).

Complications. (a) Less subject to ascending infection and electrolyte imbalance but can occur if loop too long. (b) 'Wet' ileostomy must be managed by patient – similar in principle to faecal ileostomy. (c) Intestinal obstruction due to ileal loop stenosis at area of anastomosis; later herniation of bowel through unclosed opening in mesentery.

(iv) ISOLATED RECTOSIGMOID BLADDER. Avoids mixing of urine and faeces. Ureters transplanted into sigmoid colon as above, or into rectum, and bowel above this area divided. Proximal end brought out on to skin as faecal colostomy and distal end closed to create 'bladder'. Patient therefore has control over urinary output via anus, and has a 'dry' colostomy which is easier to manage than a 'wet' ileostomy. Lower pressure builds up in rectosigmoid bladder when it contains only urine and reflux up ureters is less likely hence infection is less.

Pre-operative preparation. Total cystectomy. Specific.

(a) Bowel preparation as for ileostomy.

(b) Investigation of renal and ureteric function.

(c) Psychological preparation as for ileostomy and colostomy.

(d) Ryle's tube in situ (preventive measure for paralytic ileus).

(e) Base lines for future comparison established — haemoglobin, white cell count, serum electrolytes, urine microscopy and culture, blood urea. weight.

Post-operative care. Specific.

(a) Observations for early signs and symptoms of haemorrhage, paralytic ileus and degree of shock.

(b) Urinary output — amount and abnormalities, e.g. pus, blood, albumin. Urine may be passed via rectal catheter in method (ii) above for 2–4 days to avoid abdominal distension. Patient then encouraged to empty bowel 2–3 hourly. If rectal tube becomes blocked, gentle irrigation with 60–90 ml water may be necessary to dislodge faeces. (Larger amounts may drive bowel contents into ureters.)

(c) Ryle's tube and intravenous feeding if paralytic ileus suspected otherwise fluids commenced on demand.

(d) Electrolyte balance. Routine check daily at first. Nurse and patient must be aware of early signs and symptoms of electrolyte imbalance and must report same immediately.

(e) Care of colostomy, ileostomy and ureterostomy (similar to ileostomy).

CONDITIONS OF URETHRA

CONGENITAL

Hypospadias

Failure of fusion of ventral (inferior) folds so that terminal orifice may appear on under surface of penis or on perineum.

Types. (1) Coronal. Most common form. Opening in inferior aspect of glans penis. Prepuce incomplete on ventral surface giving hooded appearance on dorsum. Treatment not usually required.

(2) Penile. Opening appears along shaft of penis. Hooded prepuce. Tight fibrous bands (remnants of corpus spongiosum) produce a downward curvature of penis (chordee).

(3) Perineoscrotal. Less common. Opening between ununited halves of scrotum. Penis small with well marked chordee. Associated with undescended testes. Sex may be hard to determine in this condition.

Treatment 1. MEATOTOMY. Sometimes necessary for pinhole meatus.

2. STRAIGHTENING OF PENIS. 18 months to 3 years. Fibrous bands dissected and skin on ventral surface increased by grafting skin from redundant dorsal prepuce.

3. RECONSTRUCTION OF URETHRA. 5–7 years. Various techniques to create new urethra from complete skin tube, and to bury skin tube subcutaneously in penis. Skin taken from body of penis or prepuce or by free graft from area of body which is hairless. Urethrostomy tube drains bladder for 10 days and perineal fistula heals 4–5 days later.

Epispadias

Corpora cavernosa fail to fuse and urethra opens on dorsum of penis.

Types. Severe form associated with ectopia vesicae (congenital failure of fusion of abdominal wall and anterior wall of bladder. Pubic bones absent. Dorsal roof of urethra and dorsal part of sphincters absent). Milder form. Shortened urethra with dorsal curvature of penis.

Treatment. Correction of incontinence by reconstructing sphincters. Straightening of penis and urethroplasty as above. Diversion of urinary flow if incontinence cannot be controlled.

INJURY

Causes. Associated with fractured pelvis – membranous urethra. Straddle injuries – bulbous urethra. Instrumentation – pendulous urethra.

Types. (1) MEMBRANOUS URETHRA. Frequently occurs at junction of prostatic part and membranous part. Usually complete.

365

Signs and symptoms. Urethral bleeding. Retention of urine. Pain in lower abdomen or perineum. Swelling above pubis due to extravasation and/or haematoma. Soft swelling in region of prostate on rectal examination — haematoma and/or extravasation.

Investigations. Attempt made at urethral catheterization. Urethrogram — passage of opaque dye into urethra via catheter. Cystogram to exclude bladder damage.

Treatment. (a) Treat accompanying shock and haemorrhage. (b) Pass catheter into bladder if possible. Leave in situ 14—21 days to allow rupture to heal. (c) If urethra does not permit passage of catheter, supra-pubic incision to explore area. Bougies passed and then Foley bag. Repair carried out over bulb of Foley bag. Supra-pubic area drained with small tube which is removed in 48 hours. Traction (about ½ kg) applied to Foley catheter to pull prostate gland downwards and relieve tension on repair during healing. Catheter left in 14—21 days. (d) Periodic passage of bougies for 12 months to prevent stricture.

(2) BULBOUS URETHRA. *Signs and symptoms.* Urethral bleeding. Extravasation of urine and bleeding into scrotum and penis. Local pain. Mass present in perineum. Later bruising of perineal and scrotal skin.

Treatment. (a) If patient can micturate and there is no evidence of extravasation — no treatment. (b) Passage of catheter which is left in situ 2—3 weeks. (c) Surgical repair over splinting catheter if (b) unsuccessful. (d) Drainage of extensive perineal haematoma and extravasation. (e) Periodical passing of urethral sounds to prevent stricture.

(3) PENDULOUS URETHRA. *Signs and symptoms.* During instrumentation — pain and bleeding.

Treatment. As in (2) above.

STRICTURE

Annular or generalized narrowing of urethra.

Causes. (1) Congenital. (2) Acquired following: (a) urethritis. Commonly gonorrhoea but less common since advent of sulphonamides; (b) irritation from indwelling catheter especially rubber or gum elastic types; (c) trauma; (d) late complication of plastic surgery for hypospadias and prostatectomy.

Signs and symptoms. Difficulty in starting micturition (hesitancy). Poor stream. Dribbling after completion. Chronic or acute retention.

Diagnosis. Confirmed by passing sounds or bougies.

Investigations. Before treatment determine site and size of stricture and presence of false passages. Urethrogram to show length and tortuosity of urethra.

Treatment. 1. DILATATION OF URETHRA. Metal dilators of gradually increasing size passed under local anaesthetic at weekly or fortnightly intervals. Scale ascended until patient complains of discomfort or surgeon considers dilatation adequate. Care taken not to overstretch urethra as further fibrosis will occur. Last dilator left in for 5 minutes to gain maximum benefit. Meatotomy may be necessary if passage of larger dilators impeded by size of meatus.

2. SURGERY. Division of urethral stricture provides temporary relief but stricture recurs unless followed up by dilatation.

PHIMOSIS

Prepuce (foreskin) abnormally tight, adherent to glans penis and cannot be retracted.

Complications. Infection of glans penis (balanitis). Meatus may become pinpoint in size and make micturition difficult.

Treatment. (1) Gentle separation of adhesions with probe to free meatus. (2) Dorsal slit in prepuce. (3) Circumcision.

PARAPHIMOSIS

Tight prepuce retracted behind glans and unable to be drawn forward again.

Causes. (1) Following erection. (2) Following retraction to cleanse glans prior to instrumentation or while catheter in situ. (3) Mother who has been advised to pull prepuce back in order to 'stretch' it.

Pathology. Inner layer of prepuce beyond constriction swells rapidly and prevents reduction by formation of oedematous collar. May result in gangrene of prepuce and glans if not relieved.

Treatment. (1) Manipulative reduction may be attempted first — squeezing glans with hand or bandage to dispel some of the

367

oedema and withdrawing constriction up as far as possible. After few minutes sufficient oedema may have been dispelled to allow reduction. (2) Injection of hyaluronidase may dispel oedema sufficiently. (3) Dorsal slit under general anaesthetic. (4) Circumcision advised at a later date.

BALANITIS

Inflammation of epithelial surface of glans penis.

Causes. Poor hygiene – failure to clean under foreskin. Phimosis which prevents hygiene. Inadequate cleansing when catheter in situ.

Signs and symptoms. Discharge – often purulent. Irritation or burning pain at tip of penis. Glans appears red and may be ulcerated.

Treatment. Daily bathing. Application of hydrocortisone cream. Circumcision. Chronic balanitis thought to be pre-cancerous. Biopsy always indicated.

NEOPLASM OF URETHRA

Incidence. Uncommon. Benign and malignant.

Caruncle

Benign tumour of urethral meatus.

Incidence Most common in menopausal females.

Types. Papilloma, angioma, granuloma.

Signs and symptoms. Red, raspberry-like tumour. Painful and tender.

Diagnosis. Confirmed by biopsy.

Treatment. Transurethral resection. May be difficult because of vascularity.

Carcinoma

Types. Squamous epithelioma most common.

Cause. Chronic balanitis appears to be pre-cancerous condition.

Site. Usually begins in glans penis and therefore hidden by prepuce. detection of early case is rare. Transitional cell carcinoma may arise in posterior urethra – similar to bladder cancer.

Signs and symptoms. Offensive and blood-stained discharge from prepuce. Patient may not seek treatment until cancer has fungated through skin.

Diagnosis. Confirmed by biopsy and urethrogram.

Treatment. (1) Irradiation for early growths. By surface irradiation or needle implantation. (2) Partial or complete amputation of penis. (3) Transurethral resection (posterior urethral growth) or, in advanced cases, total cystectomy with removal of prostate and urethra.

SURGERY OF URETHRA AND PENIS
Circumcision

Removal of prepuce.

Indications. (1) Religion or custom. (2) Phimosis. (3) Paraphimosis. (4) Balanitis.

Operation. BABIES. Usually not under anaesthetic. Adhesions separated with blunt dissector. Prepuce pulled forward beyond glans. Artery forceps applied and prepuce cut off distal to forceps. Forceps removed and slit made in deeper layer over glans. Corners trimmed. Bleeders ligated. Cut edges secured with 3—4 fine catgut sutures. Dressing of tincture of benzoin applied leaving meatus exposed. No special post-operative care except cleanliness.

OLDER CHILDREN AND ADULTS. Under local or general anaesthesia. Prepuce not elastic enough to draw forward. Slit back to attachment behind glans and excised. Five or six individual catgut sutures inserted.

Post-operative care. Congestion and erection cause considerable pain. Sedation with barbiturates usual. In severe cases oestrogen extracts may be indicated.

Amputation of penis

1 **Partial**. When growth confined to gland and prepuce.

OPERATION. Two flaps of skin retained after amputation, inferior longer than superior. Inferior folded over stump and hole made in it for urethra to protrude below suture line. Self-retaining catheter 4—5 days. Sutures widely spaced to allow free escape of blood to prevent haematoma under flaps.

COMPLICATIONS. Stenosis of urethral meatus — periodic dilatation necessary.

2. **Total amputation.** INDICATIONS. Spread of growth along penis. Short penis.

OPERATION. Metal bougie passed into urethra. Incision encircles base of penis and is carried backwards. dividing the scrotum into two halves, to perineum. Urethra dissected out from bulb of penis and divided 5 cm from its emergence from perineal membrane. Remainder of penis removed. Wound closed so that posterior part is approximated round urethral stump. End of stump split and sutured to skin edges. Catheter left in situ for several days. Perineal meatus functions well and shows little tendency to stenose.

CONDITIONS OF PROSTATE GLAND

Benign senile hypertrophy

Physiological hyperplasia (affects peri-urethral glands of prostate rather than true prostatic substance).

Cause. Probably degenerative change due to hormonal imbalance occurring at middle age.

Pathology. Middle lobe most commonly enlarged. Expands into bladder and has 'ball valve' effect at bladder neck. The greater the intravesical pressure attempting to overcome the obstruction the more firmly the lobe becomes jammed into bladder neck.

If true capsule is thin, expansion of the lateral lobes can occur with no adverse effect on micturition.

Signs and symptoms. (1) Bladder neck obstruction — hesitancy and straining at beginning of micturition, loss of force and calibre of stream, terminal dribbling. Frequency and nocturia may also be present. (2) Haematuria due to rupture of dilated veins at bladder neck. (3) Acute urinary retention may be presenting symptom. (4) Chronic painless urinary retention with incontinence and/or signs of uraemia.

Investigations. (1) Rectal examination may reveal soft swelling. (2) Renal function — blood urea, clearance of urea, creatinine, concentration tests, etc., urinalysis may reveal infection, albumin or blood. (3) X-ray — i.v.p. may show complications, e.g. hydronephrosis, calculi. (4) Residual urine estimation — catheter passed immediately after micturition and amount of urine remaining measured (normal upper limit 100 ml). (5) Cystoscopy — degree of prostatic enlargement, degree of secondary changes, e.g. trabeculation from attempts to overcome obstruction.

Complications. Obstruction leads to infection — cystitis, pyelonephritis, prostatitis, epididymo-orchitis; calculi; diverticula; atony of bladder wall; hydronephrosis; kidney failure.

Treatment. Correction of any complications, e.g. infection and uraemia. Prostatectomy.

Prostatitis

Inflammation of prostate gland.

Causes. Specific infections, e.g. tuberculosis, gonorrhoea. Blood-borne spread — Staphylococci, *E. coli* (may lead on to prostatic abscess). Secondary spread from bladder neck obstruction. Allergy — occurs frequently in asthmatic patients.

Acute. SIGNS AND SYMPTOMS. Frequency, terminal dysuria, haematuria, retention. Rigors. Burning pain in perineum on defaecation.

INVESTIGATIONS. Rectal examination — mass palpated — large, asymmetrical, spongy (oedematous) tender. Urine infected and may contain albumin and white cells.

COMPLICATIONS. Abscess which may rupture into rectum, bladder or urethra. Chronic prostatitis. Recto-urethral fistula.

TREATMENT. *Conservative.* Bedrest, copious fluids, antibiotics for 5 days, e.g. intramuscular streptomycin 0.5 g, 6-hourly, tetracycline 250 mg, 6-hourly. Clearance of lower bowel. Catheterization with indwelling catheter, e.g. Gibbon's, may be necessary if retention occurs.

Surgical. Drainage of abscess (most satisfactory method via urethra with resectoscope).

Chronic. SIGNS AND SYMPTOMS. Vary, e.g. recurrent attacks of dysuria and frequency. Pain referred to tip of penis, perineum, inner aspect of thigh.

INVESTIGATIONS. Urine — purulent may contain mucus. Rectal examination — may be small and firm from fibrosis. Panendoscopy — dilated purulent prostatic ducts.

TREATMENT. Not always satisfactory. Antibiotics according to sensitivity. Symptoms may recur when drug stopped. Transurethral resection may prevent bladder neck obstruction.

Carcinoma of prostate

Incidence. High in middle aged and beyond.

Type. 'Hormone dependent.' Testosterone stimulates growth, oestrogen inhibits.

Form. Adenocarcinoma — posterior part of gland, thus involving true prostatic tissue. Scirrhous — most common form.

Spread. Slowly infiltrates gland and spreads to surrounding structures. Gland becomes fixed in position. Rectal examination — winged appearance. Lymph — early retroperitoneal spread and widespread bone metastases especially to vertebral column (lumbar spine), pelvis and occasionally ribs.

Signs and symptoms. Early — similar to those of benign enlargement. Late — those due to spread. Pain in back and legs. Oedema of one or both legs. Bone pains. Enlarged supraclavicular lymph nodes. Weight loss

Investigations. Rectal examination — firm, irregular, fixed, asymmetrical gland. Blood — full examination — low haemoglobin and anaemia with metastases. Blood urea raised with kidney damage. Serum acid phosphatase raised (normal level 2 units %. Level 5 units % confirms diagnosis). Radiological skeletal survey — bone metastases. Residual urine may be raised. Urethrocystoscopy — degree of prostatic involvement and secondary changes in bladder wall. Biopsy — with resectoscope or needle biopsy via perineum or transrectally.

Complications. Those of benign hyperplasia. Pathological fractures. Anaemia.

Treatment. Surgery   radical prostatectomy — curative. Transurethral prostatectomy — palliative. Endocrines — stilboestrol 5—15—25 mg, 8-hourly; chlorotrianisine 12 mg twice daily — less troublesome side effects, e.g. gynaecomastia, nausea, oedema. Intravenous diethylstilboestrol diphosphate — given in high dosage without side effects. Effective where metastases are troublesome and rapid relief required. Adrenalectomy or hypophysectomy sometimes performed when severe pain from metastases present. Hypophysectomy rarely performed because of danger of meningitis, cerebrospinal rhinorrhoea, diabetes insipidus or damage to optic chiasma.

PROSTATIC SURGERY

Prostatectomy

1. **Open.** (a) SUPRA-PUBIC. Enucleation of prostate gland through bladder incision.

Indications. Benign hypertrophy in younger patients in whom vesical calculi, neoplasm or diverticula suspected.

Methods. Various, e.g. Freyer's. Supra-pubic cystotomy (p. 361). Bladder retracted to enable exploration then bladder wall anchored with stay sutures. Enucleation. Damage avoided to ejaculatory ducts and urethra. Haemorrhage controlled, e.g. by temporary pack or implantation of absorbable haemostatic gauze, or by sutures in prostate bed (Harris and Thompson-Walker methods), or by Foley bag per urethram and inflating bag to exert constant even pressure on prostate bed. Wedge resection at posterior bladder neck avoids later obstruction to micturition from prominent shelf overhanging prostatic capsule and promotes early restoration of micturition. Closure of bladder. Supra-pubic tube may be left in situ if danger of haemorrhage, or if infection present. Self-retaining supra-pubic catheter, e.g. Malecot, de Pezzer or wide bore polythene catheter, e.g. whistle-tip may be sutured in position. Otherwise bladder may be closed and drained via urethral catheter (Wilson-Hey method often used, i.e. catheter passed retrograde – from bladder to exterior – to avoid introducing infection into bladder from urethra). Foley or whistle-tip catheter may be used. Internal end fixed with a suture passing through its tip and brought out through abdominal wall. Small corrugated drain left in cave of Retzius.

(b) RETRO-PUBIC OR MILLIN'S OPERATION. Removal of prostate gland via incision made in its capsule.

Indications. Benign hypertrophy with no associated complications.

Operation. Preceded by cystoscopy to exclude bladder complications. Vertical or transverse supra-pubic incision. Peritoneum stripped upwards and retro-pubic space opened. Prostatic capsule exposed, incised, gland enucleated. Haemostasis by temporary gauze packing. Wedge resection of posterior bladder neck as above. Urethral catheter inserted. Capsule closed with continuous close sutures. Small drain tube left in against suture line. Wound closed.

2. **Transurethral resection**. Removal of prostatic tissue via a resectoscope inserted through urethra.

Indications. Cases of obstruction without gross enlargement, e.g. small fibrous gland; enlargement of middle lobe only; carcinoma (partial removal does not appear to activate growth or to cause dissemination).

Operation. Patient placed in lithotomy position. Diathermy plate fixed to leg or buttock. Meatotomy and urethral dilatation may be necessary prior to passage of wide bore resectoscope. Anaesthetic may be spinal or general depending on patient's condition.

Resectoscope sheath with obdurator in position is passed. Obdurator removed and replaced with telescope and electrode carrier. Continuous irrigation with sterile water commenced to keep field clear of blood and debris. Loop of wire or circular punch activated by diathermy current. Can be used for cutting or coagulation.

Dangers. Damage to bladder neck or urethra. Acute renal failure due to haemolysis if water is forced into venous sinuses opened during surgery (may be prevented by using isotonic solution, e.g. glycine instead of water for irrigating).

3. **Perineal prostatectomy**. Removal of prostatic tissue via perineal incision. Rarely employed because of high risk of infection. Some surgeons advocate it for resection of early carcinoma. Method similar to open prostatectomy, through ∩ shaped incision in perineum.

4. **Radical prostatectomy**. For early carcinoma. Open prostatectomy as above. Removal of entire prostate gland within its fascial sheath, seminal vesicles, and bladder neck. Outlet of bladder anastomosed to remaining urethra over a catheter. Part of bladder may also have to be removed necessitating transplantation of ureters higher on to bladder or into rectum or skin.

PRE-OPERATIVE PREPARATION. Majority of patients in older age group. Special attention needed to ensure that they present for surgery in optimum physical and psychological condition.

Admission. Several days pre-operatively to: (a) adjust to hospital environment; (b) improve general condition, e.g. uraemia, anaemia, cardiovascular conditions, chronic lung conditions, constipation, oral sepsis, pressure sores; (c) allow time for investigations.

Investigations. Urine. Ward test, microscopy, culture for organisms and sensitivity, estimation of residual urine. Blood. Full examination especially haemoglobin and white cell count. Serum electrolytes to correct any imbalance and to act as base line for future comparison. Blood urea. Acid and alkaline phosphatase. Renal function tests. Radiography — chest and intravenous pyelography. Rectal examination for size and state of prostate gland and to exclude impacted faeces. Cystoscopic and retrograde pyelogram. E.c.g. may be necessary in elderly patients.

Catheterization. If patient presents with acute retention or chronic retention with overflow, catheterization with continuous or intermittent drainage may be necessary. Care taken to prevent ascending infection by (a) strict aseptic technique and sterile equipment; (b) closed drainage into underwater seal bottle containing antiseptic, e.g. formalin 40%; (c) care taken when changing bottle, e.g. end of tubing clamped and wrapped in sterile towel, connections immersed in antiseptic lotion before being reconnected; (d) cleansing of meatus with, e.g. aqueous chlorhexidine 0.05%, hydrogen peroxide or pHisoHex, 3 times daily; (e) antibiotics or urinary antiseptics may be given parenterally.

Exercises. Ambulation encouraged. Deep breathing — to treat existing chest conditions and prevent post-operative complications. Leg exercises to prevent deep vein thrombosis which is common in this age group and aggravated by lithotomy position.

Smoking discouraged.

Diet. Nourishing but light. Copious fluids to aid renal function and lower blood urea.

Skin preparation. Abdominal, pubic and perineal areas.

POST-OPERATIVE CARE. Specific.

(a) *Drainage.* Establishment of urinary drainage immediately after surgery.

(b) *Observations.* Routine for degree of shock and early signs and symptoms of haemorrhage (see later).

(c) *Fluid balance chart.* Output — careful checking of tubing for kinking, sagging, twisting, and amount and colour of output. Abdomen palpated for bladder distension. Intake — intravenous infusion — blood may be necessary, diuretic (see later) in 5%

dextrose for 6–24 hours until patient tolerates oral fluids (3–3½ litres daily).

(d) *Physiotherapy.* Chest and leg exercises commenced immediately on recovery of consciousness and continued until full ambulation achieved.

(e) *Ambulation.* Out of bed on first post-operative day and encouraged to exercise a little more each day. Discouraged from merely sitting in chair (increases risk of deep vein thrombosis).

(f) *General measures.* Hygiene – special care because of age. Prevention of pressure sores. Mouth and eye care. Bowels – avoid constipation, straining may cause haemorrhage in prostatic fossa. Rectal examination to discover impacted faeces if patient has spurious diarrhoea.

(g) *Diet.* Normal. May have to be soft foods if chewing difficult.

(h) *Dressings.* Left undisturbed unless evidence of infection or urinary drainage from wound. Sutures removed 7–10 days.

(i) *Drain tubes.* (i) Cave of Retzius – drains into small dressing, usually shortened and removed 48–72 hours. (ii) Supra-pubic catheter – 36 to 48 hours. Usually drains into bedside bottle or bag. (iii) Urethral catheter removed when supra-pubic wound has been dry for 5 days. In closed operations, removed when there is no evidence of haemorrhage usually about 72 hours.

Micturition. Difficulties may arise due to muscular atony or disuse of sphincter. Patient needs constant reassurance that the difficulties are temporary, e.g. burning pain (due to instrumentation of urethra), dribbling, urgency, incontinence, and can be overcome by: (i) 2-hourly micturition, gradually lengthening the interval; (ii) exercises to strengthen perineal floor and improve action of sphincters; (iii) avoidance of leaving a urinal in situ. If patient is incontinent, penile clamp may be used as temporary measure. Nurse must ensure that if bedlinen becomes soiled it is changed immediately without embarrassment to the patient; (iv) measurement of residual urine. If over 100 ml, catheter reinserted and intermittent drainage reinstituted for 1–2 days then removed and patient given further trial of micturition.

DISCHARGE. 8–10 days if no complications. Patient warned to report any haematuria.

Complications. (a) HAEMORRHAGE AND CLOT RETEN-

TION. Any bleeding into bladder must be flushed out otherwise: (i) haemorrhage will continue (bleeding in bladder mainly controlled by action of muscles on ends of bleeding vessels), and (ii) clots may block urinary outlet causing acute retention.

Preventive measures. (i) Induce diuresis — e.g. mannitol or urea. Good urinary output achieved by reduction of reabsorption in tubules thus excluding need for bladder washouts. Dosage — mannitol up to 200 g, urea 120 g daily. Usually requried for first 6—24 hours only. Given intravenously in 5% dextrose.

(ii) Bladder irrigation — sterile normal saline. Must be closed circuit. Need for continuous irrigation now considered unnecessary and may prolong bleeding. Sterile irrigation apparatus set up and clamped off. If drainage from bladder is sluggish or heavily blood stained tubing is unclamped and bladder flushed out.

(iii) Copious fluid intake (3—3½ litres) daily encouraged. Oral intake started as soon as possible.

(iv) Prevention of infection to avoid secondary haemorrhage.

Clot retention avoided by above measures and constant observation of tubing to avoid kinking and interruption of flow. Clamps and spigots never used. If drainage sluggish — 'milk' tube to try and clear clot from catheter. Narrow tubing and graduated glass connections avoided. Signs and symptoms of clot retention. Those of internal haemorrhage. Urinary drainage stops or is sluggish and heavily blood stained. Supra-pubic pain and desire to micturate. Blood stained drainage around catheter. Distended abdomen.

Treatment. (i) Gentle bladder washout with, e.g., sterile sodium citrate 3.8% to break up clots. Not more than 90 ml fluid instilled if gentle suction on syringe brings no return. Doctor notified. Analgesic given, e.g. morphia 15 mg. Catheter changed to one with wider lumen, e.g. whistle-tip, and further bladder washout performed.

Evacuation of clots in theatre with resectoscope sheath and Ellik evacuator. Spinal or general anaesthesia. Blood transfusion.

In severe cases still uncontrolled by above measures ligation of internal iliac arteries may be necessary.

(b) PREVENTION OF INFECTION. (i) Wound infection — usual measures plus maintenance of sterile urine; (ii) ascending urinary infection; (iii) epididymo-orchitis – prevented by ligation of vas deferens at operation.

Observations. Rise in temperature; signs and symptoms of wound inflammation (p. 38); pus in urine; swollen, tender, painful scrotum.

Treatment. See appropriate sections. May result in secondary haemorrhage.

(c) SUPRA-PUBIC FISTULA. Prevented by treating infection pre-operatively, ensuring free drainage from urethral catheter at all times, removal of supra-pubic drain tube in 36–48 hours, retaining urethral catheter for 5 days after supra-pubic wound is dry.

(d) RENAL FAILURE – from reflex anuria following relief of obstruction.

(e) STRICTURE OF URETHRA – may occur months later. Due to (i) size of instrument passed during surgery; (ii) infection.

(f) GENERAL COMPLICATIONS. Pulmonary especially pneumonia; vascular especially deep vein thrombosis.

(g) STENOSIS OF BLADDER NECK (especially if wedge resection not performed at operation (p. 373)). Retention of urine occurs. Residual urine must be measured and further resection of tissue performed.

(h) IMPOTENCE AND STERILITY. If vas deferens is tied ½–⅔ of ejaculate removed and impotence may result from poor stimulus.

CONDITIONS OF THE SCROTUM AND CONTENTS

Hydrocele

Collection of fluid within tunica vaginalis.

Causes. (1) Congenital. Failure of vaginalis to close from general peritoneal cavity. (2) Acquired – injury, torsion of testis, inflammation of epididymis or testis, tumour of testis.

Signs and symptoms. Painless. Patient may complain of dragging sensation if fluid collection is large. Fluid is clear, colourless or straw coloured. Scrotum can be transilluminated.

Treatment. Wearing of suspensory bandage. Aspiration if fluid develops suddenly in young male to exclude testicular neoplasm. Periodic aspiration if dragging sensation troublesome. Surgery if collection gathers rapidly after aspiration, parietal layer of vaginalis excised.

Varicocele

Varicosity, i.e. dilation and tortuosity of veins of testis.

Causes. (1) Idiopathic. (2) Associated with venous obstruction due to renal neoplasm.

Pathology. Mainly occurs on left side. May result in congestion of testes and infertility.

Signs and symptoms. Scrotal swelling involving spermatic cord. Aching pain. Scrotum feels like 'bag of worms'.

Treatment. None unless infertility is cause for concern. Ligation of main veins high in inguinal canal. May be done under local anaesthetic.

Mal-descent of testes

1. Arrest of testes in normal path of descent (cryptorchidism).

2. Displacement from normal route (ectopic testis).

Cause. (1) Anatomical abnormality (hernia, fascial bands). (2) Developmental fault (thought to be due to lack of stimulation from anterior pituitary gland hormones).

Complications. (1) Spermatogenesis depends on temperature of testes being lower than that of body generally. If testis remains out of scrotum after age 6 years it may not mature. (2) Inguinal hernia. (3) Torsion of testis. (4) Malignancy of testis — 10 times more common following this condition.

Signs and symptoms. One or both testes absent from scrotum. Under-development of scrotum on side of missing testis. Testis may be palpable above scrotum.

Treatment. Hormone therapy if cause (2) above. Orchidopexy. Orchidectomy if atrophy of testis evident.

Torsion of testis

Twisting of spermatic cord or of attachement of testis to epididymis.

Cause. Developmental anomaly.

Pathology. Loss of blood supply leads to infarction and atrophy of testis.

Signs and symptoms. Sudden onset of severe lower abdominal pain with vomiting. May arise spontaneously or follow physical exercise, mild trauma. Testis becomes hard, swollen and tender. Lies higher in scrotum due to shortening of cord. Scrotal skin red and oedematous. Secondary hydrocele develops.

Treatment. Surgical detorsion — emergency operation. May be achieved by manipulation under anaesthesia. If this fails — open operation. Orchidectomy if testis necrosed.

INFECTION
Orchitis
Inflammation of testis.

Causes. (1) Complication of acute specific infections, e.g. mumps, typhoid. (2) Spread of infection from epididymis.

Signs and symptoms. Painful swelling of testis. Pyrexia. Parotitis. Leucocytosis.

Complications. Atrophy. Infertility.

Treatment. Infiltration of 1% procaine into spermatic cord. Bedrest. Copious fluids. Analgesics. Cold compresses. Scrotal support.

Epididymitis
Inflammation of the epididymis.

Causes. 1. Non-specific infections spreading from urethra, prostate or vas deferens. Complication of urinary tract infection, prostatic obstruction, surgery of lower urinary tract, instrumentation via urethra. May be spread from testis.

2. Specific infections. Tuberculosis, syphilis, gonorrhoea. Spread to testes common.

Signs and symptoms. Intense pain associated with marked swelling and redness on affected side of scrotum. Pyrexia — up to 40°C. Epididymis tender but testis normal at first. Later testis also affected. Spermatic cord thickened. Secondary hydrocele may develop and obscure symptoms. Secondary cystitis causes infected urine.

Treatment. Bedrest. Scrotal support. Analgesics. Appropriate antibiotic. Copious fluids. Cold compresses. Procaine 1% injected into cord may hasten resolution.

NEOPLASM

Benign

Very rare, e.g. interstitial cell tumour.

Pathology. Androgens and oestrogens secreted. Causes virilism in boys and gynaecomastia in adults.

Malignant

Rare.

Incidence. 20–35 years.

Types. Seminoma. Teratoma. Lymphoma.

Spread. Local infiltration with lymphatic and vascular invasion. Lung, bone and liver metastases common.

Causes. Thought to be associated with hereditary factor, trauma, mal-descent of testes, benign growth becoming malignant.

Signs and symptoms. Painless swelling of testis increasing rapidly. Haemorrhage may cause pain and tenderness (may simulate epididymo-orchitis or torsion of testis). Gynaecomastia, impotence, reduced libido (interstitial cell involvement). Usually associated with secondary hydrocele.

Treatment. Simple orchidectomy via inguinal incision followed by radiotherapy. (Seminomas are radiosensitive.)

Radical orchidectomy with block dissection of pelvic and para-aortic lymph nodes. Contra-indicated if metastases present. Technically difficult. High mortality rate.

SCROTAL SURGERY

Orchidectomy

Removal of one or both testes.

Indications. Malignancy. Infarction and atrophy.

Operation. Inguinal incision. Canal opened. Spermatic cord divided between ligatures. Testis freed from scrotal attachments and removed. Precautionary drain tube left in situ from scrotum. Canal and wound closed with sutures.

Orchidopexy

Fixation of mal-descended testis in scrotum.

Operation. Inguinal incision. Canal opened. Spermatic cord explored and any fascial bands or adhesions freed. Testis brought down into scrotum and fixed by various means, e.g. stitch passed through tunica albuginea and lower pole of testis. Stitch brought out through lower end of scrotum and anchored to skin of thigh by tying over a piece of rubber tubing. (Too great tension must be avoided or atrophy may occur.)

SPECIAL INVESTIGATIONS
X-ray

1. **Intravenous pyelogram.** Visualization of calcyes and pelvis of kidney after intravenous injection of contrast medium. Also indicates function of kidneys. Contra-indicated in failing renal function with high blood urea.

PREPARATION. Bowel preparation as for barium enema to rid bowel of obscuring shadows from faeces and gas. Test dose of medium to exclude allergy or hypersensitivity. No oral food or fluids for 6 hours.

METHOD. Medium given by intravenous injection (Hypaque 50%, Urographin 76%). Series of films taken. Normal excretion follows pattern — calcyes, pelvis, ureters, bladder. Medium should appear in kidney within 2–3 minutes and should have passed into lower urinary tract within 25 minutes. Bladder emptied immediately after X-ray.

AFTERCARE. Observations for reaction to medium. Flushing, coughing, sneezing from too rapid administration. Allergic reactions — urticaria, bronchospasm, anaphylactic shock and collapse (rare). Prevented by test dose on day before and asking patient about history of allergy — hay fever, asthma.

2. **Retrograde pyelography.** Contrast medium introduced into ureters and pelves of kidneys via long thin ureteric catheters passed through cystoscope.

INDICATIONS. Mainly to confirm or support diagnosis made by intravenous pyelography or renal arteriogram. Does not show kidney function but gives clearer outline of kidney. Can be done on one or both kidneys. Only method of obtaining specimens of urine from one kidney.

METHOD. Cystoscope passed under general or local anaesthesia. Patient prepared as above. Ureteric catheters introduced into bladder. Ureteric orifices located and catheters passed into ureters. Cystoscope removed. Medium injected via catheters.

X-ray taken preferably when patient is conscious. Correct amount of medium gauged by patient's response (experiences backache or loin pain when filling of renal system complete. Amount varies 5–20 ml).

3. **Cysto-urethrogram.** Passage of medium via urethral catheter and screening performed as patient micturates.

INDICATIONS. Bladder conditions — diverticula, changes in bladder neck; stricture of urethra, dilation, trauma; vesico-ureteral reflux; control of micturition.

PREPARATION. Catheter passed with strict aseptic precautions.

MEDIUM, Umbradil, Urumbrin, sterile barium sulphate.

METHOD. Medium instilled. Patient sits behind fluoroscope screen on chair similar to commode. X-ray taken before patient voids, while bearing down but not voiding, during act of micturition.

Endoscopy

1. *Urethroscopy.* Examination of urethra under direct visualization.

2. *Cystoscopy.* Examination of bladder similarly.

3. *Panendoscopy.* Examination of urethra and bladder.

INDICATIONS. Diagnostic — neoplasm; trauma; stricture; infection; diverticula; calculi; prostatomegaly.

Investigations. Renal function assessed by renal catheterization of one or both kidneys. Type of prostatectomy to be performed.

CONTRA-INDICATIONS. Acute nephritis. Advanced renal failure.

PREPARATION. May be done under local but more commonly under general anaesthesia. Routine pre-operative preparation. Pubic area not shaved unless ordered.

METHOD. Position — lithotomy, for cystoscopy. Cystoscope with obdurator in situ passed gently into bladder. Urethral meatomy and dilation may be necessary before cystoscope passed. Obdurator removed. Bladder irrigated with sterile water either from syringe or overhead irrigator until returned clear. If patient conscious, bladder capacity recorded by filling bladder until patient complains of slight discomfort. Telescope attached to cystoscope and systematic examination of bladder carried out. Continuous irrigation may be carried out during investigation but about 240 ml water kept in situ to ensure opening of rugae. Renal function may be tested by injecting intravenously a brightly coloured dye which will be seen coming from ureteric openings. Ureteric catheters may be inserted to collect separate specimens from each kidney. These may be left in position and drained into receptacles attached to patient's thighs.

AFTERCARE. Routine post-anaesthetic care. Ensure that catheters drain into correct receptacles and specimens labelled and sent to laboratory when completed. Ureteric catheters removed slowly and carefully.

Renal function tests

1. **Urea clearance.** Assessment of kidney's ability to excrete a given amount of urea in a certain length of time.

METHOD. Intake restricted to 150 ml water from 10 p.m. Patient empties bladder next morning, e.g. 6 a.m. This specimen is discarded. One hour later patient empties bladder. Specimen saved and labelled 'Pre-urea specimen'. Blood collected for blood urea. Exact time of collection recorded on both specimens. Patient then drinks 15 g urea in 120 ml water. 8 a.m. urine collected. 9 a.m. urine and blood collected. 10 a.m. urine collected. Test finished. Patient given breakfast. All specimens clearly labelled and exact time of collection clearly recorded and sent to laboratory.

2. **Water concentration – dilution test (Fishberg).** Assessment of kidney's ability to concentrate a given amount of water in a certain time.

METHOD. Intake restricted to 150 ml water from 10 p.m. Bladder emptied in morning, e.g. 6 a.m., and this specimen discarded. 7 a.m. bladder emptied completely and patient given 1 litre of water to drink. Specimens collected at hourly intervals for 3 specimens. All specimens saved, labelled and sent to laboratory. Patient given breakfast. Exact time of passing specimens is important and recorded. Specific gravity of each specimen may be taken in ward.

3. **Dye excretion test.** e.g. PSP (phenol red). Assessment of secretory ability of kidneys and measurement of residual urine.

METHOD. Normal fluid intake before and during test. 7 a.m. 1 ml of dye given by intravenous injection. 7.30 a.m. urine collected — should contain 50–60% of the dye. 8 a.m. urine collected — should contain 10–15% of the dye. (If more than 15% of dye in second specimen the amount of residual urine can be estimated.)

Further Reading

Farrow, R. & Forrest, D. (1974) *The Surgery of Childhood for Nurses*. 4th edn. Edinburgh: Churchill Livingstone.

Mann, T. S. (1969) *Accident Surgery for Nurses*. Churchill Livingstone.

Moroney, J. (1975) *Surgery for Nurses* 13th edn. Edinburgh: Churchill Livingstone.

Naylor, A. (1971) *Fractures and Orthopaedic Surgery for Nurses and Physiotherapists*. 6th edn. Edinburgh: Churchill Livingstone.

Norris, W. & Campbell, D. (1976) *A Nurse's Guide to Anaesthetics, Resuscitation and Intensive Care*. 6th edn. Edinburgh: Churchill Livingstone.

Poweil, Mary (1976) *Orthopaedic Nursing* 7th edn. Edinburgh: Churchill Livingstone.

INDEX

387

390

392